Transformative Learning in Healthcare and Helping Professions Education

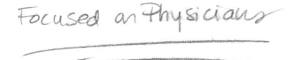

Focused on Physicians

A volume in
Adult Learning in Professional, Organizational, and Community Settings
Carrie J. Boden, *Series Editor*

Transformative Learning in Healthcare and Helping Professions Education

Building Resilient Professional Identities

edited by

Teresa J. Carter
Virginia Commonwealth University

Carrie J. Boden
Texas State University

Kathy Peno
University of Rhode Island

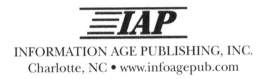

INFORMATION AGE PUBLISHING, INC.
Charlotte, NC • www.infoagepub.com

Library of Congress Cataloging-in-Publication Data

A CIP record for this book is available from the Library of Congress
http://www.loc.gov

ISBN: 978-1-64113-679-2 (Paperback)
        978-1-64113-680-8 (Hardcover)
        978-1-64113-681-5 (ebook)

Printed in the United States of America

CONTENTS

PART I

TEACHING AND LEARNING FOR CHANGE

PART II

DEVELOPING A PROFESSIONAL IDENTITY

PART III

BUILDING CAPACITY FOR RESILIENCE

PART IV

CARING FOR SELF AND OTHERS

Developmental

FOREWORD

It is a delight to write the Foreword to this edited collection, *Transformative Learning in Healthcare and Helping Professions Education: Building Resilient Professional Identities*. This is an important book, and very timely, given that there has been increased attention to issues of burnout and compassion fatigue among healthcare professionals (Sternberg, 2016). Hence, it is incumbent that educators who facilitate programs for emerging or current health professionals are aware of the power of transformative learning, especially as it relates to building resilient professional identities. As one who facilitates such programs for health professionals and who has written with a colleague (see Tisdell & Palmer, 2018) about their need for self-care, I can attest to the importance of this text right at this time.

Developing a resilient professional identity, and the power of transformative learning in doing so, is a lifelong process as any form of development involves constant change. Professional identity changes over time, as developmental tasks are different at various life stages. For example, in the earliest stages, we are developing expertise in our areas of practice as we move from novice to expert (Benner, 2000). In our mid-level stages, we might take on more formal administrative or teaching roles as we pass our knowledge on to others, while at our later stages of professional development, we might be leaders in our field, developing a legacy of leadership in others. Of course, the formation of a professional identity also intersects with our personal lives as we try to balance professional responsibilities with the demands of our family, friends, and community commitments, aging bodies and spirits, and changes in our health and energy levels. Further,

Transformative Learning in Healthcare and Helping Professions Education, pages ix–xii
Copyright © 2019 by Information Age Publishing
All rights of reproduction in any form reserved.

at every stage of our lives we need to deal with the constant changes and lifelong learning demands brought about by technology, globalization, political climates, and agendas that affect how we do our jobs and live out our lives. All these things affect our health, attitudes, our view of the world, and our sense of self. Building resilience in dealing with change is key to fostering well-being, and should be a part of personal and professional identity formation. This book helps show how many in healthcare and the helping professions seek to do so.

Negotiating one's professional identity at every stage presents choices to be made and challenges to be addressed as one begins to consider the values, norms, and beliefs associated with a professional discipline. Some dilemmas are personally disorienting, such as those we face when an unexpected health crisis, divorce, or job change occurs. Others involve the ethical decisions we are faced with in caring for the patients and clients who are dependent upon us for their own health and well-being. Even life events that are positive and actively chosen and planned, such as a new job or a new marriage, can be disorienting. It is in how we deal with these disorienting dilemmas and unpack our prior assumptions about what it means to work as a professional that we are presented with opportunities for transformative learning (Cranton, 2016; Mezirow, 2000; Taylor & Cranton, 2012)—opportunities that can also build resilience and facilitate our ongoing development.

This book presents multiple stories of resilience, transformative learning, and professional identity formation of those in healthcare and the helping professions. Some stories focus on the transformative learning of the authors themselves, as they have negotiated various disorienting dilemmas and confronted unconscious assumptions, leading to their resilience and overall professional development. Other stories focus on how educators in healthcare and the helping professions have tried to facilitate transformative learning among learners in medical education and other professional education settings.

Many of the stories are about shared vulnerability that leads not only to transformative learning among students and trainees, but also to leadership development that can promote a legacy of learning. As Brene Brown (2018) discusses, those who can share their expertise while also sharing their vulnerability can build a community of co-learners and leaders also willing to do so—an important leadership development strategy, as well as a vehicle of transformative learning. Educators as leaders of those who are learning to be healthcare and helping professionals can offer examples to others, not only of their expertise but also of how to create a meaningful life that is full of heart and soul. The stories in this volume present examples of transformative learning that draw upon not only the cognitive dimension of learning, but also the emotional, spiritual, embodied, and metaphoric dimensions as well. My former colleague Patricia Cranton (2016) refers to this as an *integrative perspective* of transformative learning. In such a perspective, learners confront underlying assumptions and create new meaning schemes, or new ways of seeing, by drawing upon multiple ways of knowing.

Dr. Patricia Cranton was a major figure in describing how transformative learning can be realized by students, as well as their educators. Hence, I could not help but think about her and how much she would enjoy this book and would testify to its importance for those in healthcare and the helping professions. Here I thought I would close this forward by saying something about her in relation to this text, as she died unexpectedly in the Summer of 2016. I had the pleasure of teaching with Dr. Cranton from 2005–2011 while she was a professor at Penn State University–Harrisburg where I teach, though I remained in close touch with her in the years after she left and moved back to Canada. One story of Patricia that I share here I have shared in different contexts, including conferences and other written venues. Some of the chapters in this book remind me of Patricia and how an integrative perspective of transformative learning suggests using multiple ways of knowing to help people see in new ways.

When Patricia came to interview at Penn State University–Harrisburg in the early Spring of 2005, someone asked if she had a metaphor to describe herself as a teacher and scholar. Without missing a beat, she explained that she was also a photographer, and she went on to describe one of the photos she had taken that perhaps captured what we were asking. She described a photo of rocks at the bottom of a creek bed, rocks and stones of many sizes and shapes (much like the variety in her students) made visible by the light streaming through the water. She explained that the light acted as a lens that gave a particular perspective on the beauty of each rock. Her job as a teacher and a scholar was to help students get in touch with how they see the world through a lens, the light or *perspective* through which they see, and to examine what assumptions were embedded in that perspective. Further, she wanted her approach to teaching to be as fluid and transparent as the water, which is partly what she thought it meant to be an authentic teacher.

Dr. Patricia Cranton was indeed an authentic teacher, not only by how she taught in formal classroom settings, but in also how she lived her life. She often shared some of her own personal stories in her writing and with her students in classrooms and less formal settings to illustrate points about transformative learning. In this sense, she lived through an integrative perspective on transformative learning. Hence, in working with healthcare and helping professionals in educational settings to facilitate self-care and well-being, we, too, can promote an integrative perspective on transformative learning to help learners deal with burnout and compassion fatigue and promote the development of a resilient professional identity.

We need to encourage these professionals in training to get in touch with their assumptions, to live integrated lives that do not separate their personal and professional identities, but marry the two. We need to help them examine how they can make conscious choices when faced with disorienting dilemmas, and how they can embrace the contradictions in their lives that will open them to newly revised meaning. We need to encourage them to draw on multiple ways of knowing so that they can continually come into new ways of seeing at every stage of their personal and professional development. Indeed, this is a lifelong process, but doing so promises to help build resilience and foster well-being. The stories shared in this book offer many examples of this integrative perspective, and, hopefully, they will lead to further conversations on transformative learning and the building of a resilient professional identity. I look forward to these continued conversations and hope they lead to better coping and further well-being in the pursuit of exciting careers in healthcare and the helping professions.

—**Elizabeth J. Tisdell**
Professor of Lifelong Learning and Adult Education
Penn State University–Harrisburg
Harrisburg, PA

REFERENCES

Benner, P. (2000). *From novice to expert: Excellence and power in clinical nursing practice.* Menlo Park, CA: Addison Wesley.

Brown, B. (2018). *Dare to lead: Brave work. Tough conversations. Whole hearts.* New York, NY: Random House.

Cranton, P. (2016). *Understanding and promoting transformative learning* (3rd ed.). Sterling, VA: Sylus.

Mezirow, J. (2000). *Learning as transformation: Critical perspectives on a theory in progress.* San Francisco, CA: Jossey-Bass.

Sternberg, S. (2016, December 15). National academy to tackle burnout in medicine. *US News and World Report.* Retrieved from https://www.usnews.com/news/national-news/articles/2016-12-15/national-academy-to-tackle-burnout-in-medicine

Taylor, E., & Cranton, P. (Eds.). (2012). *The handbook of transformative learning.* San Francisco, CA: Jossey-Bass.

Tisdell, E., & Palmer, C. (2018). Adult development in health professions education in a changing health care context: The need for self-care. *New Directions for Adult and Continuing Education, 2018*(157), 17–26.

PREFACE

This is a very positive book. It is positive because the professionals who have authored its chapters have drawn upon personal experiences with students, residents, and trainees in healthcare and the helping professions to offer hopeful and practical strategies for addressing burnout and fostering resilience, two recurrent themes present in the literature today. It is positive because it "unpacks" the process of professional identity formation with thoughtful descriptions of learners engaged in becoming that which they are studying. It is noteworthy for the wide variety of professional backgrounds addressed, and the specific challenges that learners in training may encounter as they navigate the complex road toward professional practice. It has been gratifying for us to construct because of the authentic voices of authors who offer insight into what it means to build a *resilient* professional identity from their own experiences and the possibilities for transformative learning in doing so.

As editors, we have attempted to create a volume that draws from practical experience as well as from the literature to bridge two practice worlds. These are the world of educators familiar with Mezirow's transformative learning theory, and the professional practice world of those whose mission it is to help and to heal. The result, we hope, will be informative and useful, enabling readers to appreciate daily struggles as well as triumphant moments of professional life. The firsthand experiences presented by these authors were purposefully encouraged by us to enlighten, challenge, and provide guidance; in short, to let learners know that they are not alone in what may sometimes feel like an uphill climb in professional preparation.

Transformative Learning in Healthcare and Helping Professions Education, pages xiii–xv
Copyright © 2019 by Information Age Publishing
xiii

This book is intended primarily for two audiences: professional students and trainees in healthcare and the helping professions, and the professionals who are their teachers, mentors, and role models. We think it is well-suited as a supplemental text for courses involving interprofessional learners, those who are studying together to improve their ability to collaborate and provide better care for patients and clients. We envision that it might be a useful volume for longitudinal courses that span the curriculum in medical education and in other health professions disciplines, as well as a resource for those who are studying in the helping professions of teaching, counseling, and social work. Since each chapter is a "stand-alone" in content and focus, it should serve well as a reading assignment to facilitate small group dialogue on the nature of burnout and compassion fatigue, as well as to provoke ideas for strategies to cope with these all-too-common dilemmas of professional training. We hope it will help professionals in training to realize the journey involved in their own professional identity formation.

Specific chapters may work well to introduce the challenges of career decision-making, and the self-examination needed by learners to discover the field best suited for them to provide a good fit, as well as to understand what is really involved in helping others. Other chapters address the need for self-care by encouraging professionals in training to dig deep into the reservoirs of their own experiences to reflect on the need to maintain a positive focus, realize personal strengths, and discover how to bring the best of who they are to their work and studies. The organizational focus of the chapter on Appreciative Inquiry (Chapter 13) illustrates what some have already discovered about how individuals and institutions change to create work climates that bring out the best in people on a daily basis.

Faculty developers may find the book useful for courses, seminars, and workshops to support teaching and learning in the professions. Throughout, the emphasis has been to integrate the extant literature on resilience and professional identity formation with firsthand experience from professional educators and trainees to support professional development. Our goal is to introduce the need for transformative learning among the next generation of healthcare and helping professionals, and to provide ideas, resources, and strategies for doing so.

Transformative learning, as defined by Jack Mezirow, has become the predominant theory of adult learning today. It is all about how adults can revise the meaning they make of their experiences to realize perspectives that are more open to alternative viewpoints, more discriminating among them, and more integrative of a broader range of experience in the world. It is a developmental theory based upon the adult's capacity to revise frames of reference that are no longer working well for the individual to help realize one's full potential. This book illustrates the significant role of relationships with peers, teachers, family, and friends who help facilitate transformative learning by challenging as well as supporting learners through difficult experiences. This focus on what it takes to build a resilient professional identity is one that supplements, but does not attempt to replace, the current emphasis on competency-based education so needed by tomorrow's professionals in healthcare and the helping disciplines.

This book is divided into four sections: "Teaching and Learning for Change" (Part I), "Developing a Professional Identity" (Part II), "Building Capacity for Resilience" (Part III), and "Caring for Self and Others" (Part IV). In the section entitled "Teaching and Learning for Change," authors illustrate the significance of educational experiences that situate learners in practice worlds so that they come to realize that they are part of something much larger than themselves. Charity Johansson explores what it means to provide help for another person, and the reality that helping is much more complex than providing advice or recommendations based upon expert knowledge. Judith Livingston and Marsha Griffin introduce readers to a powerful learning experience in an elective rotation at the Texas-Mexico border for medical students and residents. At Community for Children, future pediatricians learn leadership skills by advocating for social justice and the rights of children during a time of crisis in immigration. They introduce learners to the pedagogy of privilege and an epistemology of empathy by caring for children unable to advocate for themselves.

In another rotation experience for medical and health professions students, Scott Armistead accompanies students to two different countries in Africa and discovers some of the ethical and moral challenges within global health electives that can either foster or inhibit transformative learning. In an introduction to situated learning and the communities of practice in which healthcare and helping professionals learn and work, Terry Carter and Bryan Adkins describe the anthropological origins of these concepts that explain how professionals acquire tacit knowledge by absorbing the norms, values, and communal meanings associated with belonging to a profession. These four chapters highlight the contribution of formal, as well as informal and incidental learning. They illustrate how professional identities are fostered through experiences that challenge pre-formed beliefs, and how these can be transformed to enable professionals in training to become more resilient as they acquire the knowledge and skills needed in their work.

In the second section of the book, "Developing a Professional Identity," five chapters describe specific experiences that facilitate the transformation of a lay person into a healthcare or helping professional. Doug Franzen draws upon his experience in interviewing students and reviewing hundreds of residency program applications to reveal the physician archetype, an internal image that students hold about what a physician is or should be, and how this influences career choice and specialty decision-making.

In the chapter on learning from mentors and role models, Terry Carter invites current and former physician colleagues from Virginia Commonwealth University to share their personal stories of the important lessons they have learned that influence how they practice medicine and approach teaching and learning of their junior colleagues in training.

In a unique story of personal transformation, medical student Chris Brown describes the dual influences of volunteering with the homeless population and participating in an international/intercity, rural preceptorship program to foster a commitment to the underserved during his career. In a case study of a science teacher, Elaine Mangiante offers an engaging look into how a professional identity is created and evolves over time, as well as the experiences that promote lifelong learning for both teacher and students. The last chapter in this section alters traditional views of remediation for medical students and residents to illustrate how professional identities can be formed and resilience bolstered through novel strategies that motivate learners to achieve their potential. These chapters put flesh on the bones of professional identity formation by describing learning processes that develop self-awareness among learners who become fully cognizant of their roles as society's helpers and healers.

The third section of this book, "Building Capacity for Resilience," illustrates how professionals in training can use the experiences of their colleagues in practice settings, as well as their own, to enhance resilience during a career. Christine Norton and colleagues worked with the State of Connecticut's Department of Children and Families Wilderness School to introduce an outdoor adventure therapy program for social workers who were experiencing vicarious trauma and burnout from the intensity of their work with abused and neglected children. Their experiences in learning how to recover from a stressful work situation provide a model of strength for others. Patty Wunsch and Mike Webb, both dental school educators, openly describe how they were affected by traumatic events that occurred at work, one involving patient care, and the other, a leadership role challenge. Both of these instances illustrate potentially career-damaging adversity in a practice setting that can occur for professionals without warning. The story of how each of them came to discover personal strengths needed to foster resilience offers evidence of transformative learning as well as the human capacity to respond with courage and fortitude. It was through the help of supportive relationships that they were able to respond in ways that were personally and professionally restoring. In a chapter on building resilience among health professions trainees, Wendy Ward, Carrie Boden, and Ashley Castleberry explore unforeseen events that challenge students and trainees with sudden setbacks. The words and stories of these learners describe well what it means to develop a resilient professional identity while in training. In the final chapter of this section, Marion Nesbit and Terry Carter bring complementary concepts within psychology and organization development to the fore to illustrate the potential for positive organizational change with Appreciative Inquiry. Frequently adopted by healthcare professionals and others in the helping professions, this strategy explores how questions that inquire into times when both individuals and organizations were at their best can revitalize a culture, promote resilience, and support a climate of well-being.

The final section of this book, "Caring for Self and Others," addresses the need for self-care so that professionals can continue to care for others. Nurse educator Mary Falk narrates an autoethnographic account of personal transformation in her experiences with a heart transplant patient. She discovers the paradoxical relationship between caring for others and restoring one's ability to remain resilient in the face of compassion fatigue. In making a case for self-care, Amanda Minor describes the challenges of vicarious trauma and secondary traumatic stress among mental health professionals, offering multiple strategies for self-care and the imperative for helping professionals to care for themselves to promote their own well-being. In the final chapter of the book, Canadian scholar Maureen Coady explores a longitudinal study of professionals engaged in a community-based health education program that was offered to diverse communities within Nova Scotia over 6 years. Her chapter beautifully illustrates the challenges for interprofessional teams when learning to work together to improve the health of a community, while also bootstrapping themselves into the role of educators. It was in learning to care for others as a team that these healthcare professionals developed relationships built upon respect and collaboration to foster their own transformative learning.

We hope our book provides insight for professionals in practice as well as those in training. When we began this project, it was with the idea that there was a connection between resilience and the formation of a professional identity that could support and be promoted by transformative learning. Little did we realize it would foster our own learning as we experienced the compelling stories of colleagues and learners within these disciplines. We express our gratitude and thank the authors for bringing us their stories to share with you.

ACKNOWLEDGMENTS

We are indebted to the many professionals who have contributed to this work as authors, and wish to thank them publicly for their exceptional stories borne of the hardships, triumphs, and commitments made to others in their daily work. Their extraordinary insights offer strategies to promote resilience, form professional identities, and provide opportunities for transformative learning in professional learning contexts. Drawing upon the work that they do every day to teach, mentor, and serve as role models for learners, we see clearly that tomorrow's healthcare and helping professionals are in good hands. The evidence of this is borne out in the chapter on vulnerable populations written by our student author (see Chapter 7). We believe the experiences recounted here can benefit countless other professionals in training, as well as their educators, by strengthening resolve and commitment when needed, and emphasizing the relational capacity that fosters meaning in work. For this reason, we dedicate this book to all professionals in training and in practice within the helping and healthcare disciplines.

Each of us as co-editors also depends upon a host of others who have made publishing this book possible, and we acknowledge their contributions here.

Terry: I wish to thank the medical students in my Heart Groups at VCU—you are my inspiration. I stand in awe of faculty members in the School of Medicine and in the health professions at VCU who shared insight into their practice world to give me a window into the lives of healers as educators; thank you for inviting me in to better understand what you do.

Transformative Learning in Healthcare and Helping Professions Education, pages xix–xx
Copyright © 2019 by Information Age Publishing
All rights of reproduction in any form reserved.

Learning from you has been a tremendous joy and having you participate in my classes, even more so. I also wish to acknowledge colleagues in the Entrustable Professional Activities pilot project of the AAMC. You have taught me more about the complexities of teaching and learning in medicine than I ever thought possible. I thank Carrie Boden and Kathy Peno for supporting me in undertaking this work and for their willingness to recruit some wonderful contributors. Finally, no words can adequately express my gratitude for the love and support of my husband, Rob. Your understanding and patience made this book possible.

Carrie: I am grateful for the opportunity to collaborate with Drs. Terry Carter and Kathy Peno, whose great minds have shaped my thinking and generous hearts have opened my own. I appreciate the stories and scholarship of the contributors, whose vulnerability, creativity, hope, and right action inspire me to improve my practice. It is an honor to make a living working with people and ideas and to have the opportunity to dialog with colleagues in the extended way this volume affords. For this, I am grateful. Finally, I wish to acknowledge all of the teachers, healers, and helpers—those known to me and unknown—who find themselves in places that need them and are doing good work that transforms individuals, communities, workplaces, cities, and more. May you be resilient and thrive.

Kathy: I begin by thanking the authors for sharing their stories and experiences which have encouraged me to reflect on my own teacher–student interactions, my teaching style, and my need to engage in self care. I wish to thank my graduate students who challenge me daily to reflect on my practice and grow as a teacher, mentor, and practitioner. I am thankful that even though I am in the final stage of my career, they challenge me to remain a lifelong, reflective learner and practitioner. Finally, I am humbled by the opportunity to collaborate with two amazing women, Dr. Terry Carter and Dr. Carrie Boden, whose depth of knowledge, experience, and commitment to the field of adult learning is inspirational.

INTRODUCTION

The Role of Transformative Learning in Building a Resilient Professional Identity

Teresa J. Carter
Virginia Commonwealth University School of Medicine

Carrie J. Boden
Texas State University

Kathy Peno
University of Rhode Island

ABSTRACT

Professional learners, and the educators who prepare them for practice, are facing unprecedented challenges in the nature of their work as society's healers and helpers. In healthcare professions, work-related stress and burnout are at such high levels that leading scholars perceive a public health crisis. Students in professional healthcare fields are not immune from similar pressures, with levels of stress, burnout, and depression that far exceed those in the general population. In teacher and counselor education, demands for accountability abound, along with national debates about how best to assess teacher performance and improve educational outcomes. Other profession-

Transformative Learning in Healthcare and Helping Professions Education, pages xxi–xxxvii
Copyright © 2019 by Information Age Publishing
xxi

als, including counselors, therapists, and social workers, find practice environments increasing in complexity as they interact with greater numbers of specialists in diverse communities of practice. Today's professional learners will
need to develop a resilient professional identity to thrive in these demanding,
but rewarding, careers. The chapters in this book offer positive and growth-
enhancing strategies to support teaching and learning, enhance professional
identity formation, build capacity for resilience, and learn to care for self and
others. We share them for what they contribute to the potential for well-being
among trainees and professionals in healthcare and the helping professions.

Today's professional learners, and the professional educators who prepare
them for practice, are facing unprecedented challenges in the nature of
their work as society's healers and helpers. In the professions of medicine,
nursing, and other healthcare disciplines, the demands of practice have
grown considerably in recent years, along with the associated costs of providing care. In professional training for therapeutic professional services,
including social work, counseling, and in teacher education, universities
are under pressure to elevate the standards of professional preparation,
hold costs down, and attract the best faculty talent to educate learners in
these challenging disciplines. As a nation, we are asking more of our professional care providers, demanding greater accountability from them, ex-
pecting improved quality and enhanced safety of care, and subjecting them
to increasing liability for malpractice in a litigious society. In short, the road
to professional practice is one of challenges for all involved.

For these reasons, and others related to the workload and debt load that
professional students incur while pursuing their education, stress, burnout, depression, and related problems are on the rise for many. Medical
students, residents, nurses, and others in the health professions seem particularly prone to depressive symptoms and their consequences in rates
much higher than their counterparts in the general population (Dyrbye
et al., 2012; Johnson et al., 2017; Rotenstein et al., 2016; Schwenk, Davis,
& Wimsatt, 2010; Shanafelt et al., 2015), with more than half of U.S. physicians experiencing professional burnout (Shanafelt et al., 2015). Clearly,
something more is needed to help professional learners and their educators understand and cope with the present situation, and that "something"
is most likely going to have to come from within, rather than in the form of
externally supplied relief.

As learners form their professional identities by absorbing the values, beliefs, and underlying assumptions of the roles they are to assume in society,
the need to develop a *resilient* professional identity has never been greater
than it is for those in training today. Not only must learners grow cognitively
and emotionally during professional training, but they will also need to
generate their own internal sources of strength and resilience to cope with
the difficulties of practice environments. Kegan (2000) elegantly described

needs for learning of this magnitude as an epistemological shift that transforms, rather than forms. His constructivist-developmental approach to learning describes the insufficiency of instrumental, cause-and-effect knowledge acquisition upon which most competency-based education relies. In Kegan's schema, fully developed learners have an internalized set of values and beliefs that they adhere to, but they also have the capacity to reflect on experience, consider alternative perspectives, and enlarge their own worldview when it is no longer functional and limits growth. This perspective on transformative learning described by Kegan offers a missing piece when considering professional identity formation (PIF) by allowing for the possibility of professional identity *trans*formation (Wald, 2015).

TRANSFORMATIVE LEARNING THEORY

Within adult learning theory and practice, transformative learning has become a major theoretical perspective to help adult learners realize their ability to revise the meaning of experience when present frames of reference are no longer serving them well (Dirkx, 1998; Taylor, 2008). Since early descriptions of a perspective transformation (Mezirow, 1978), this theoretical stance has served as a framework for understanding how adults can learn to revise underlying assumptions, alter dysfunctional belief systems, and become more critically reflective and open to alternatives for thinking and acting in the world (Cranton, 2016; Taylor, 2008).

Transformative learning theory, first posited in the 1970s by Mezirow (1978), has developed and evolved over the past 4 decades to encompass a greater role for relationships in learning and other ways of knowing beyond Mezirow's largely cognitive approach to individual change. Several elements of the theory have remained relatively unchanged, however, since original description of a perspective transformation. Central to the theory is the idea that knowledge is socially constructed and involves revision in the meaning that an adult makes of experience. Mezirow's (1991) ideas had their origins in the work of many renowned scholars and writers, and over the decades, the theory has become more sophisticated and nuanced in elaborating upon the unique features of learning in adulthood.

Drawing upon the seminal work of Habermas (1987), Mezirow (1991, 2012) categorized knowledge as occurring in two domains: instrumental (cause and effect or task-oriented learning), and communicative, which involves feelings, emotions, and intentions expressed through communicative acts and words. Mezirow believed that transformative learning could potentially occur through either, but was far more likely to involve the communicative domain. When either instrumental or communicative learning resulted in a revised perspective, Mezirow perceived this as emancipatory, freeing the person from previously held beliefs or assumptions that were limitations to growth and personal development. With the concept of emancipatory learning, Mezirow also drew upon Freire's (1970) concept of conscientization, or the development of a critical consciousness (Baumgartner, 2012; Tan & Nabb, 2012). Mezirow asserted that it was only in adulthood that a person is capable of revising beliefs, values, and assumptions that had been assimilated uncritically in childhood from caregivers and significant others.

By reflecting on the meaning of experience and engaging in critical reflection and self-reflection, Mezirow (1991, 2012) argued that less functional beliefs and assumptions can be revised to include alternative frames of reference and viewpoints that are more expansive and discriminating of experience. He also described the nature of reflection in transformative learning as either objectively or subjectively interpreted. Objective reframing of the meaning of experience occurs through critical reflection on the assumptions of others encountered in task-oriented problem solving or by applying reflective insight from someone else's narrative to one's own experience (Mezirow, 2012, p. 87). Subjective framing, however, he believed to consist of critical self-reflection, in which an individual reflects upon the nature of personal experience to reexamine one's own underlying assumptions to determine if they are still valid. Mezirow also indicated that transformative learning requires a decision to act upon revisions in meaning, whether that action is immediate or future-oriented. Often difficult or troubling in nature, this change in perspective holds the potential to result in a revised worldview, freeing the individual from outdated, unworkable assumptions.

As Clark (1993) described, adults are different after experiencing transformative learning in ways that they and others can also recognize. Thus, transformative learning is not an everyday occurrence, but a relatively rare experience, and a significant one in the lives of adults. Since transformative learning is usually an intense, personal experience, Mezirow (1991, 2012) initially described the catalyst for such learning as a "disorienting dilemma" and outlined his observations of a 10-step process of how it occurs. Since these early descriptions, the actual learning process has been found to be more recursive in nature for some individuals, and often incremental, so that the change in perspective occurs over time rather than as a dramatic, one-time learning experience (Courtenay, Merriam, Reeves, & Baumgartner, 2000). Other scholars have described less rational, more intuitive and emotion-driven or somatic way of knowing that characterize the transformative learning of some learners (Clark, 2012; Dirkx, 2008; Stroud, Prindle, & England, 2012).

Taylor (2006, 2009) describes teaching for transformation as teaching for change. As such, it is much easier to describe the outcomes of transformative learning than it is to realize it in practice, or to know how to help learners accomplish the change involved. Taylor notes that teaching with the potential for transformative learning is not to be taken lightly, since it requires intentional action on the part of the educator, genuine concern for the learner's development, and a willingness to take some personal risk (Taylor, 2006, p. 1). Opportunities to encourage learners to engage in transformative learning can be provoked by the questions educators ask and through guided exercises that engage students in reflective practices. Even then, as he notes, there are no guarantees that the best intentions will foster learners' growth and development. Ettling (2006) cautions educators to be aware of the ethical dimensions of fostering transformative learning by appreciating the challenges involved and the skills needed:

> How does one decide how far to engage students in the practice of looking at underlying assumptions and beliefs?. . .Is it justified to pose real-life dilemmas that force examination of one's life story and lived assumptions? And do adult educators have the expertise to lead participants through the transforming experience? (p. 63)

Cranton (2006) provides several strategies for educators to develop authentic relationships with learners that will support critical reflection on assumptions and values of practice, including Dirkx's (2000) advice to pay attention to the everyday occurrences by having learners recognize, name, and understand the meaning of what they may be taking for granted. These strategies for educators include becoming aware of characteristics and preferences of learners by realizing that they may be very different from their own, developing a relationship with learners that is genuine and open, and engaging in critical reflection and self-reflection about one's own teaching practices (Cranton, 2006, p. 7). In the last 20 years, research on transformative learning has evolved into many different approaches including the cognitive-rational, neurobiological, psycho-developmental, structural-developmental, race-centric, and planetary approaches (Boden-McGill & Kippers, 2012; Fisher-Yoshida, Geller, & Schapiro, 2009; Taylor, 2008).

We believe the capacity for transformative learning can improve resilience and coping strategies for those in healthcare and the helping professions. Fostering transformative learning can become a developmental goal of professional educators whenever circumstances and the readiness to learn are apparent within the learner. By attending to these opportunities as they arise, educators can help learners form resilient professional identities to cultivate a helping professional who knows how to generate self-care as well as provide care to others.

TRANSFORMATIVE LEARNING AND
THE BUILDING OF A RESILIENT PROFESSIONAL IDENTITY

In our examination of PIF, resilience strategies, and the potential for transformative learning, we examined the literature of multiple disciplines to discover an intersection of theory with practice. There are many challenging questions about learning in healthcare and the helping professions, since socialization into a professional discipline is viewed as a complex process, one that is rarely overtly taught (Beddoe, Davys, & Adamson, 2013; Cruess, Cruess, Boudreau, Snell, & Steinert, 2015; Johnson et al., 2014; Trede, Macklin, & Bridges, 2012; Wald, 2015). In professional education, experiences in both classroom and clinical environments often generate potential opportunities for transformation (Marlowe, 2016). Examples include formal and informal assessments, critical incidents (Brookfield, 1990), unexpected consequences from actions, patient care situations, medical errors and "near misses" [safety incidents], role modeling, and mentoring episodes (Carter et al., 2016) and reflection. During encounters with the hidden curriculum (Hafferty, 1998; Hafferty & Franks, 1994), learners tacitly acquire the underlying values and beliefs by observing the behaviors of others. By incorporating the tools of critical reflection and questioning of underlying assumptions throughout professional development, learners may uncover instances of the hidden curriculum in practice environments and use these to align personal and professional values. Ultimately, this may lead them to develop authentic professional identities and the skills of reflective practice (Cranton & King, 2003).

Professional Identity Formation

All aspiring professionals, whatever their discipline, enter the learning environment with a *personal* identity; what happens during the years of their training is formation of a *professional* identity (Cruess et al., 2015; Goldie, 2012; Trede et al., 2012; Wald, 2015). Goldie (2012) defines professional identity within medical education as a dynamic construct that is relational, situated, and embedded in relations of power, yet negotiable. Irby and Hamstra (2016) cast PIF as one of three major approaches in the development of professionalism in medical education. The first of these approaches is a virtue-based construct that focuses on the development of moral character and humanistic habits of heart. The second, a behavioral framework that emphasizes milestones, competencies, and measurement of observable behaviors, has dominated competency-based health professions education in the last decade and continues to do so, with professionalism as an underlying competency needed to develop *entrustable* learners

(Association of American Medical Colleges, 2014). By contrast, the third approach toward PIF is a focus on the socialization of learners into a community of practice: "The good physician integrates into his or her identity a set of values and dispositions consonant with the physician community and aspires to a professional identity reflected in the very best physicians" (Irby & Hamstra, 2016, p. 1606).

The concept of a professional identity may be more obvious in the health professions literature in which it has emerged as a major discourse in recent years (Cruess et al., 2015; Goldie, 2012; Irby & Hamstra, 2016; Wald, 2015); however, we found evidence that other professional programs of study, such as teacher education, social work, and counselor education, all view the development of a professional identity as a unique and essential outcome of professional preparation (Buchanan, 2015; Hong, Greene, & Lowery, 2017; Lamote & Engels, 2010; Oliver, 2013; Owens & Neale-McFall, 2014; Stenberg, 2010; Trede et al., 2012; Wiles, 2012; Woo, Henfield, & Choi, 2014).

Stenberg (2010) views high-quality teaching as that which requires self-awareness into the sources of the teacher's pedagogical decision-making (p. 331). The risk for teachers who have not yet examined their own underlying assumptions includes stereotypes, fixed beliefs about teaching that may be inaccurate, and fears or misunderstanding of the power dynamics involved in the teacher–learner relationship (Stenberg, 2010). Stenberg viewed the development of a teacher's professional self-knowledge as "identity work," including self-reflection on life experiences. Other examinations of PIF address the complex interprofessional roles of social workers in healthcare and helping professions that enable them to function as boundary-spanners whose work crosses and intersects with multiple communities of practice (CoPs) as they form a professional identity (Oliver, 2013). Whatever the discipline, acquiring the beliefs, values, and assumptions that one associates with a professional field of practice is a complex journey which entails significant learning over many years, depending upon the discipline and educational requirements for certification or credentialing (Cruess et al., 2015; Wald, 2015). We believe that the nature of this learning can become transformative, rich with possibilities for enhancing careers that are among the most demanding in society, but also among the most rewarding.

The Need for Strategies to Promote Resilience

Why the emphasis on building a *resilient* professional identity among students in healthcare and the helping professions? These learners are among the most vulnerable to stress-related illnesses, depression, and burnout in our society. This appears to be particularly true for those in

Collectively and individually, professional learners and providers of care need strategies for remaining resilient in spite of adversity to ensure their own well-being and to cope with the demands of their roles as healers and helpers. Learners in these demanding disciplines will require the capacity for lifelong learning and reflective practices that allow them to revisit tacitly acquired ways of being to address the caregiving challenges of professional work. Transformative learning, when it occurs, can serve as a means to revise beliefs and assumptions (Mezirow, 1990, 1991) to bolster resilience strategies and create protective approaches to manage stress as part of a robust professional identity. Scholars have found that developing resilience is key to enhancing quality of care, quality of caring, and sustainability of the healthcare workforce (Epstein & Krasner, 2013).

Many in healthcare and helping fields view resilience as a skill that can be developed, rather than as a personal trait (Epstein & Krasner, 2013; McAllister & Lowe, 2011; Stephens, 2013). Cultivating specific skills, habits, and attitudes that promote resilience is possible for professional learners as well as professionals already immersed in practice environments. However, these skills are not easily developed, nor will they be sustained, without ample support systems, institutional commitment, and opportunities for learning (Gillman et al., 2015). The benefits to institutions, in addition to promoting the well-being of students and trainees, include creation of a culture of safety by reducing medical errors, stress, and burnout as factors that contribute to attrition among faculty (Epstein & Krasner, 2013).

Practice-Based Learning in a Community of Practice

Among the resources available for learners and practitioners are relationships and support networks created by informal CoPs within today's institutions (Lave & Wenger, 1991, Wenger, McDermott, & Snyder, 2002). When learners enter a new field of professional study or practice, rarely do they have full appreciation of what it means to be socialized into the learning community. Communities of practice are largely invisible to an outsider since membership is rarely displayed or even needed, but those who are within the community are well aware of the shared practices, norms, language, and worldview shared by members.

Professional learners are newcomers on the periphery of practice. Many are simultaneously members of multiple of these naturally-occurring entities that form around shared practices, negotiated meanings, and a common purpose. Some professionals, particularly social workers and others whose work intersects with multiple disciplines (Oliver, 2013), find that they must cross many different CoPs to share their knowledge and accomplish their tasks. Learning that occurs within a CoP is culturally transmitted through the norms and the actions of everyday work. This learning consists of the use of tools, symbols, acronyms, and accepted knowledge of "how things get done around here" that are part of the daily routine (Lave & Wenger, 1991). As such, the learning of professional students is not only socialization into what it means to be a doctor, nurse, teacher, or other professional, but the work itself is less often taught than it is tacitly acquired. Initially, novice learners assume lesser roles within the practice environment including observation and peripheral tasks, and then they gradually acquire increasing membership, progressively developing the expertise, knowledge, and skills associated with competent practice. One of the more underappreciated resources for promoting resilience can be found within the developmental relationships fostered within a CoP and the learning potential of mentors and positive role models that exist within these communities.

Mentors and Role Models

Although mentoring relationships can be found in a variety of formal and informal environments to support professional learning (Peno, Mangiante, & Kenahan, 2016), it is far more likely for students in healthcare and helping professions to experience role modeling in classroom and clinical settings. In healthcare, role modeling has been considered the primary mechanism for passing on tacit knowledge within the hidden curriculum (Gofton & Regehr, 2006; Hafferty & Franks, 1994) and an untapped educational strategy among physicians to promote ethical behavior (Goldie, 2012; Kenny, Mann, & MacLeod, 2003). Role models can be positive examples of how to act as a professional within the discipline, or negative ones of what not to do. Both yield experiences from which a trainee can learn. Positive role models serve as exemplars of outstanding professional practice, while negative role models leave long-lasting impressions that learners recall about behaviors they do not want to emulate when working with patients, students, or colleagues (Carter et al., 2016).

In today's professional learning and work environments, peer relationships also remain strong influences for what is learned and how trainees adopt the norms of acceptable behavior within the community (Marlowe & Carter, 2016). Often those who are involved in supervising a professional student are not much older than the learner. This is true of teaching assistants and advanced trainees in health professions education, including residents in clinical settings. Within academic medicine, role modeling has been considered the primary mechanism for fostering PIF (Cruess et al., 2015; Goldie, 2012) and the lack of positive role models has been identified as a significant issue within the hidden curriculum meriting attention (Gofton & Regehr, 2006; Holmes, Harris, Schwartz, & Regehr, 2015).

Influences of the Hidden Curriculum

What is meant by the "hidden curriculum?" Hafferty (1998) defined it as the set of influences outside the formal curriculum that transmit cultural norms and values to learners. By definition, then, CoPs become carriers of learning through the hidden curriculum. Vicarious learning by observing others was first described by Bandura (1986) in developing his theory of social learning. Scholars who have examined the formation of a professional identity (Bandini et al., 2017; Beauchamp & Thomas, 2009; Cruess et al., 2015; Goldie, 2012) view the hidden curriculum as a major contributor to learner socialization. How learners make sense of both clinical and nonclinical experiences that contradict or undermine what is being taught to them in formal learning settings and through informal means becomes the issue for educators who must strive for congruence between what is taught and what is learned (Goften & Regehr, 2006; Holmes et al., 2015).

Many who supervise and instruct professional learners remain unaware of how their actions exert shaping influences on those who are newcomers to the profession. Some see this as the dilemma of the hidden curriculum's challenge to professional education and the need for culture change, but also recognize the difficulty involved in effecting change of this magnitude (Holmes et al., 2015). Others assert that the power differential between learners and educators makes it unlikely that learners will challenge authority figures, even when educators demonstrate unprofessional behavior in practice settings (Brainard & Brislen, 2007).

Thus, the hidden curriculum poses a distinct challenge for development of professional identities that will be resilient to the stresses and strains of today's work world. Many learners will learn and retain behavioral traits and ways of being that they absorb as acceptable because they see them modeled by others until they encounter instances in which these behaviors no longer serve them well. When this happens, the opportunity to engage in learning that will transform the learner's professional identity arises. In this way, learners can develop greater capacity for resilience and the ability to bounce back from adversity.

Building Resilient Professional Identities

As adult educators who work in adult education and healthcare professions, we see the challenges faced by today's professionals in training.

We join our colleagues who teach professional learners in sharing their concerns about the stressors and strains within current educational and practice environments. Some describe these stressors as at the breaking point for professionals in training and in work practice, and others point to a looming crisis (Rappley et al., 2016). In response, we have sought colleagues to share their unique insights from a multidisciplinary perspective to contribute the chapters that follow. We asked that they consider the constructs of resilience and PIF in the socialization of learners into a community of practice, with a focus on what might be valuable, positive, and developmental if the learning experience for professionals were also to provide opportunities for transformation. The insights they have provided astound us for their potential to engage learners in transformative learning and build resilient professional identities. Their shared vision for learners is to deepen their self-understanding, reflect critically upon previously acquired beliefs and assumptions, and arrive at the threshold of professional practice as competent, caring healers and helpers who are ready to benefit society.

REFERENCES

Association of American Medical Colleges. (2014). *The core entrustable professional activities for entering residency: Curriculum developers' guide.*Washington, DC: Association of American Medical Colleges.

Bandini, J., Mitchell, C., Epstein-Peterson, Z. D., Amobi, A., Cahill, J., Peteet, J.,... Balboni, M. J. (2015). Student and faculty reflections of the hidden curriculum: How does the hidden curriculum shape students' medical training and professionalization? *American Journal of Hospice and Palliative Medicine, 34*(1), 57–63. https://doi.org/10.1177/1049909115616359

Bandura, A. (1986). *Social foundations of thought and action: A social cognitive theory.* Englewood Cliffs, NJ: Prentice Hall.

Baumgartner, L. M. (2012). Mezirow's theory of transformative learning from 1975 to present. In E. W. Taylor & P. Cranton (Eds.), *The handbook of transformative learning: Theory, research, and practice* (pp. 99–115). San Francisco, CA: Jossey-Bass.

Beauchamp, C., & Thomas, L. (2009). Understanding teacher identity: An overview of issues in the literature and implications for teacher education. *Cambridge Journal of Education, 39*(2), 175–189.

Beddoe, L., Davys, A., & Adamson, C. (2013). Educating resilient practitioners. *Social Work Education, 32*(1), 100–117.

Boden-McGill, C. J., & Kippers, S. M. (2012). *Pathways to transformation: Learning in relationship.* Charlotte, NC: Information Age.

Brainard, A. H., & Brislen, H. C. (2007). Viewpoint: Learning professionalism: A view from the trenches. *Academic Medicine, 82*(11), 1010–1014.

Brookfield, S. (1990). Using critical incidents to explore learner's assumptions. In J. Mezirow & Associates (Eds.), *Fostering critical reflection in adulthood: A guide to transformative and emancipatory learning* (pp. 177–193). San Francisco, CA: Jossey-Bass.

Buchanan, R. (2015). Teacher identity and agency in an era of accountability. *Teachers and Teaching, 21*(6), 700–719.

Carter, T. J., Brock, E. L., Fulco, F. A., Garber, A. M., Hemrajani, R. H., Lee, B. B., Matherly, S. C.,... Pierce, J. G., Jr. (2016). The influence of mentors and role models on teaching and learning in academic medicine. In K. Peno, E. M. Silva Mangiante, & R. T. Kenahan (Eds.), *Mentoring in formal and informal contexts* (pp. 247–262). Charlotte, NC: Information Age.

Clark, M. C. (1993). Transformational learning. In *New Directions for Adult and Continuing Education,* 57, 47–56. San Francisco, CA: Jossey-Bass.

Clark. M. C. (2012). Transformation as embodied narrative. In E. W. Taylor, P. Cranton, & Associates (Eds.). *The handbook of transformative learning* (pp. 425–438). San Francisco, CA: Jossey-Bass.

Courtenay, B. C., Merriam, S., Reeves, P., & Baumgartner, L. M. (2000). Perspective transformation over time: A 2-year follow-up study of HIV-positive adults. *Adult Education Quarterly, 50*(2), 102–119.

Cranton, P. (2006). Fostering authentic relationships in the transformative classroom. In E.W. Taylor (Ed.), *New Directions for Adult and Continuing Education,* Spring(109), 5–13.

Cranton, P. (2016). *Understanding and promoting transformative learning: A guide to theory and practice* (3rd ed.). San Francisco, CA: Jossey-Bass.

Cranton, P., & King, K. P. (2003). Transformative learning as a professional development goal. *New Directions for Adult and Continuing Education, 2003*(98), 31–38.

Cruess, R. L., Cruess, S. R., Boudreau, J. D., Snell, L., & Steinert, Y. (2015). A schematic representation of the professional identity formation and socialization of medical students and residents: A guide for medical educators. *Academic Medicine, 90*(6), 718–725.

Dirkx, J. M. (1998). Transformative learning theory in the practice of adult education: An overview. *PAACE Journal of Lifelong Learning, 7,* 1–14.

Dirkx, J. M. (2000). After the burning bush: Transformative learning as imaginative engagement with everyday experience. In C. Wiessner, S. Meyer, & D. Fuller (Eds.), *Challenges of practice: Transformative learning in action. The Proceedings of the Third International Conference on Transformative Learning.* New York, NY: Teacher's College Press.

Dirkx, J. M. (2008). The meaning and role of emotions in adult learning. In *New Directions for Adult and Continuing Education, 2008*(120), 7–18. https://doi.org/10.1002/ace.311

Dyrbye, L. N., Harper, W., Moutier, C., Durning, S. J., Power, D. V., Massie, F. S.,... Shanafelt, T. D. (2012). A multi-institutional study exploring the impact of positive mental health on medical students' professionalism in an era of high burnout. *Academic Medicine, 87*(8), 1024-0131.

Epstein, R. M., & Krasner, M. S. (2013). Physician resilience: What it means, why it matters, and how to promote it. *Academic Medicine, 88*(3), 301–303.

Ettling, D. (2006). Ethical demands of transformative learning. In E. W. Taylor (Ed.), Teaching for change: Fostering transformative learning in the classroom. *New Directions for Adult and Continuing Education,* Spring(109), 59–67.

Fisher-Yoshida, B., Geller, K., & Schapiro, S. (2009). *Innovations in transformative learning: Space, culture, and the arts.* New York, NY: Peter Lang.

Freire, P. (1970). *Pedagogy of the oppressed.* New York, NY: Continuum.

Gillman, L., Adams, J., Kovac, R., Kilcullen, A., House, A., & Doyle, C. (2015). Strategies to promote coping and resilience in oncology and palliative care nurses caring for adult patients with malignancy: A comprehensive systematic review. *JBI Database of Systematic Reviews and Implementation Reports, 13*(5), 131–204. doi:10.11124/jbisrir-2015-1898

Gofton, W., & Regehr, G. (2006). What we don't know we are teaching. *Clinical Orthopaedics and Related Research, 449,* 20–27.

Goldie, J. (2012). The formation of professional identity in medical students: Considerations for educators. *Medical Teacher, 34*(9), e641–e648.

Habermas, J. (1987). *The theory of communicative action* (T. McCarthy, Trans.). Reason and the rationalization of society (Vol.1). Lifeworld and system: A critique of functionalist reason (Vol. 2). Boston, MA: Beacon Press.

Hafferty, F. W. (1998). Beyond curriculum reform: Confronting medicine's hidden curriculum. *Academic Medicine, 73*(4), 403–407.

Hafferty, F. W., & Franks, R. (1994). The hidden curriculum, ethics teaching, and the structure of medical education. *Academic Medicine, 69*(11), 861–871.

Hinderer, K. A., VonRueden, K. T., Friedmann E., McQuillan, K. A., Gilmore, R., Kramer, B., & Murray, M. (2014). Burnout, compassion fatigue, compassion satisfaction, and secondary traumatic stress in trauma nurses. *Journal of Trauma Nursing, 21*(4), 160–169.

Holmes, C. L., Harris, I. B., Schwartz, A. J., & Regehr, G. (2015). Harnessing the hidden curriculum: A four-step approach to developing and reinforcing reflective competencies in medical clinical clerkships. *Advances in Health Science Education, 20*(5), 1355–1370.

Hong, J., Greene, B., & Lowery, J. (2017). Multiple dimensions of teacher identity development from pre-service to early years of teaching: A longitudinal study. *Journal of Education for Teaching, 43*(1), 84–98. https://doi.org/10.1080/026 07476.2017.1251111

Irby, D. M., & Hamstra, S. J. (2016). Parting the clouds: Three professionalism frameworks in medical education. *Academic Medicine, 91*(12), 1606–1611. https://doi.org/10.1097/ACM.0000000000001190

Jackson, E. R., Shanafelt, T. D., Hasan, O., Satele, D. V., & Dyrbye, L. N. (2016). Burnout and alcohol abuse/dependence among U.S. medical students. *Academic Medicine, 9*(19), 1251–1260. https://doi.org/10.1097/ACM.000000000000 1138

Johnson, B., Down, B., Le Cornu, R., Peters, J., Sullivan, A., Pearce, J., & Hunter, J. (2014). Promoting early career teacher resilience: A framework for understanding and acting. *Teachers and Teaching, 20*(5), 530–546.

Johnson, J., Louch, G., Dunning, A., Johnson, O., Grange, A., Reynolds, C., ... O'Hara, J. (2017). Burnout mediates the association between depression and patient safety perceptions: A cross-sectional study in hospital nurses. *Journal of Advanced Nursing,* [Epub ahead of print] https://doi.org/10.1111/jan.13251

Keidel, G. C. (2002). Burnout and compassion fatigue among hospice caregivers. *American Journal of Hospice and Palliative Medicine, 19*(3), 200–205.

Kegan, R. (2000). What "form" transforms? A constructive-developmental approach to transformative learning. In J. Mezirow and Associates (Eds.), *Learning as transformation: Critical perspectives on a theory in progress* (pp. 35–70). San Francisco, CA: Jossey-Bass.

Kenny, N. P., Mann, K. V., & MacLeod, H. (2003). Role modeling in physicians' professional formation: Reconsidering an essential but untapped educational strategy. *Academic Medicine, 78*(12), 1203–1210.

Lachman, V. D. (2016). Compassion fatigue as a threat to ethical practice: Identification, personal and workplace prevention/management strategies. *MedSurg Nursing, 25*(4), 275–278.

Lamote, C., & Engels, N. (2010, January 21). The development of student teacher's professional identity. *European Journal of Teacher Education, 33*(1), 3–18. doi .org/10.1080/02619760903457735

Lave, J., & Wenger, E. (1991). *Situated learning: Legitimate peripheral participation.* Cambridge, England: University of Cambridge Press.

Marlowe, E. P. (2016). *"I just need to get myself supervised:" Exploring transformative learning in the development of professionalism among physicians in the first year of graduate medical education.* Retrieved from ProQuest Dissertations Publishing (Order No. 10130157)

Marlowe, E. P., & Carter, T. J. (2016, June). The role of transformative learning in fostering identity development among learners in professional programs of study. *Proceedings of the 2016 Adult Education Research Conference (AERC)*, Charlotte, NC.

McAllister, M., & Lowe, J. B. (2011). *The resilient nurse: Empowering your practice.* New York, NY: Springer.

Mezirow, J. (1978). Perspective transformation. *Adult Education, 28*(2), 100–110.

Mezirow, J. (1990). How critical reflection triggers transformative learning. In J. Mezirow & Associates (Eds.), *Fostering critical reflection in adulthood* (pp. 1–20). San Francisco, CA: Jossey-Bass.

Mezirow, J. (1991). *Transformative dimensions of adult learning.* San Francisco, CA: Jossey-Bass.

Mezirow, J. (2012). Learning to think like an adult: Core concepts of transformation theory. In E. Taylor, P. Cranton, & Associates (Eds.), *The handbook of transformative learning: Theory, research, and practice* (pp. 73–95). San Francisco, CA: Jossey-Bass.

Oliver, C. (2013). Social workers as boundary spanners: Reframing our professional identity for interprofessional practice. *Social Work Education, 32*(6), 773–784.

Owens, E. W., & Neale-McFall, C. W. (2014). Counselor identity development: Toward a model for the formation of a professional identity. *Journal of Counselor Leadership and Advocacy, 1*(1), 16–27.

Peno, K., Mangiante, E. M. S., & Kenahan, R. T. (2016). *Mentoring in formal and informal contexts.* Charlotte, NC: Information Age.

Prinz, P., Hertrich, K., Hirschfelder, U., & de Zwaan, M. (2012). Burnout, depression and depersonalisation – Psychological factors and coping strategies in dental and medical students. *GMS (German Medical Science) Journal for Medical*

Education, 29(1). Retrieved from https://www.egms.de/static/en/journals/zma/2012-29/zma000780.shtml

Rappley, M., Moutier, C., West, C. P., Suchman, A., Haramati, A., & Kirch, D. G. (2016). *Creating a culture of wellbeing and resilience in academic medicine.* Association of American Medical Colleges (AAMC) Leadership Forum, Washington, DC.

Reed, D. A., Shanafelt, T. D., Satele, D. W., Power, D. V., Eacker, A., Harper, W.,...Dyrbye, L. N. (2011). Relationship of pass/fail grading and curriculum structure with well-being among preclinical medical students: A multi-institutional study. *Academic Medicine, 86*(11), 1367–1373. https://doi.org/10.1097/ACM.0b013e3182305d81

Rotenstein, L. S., Ramos, M. S., Torre, M., Segal, J. B., Peluso, M. J., Guille, C.,...Mata, D. A. (2016). Prevalence of depression, depressive symptoms, and suicidal ideation among medical students: A systematic review and meta-analysis. *Journal of the American Medical Association, 316*(21), 2214–2236. https://doi.org/10.1001/jama.2016.17324

Schwenk, T. L., Davis, L., & Wimsatt, L. A. (2010). Depression, stigma, and suicidal ideation in medical students. *Journal of the American Medical Association, 304*(11), 1181–1190. https://doi.org/10.1001/jama.2010.1300

Shanafelt, T. D., Hasan, O., Dyrbye, L. N., Sinsky, C., Satele, D., Sloan, J., & West, C. P. (2015). Changes in burnout and satisfaction with work-life balance in physicians and the general US working population between 2011 and 2014. *Mayo Clinic Proceedings, 90*(12), 1600–1613. https://doi.org/10.1016/j.mayocp.2015.08.023

Smart, D., English, A., James, J., Wilson, M., Daratha, K. B., Childers, B., & Magera, C. (2014). Compassion fatigue and satisfaction: A cross-sectional survey among US healthcare workers. *Nursing & Health Sciences, 16*(1), 3–10.

Stenberg, K. (2010). Identity work as a tool for promoting the professional development of student teachers. *Reflective Practice: International and Multidisciplinary Perspectives, 11*(3), 331–346.

Stephens, T. M. (2013). Nursing student resilience: a concept clarification. *Nursing Forum, 48*(2), 25–133.

Stroud, D., Prindle, J., & England, S. (2012). Narrative, somatic, and social/constructivist approaches to transformative learning in training programs for the helping professions. In C. J. Boden-McGill & S. M. Kippers (Eds.), *Pathways to transformation: Learning in relationship.* Charlotte, NC: Information Age.

Tan, F., & Nabb, L. (2012). Advancing transformative theory: Multifold and cyclical transformation. In C. J. Boden-McGill & S. M. Kippers (Eds.), *Pathways to transformation: Learning in relationship* (pp. 325–342). Charlotte, NC: Information Age.

Taylor, E. W. (2006). The challenge of teaching for change. In E. W. Taylor (Ed.), *Teaching for change: Fostering transformative learning in the classroom* (special edition), 109, 91–95.

Taylor, E. W. (2008). Transformative learning theory. In *New Dimensions for Adult and Continuing Education,* 119, 5–15.

Taylor, E. W. (2009). Fostering transformative learning. In J. Mezirow, E.W. Taylor, & Associates (Eds.), *Transformative learning in practice: Insights from community, workplace, and higher education* (pp. 3–17). San Francisco, CA: Jossey-Bass.

Trede, F., Macklin, R., & Bridges, D. (2012). Professional identity development: A review of the higher education literature. *Studies in Higher Education, 37*(3), 365–384.

Wald, H. S. (2015). Professional identity (trans)formation in medical education: Reflection, relationship, resilience. *Academic Medicine, 90*(6), 701–705. https://doi.org/10.1097/ACM.0000000000000731

Wenger, E., McDermott, R., & Snyder, W. M. (2002). *Cultivating communities of practice.* Boston, MA: Harvard Business School Press.

Wiles, F. (2012). "Not easily put in a box": Constructing professional identity. *Social Work Education, 32*(7), 854–866.

Woo, H., Henfield, M. S., & Choi, N. (2014). Developing a unified professional identity in counseling: A review of the literature. *Journal of Counselor Leadership and Advocacy, 1*(1), 1–15.

PART I

TEACHING AND LEARNING FOR CHANGE

CHAPTER 1

THERAPISTS IN THE MAKING

Charity Johansson
Elon University

ABSTRACT

Physical therapy students enter their highly competitive doctoral programs prepared to absorb vast amounts of knowledge, anticipating their graduation two-to-three years later as healthcare's experts in mobility. Like many others training in the "helping professions," what students often do not expect are the challenges to their understanding of who they are as professionals that they will encounter along the way. In particular, the unexamined complexities of the helping process threaten to undermine the passion and long-term resilience of physical therapists. This chapter explores three powerful assumptions that impede shared partnership in patient care: what it means to help, whose knowledge is most important, and the value of receiving care, along with the transformative possibilities that emerge from diving headlong into these assumptions and wrestling with them.

"So why do you want to be a physical therapist?" I ask the eager student perched on the chair across from me. It is a predictable interview question for prospective students applying to physical therapy educational programs and her sincere answer is almost equally predictable: "I really want to help people." "What does that mean," I counter, leaning forward as if

Transformative Learning in Healthcare and Helping Professions Education, pages 3–22

uncomprehending, "to '*help*' people?" A moment of perplexity flashes on her face, then, "I want to make people better," she explains with assurance.

I have listened for nearly 25 years to students as they make their cases for being awarded one of the limited seats in a physical therapy program's cohort for the year. Students who go into physical therapy are, for the most part, enthusiastic and good-hearted people looking forward to taking their places in a helping profession. They are eager to gain the knowledge and skills that will allow them to pass their licensing exams and begin treating patients. They bring into their training personal identities developed over at least two decades and preformed images of who they will be as therapists. They expect to work hard and study long hours to expand their existing knowledge and skills, but, like undergraduate students (Johansson & Felten, 2014), rarely do they expect to undergo any fundamental change in who they are along the way. They typically expect their education to render them better informed, to be sure, but not particularly transformed.

On the horizon, however, loom indicators that their current understanding may not be sufficient to carry them successfully through their professional careers. Burnout and compassion fatigue take their toll on a troublingly high number of physical therapists (Anderson, 2015; Balogun, Titiloye, Balogun, Oyeyemi, & Katz, 2002; Klappa, Fulton et al., 2015; Klappa, Howayek, Reed, Scherbarth, & Klappa, 2015). The end result of burnout and compassion fatigue is not merely disillusioned and dissatisfied healthcare providers, but diminished quality of care, poor patient outcomes, and, ultimately, the attrition of skilled and caring professionals from the workforce (Cimiotti, Aiken, Sloane, & Wu, 2012; Craig & Sprang, 2010; Figley, 2002; Killian, 2008; Klappa, Fulton et al., 2015; Lyndon, 2016; Najjar, Davis, Beck-Coon, & Carney Doebbeling, 2009; Passalacqua & Segrin, 2012; Potter et al., 2013; Slatten, Carson, & Carson, 2011; West et al., 2006) at a time when we are desperately in need of them.

How is it that these enthusiastic, caring, and dedicated young professionals become so disillusioned and disconnected? I believe at the heart of this conundrum lies our conflicted and unexamined sense of helping. The altruistic desire to help drives students to invest heavily of their time, energy, and money in a "helping" profession, yet little or no systematic examination is devoted to what it actually means to *help*. Why, when there are concepts of homonymous hemianopsia and paroxysmal nocturnal dyspnea to master, would we expend our precious educational currency on a word we have all understood since we were toddlers? This schism that arises between initial enthusiastic intentions and the realities of practice over time stems not only from a lack of knowledge of the workings of the human body, but also from unchallenged assumptions about our fundamental role in patient interactions. A more authentic understanding of their identities as helping professionals, on the other hand, better equips novice therapists to navigate the future challenges of patient care with fulfillment and resilience.

During their professional education, students look forward to learning more about the human body, movement pathologies, and methods of diagnosis and treatment. In sum, they expect to learn extensively about patient care. To achieve optimal, holistic outcomes, however, the reality is that the students' learning must be directed both outward and inward. For optimal patient intervention, Jensen and Paschal (2000) claim that developing practitioners must engage in ongoing self-discovery, or "critical self-reflection" (p. 42) by uncovering long-held assumptions.

Any time underlying assumptions are acknowledged, transformative learning is a possibility. It is never guaranteed, however. To foster lasting and meaningful change, educators must be intentional in designing learning activities to that end, guiding students into the inevitable frustration and confusion, through analysis and reflection, and finally into actions that bear out their new level of understanding. This chapter examines three common assumptions about professional helping roles that threaten to undermine the passion and long-term resilience of physical therapists in training. In it, I reframe frustrations in patient care as invitations to enter the transformative process, with learning strategies that challenge assumptions about helping. These exercises can serve as guides to help emerging professionals, whatever their discipline, develop a deeper, more evolved sense of themselves as professional helpers.

WHAT DOES IT MEAN TO HELP?

Dedicating one's career to helping others is certainly commendable. However, investing so heavily in one of the helping professions without deeply questioning the nature of what it means to *help* seems at the least unwise and, perhaps, ultimately, career ending. Such basic questions as, "What is help?" "Who is responsible for the outcome of my help?" "If a patient does not succeed, have I failed?" "What's in it for me when I help someone else?" are rarely asked. Is helping, in fact, as the prospective student declared, actually the same as making people better?

According to Schein (2011) in his work, *Helping: How to Offer, Give, and Receive Help*, helping is "the action of one person that enables another person to solve a problem, to accomplish something, or to make something easier" (p. 7). Helping is not simple, however, nor are the assumptions we make about it. According to Schein, helping is a complex phenomenon fraught with conscious and unconscious beliefs and expectations. Acting on these assumptions without examining them first can undermine patient interactions and set the professional up for disappointment and frustration.

Assumption: Superiority of Knowledge

When a patient or client solicits help from a professional such as a physical therapist, presumably, it is because the individual perceives the professional to possess expert knowledge and skill in the designated area. It is easy, however, for that expertise to take on a quality of superiority. As Smith (2008) notes, "The simple act of naming ourselves 'professional' can feed into an unthinking assumption that we know best" ("Does Helping Involve Seeing People in Deficit?" para. 1). This notion certainly has some basis. Professionalism is characterized by the attainment of a specialized body of knowledge and the application of that expertise on behalf of the person being helped. When afforded only surface attention, however, this seemingly benign—even benevolent—assumption can unknowingly harbor and promote negative and injurious judgments.

To be sure, the patient rarely has the same command of scientific knowledge as a doctor of physical therapy, but patients have knowledge that even the most extensively trained and expert physical therapist does not have—knowledge of their own bodies and minds and the lived experience of their health conditions. As osteopathic physician William Osler is purported to have said more than a 100 years ago, "Ask not what disease the person has, but rather what person the disease has." The best patient outcomes emerge when healthcare providers see themselves not as dispensers of knowledge but as exchangers of knowledge, collaborators who recognize the unique value and autonomy of the patient's experiences and choices. Jensen and Paschal (2000) concur. Recognizing the tendency of novice physical therapists to jump into advising and intervening, they caution that at the heart of expert clinical decision making and care is approaching the patient "as a valued and trusted source of knowledge" (p. 45).

Even for those who listen to their patients, authoritarian superiority can prevail, creating expectations for patient behaviors. Expectations, in turn, generate judgments based on whether or not those expectations are met. The degree to which therapists are comfortable telling their patients what they should do is the degree to which those therapists will tend to judge the patient who does not follow their advice.

Judgmental attitudes, whether conscious or not, are inevitably communicated at some level to patients, and outcomes are rarely the better for it. When making education recommendations for physical therapy, Jensen, Gwyer, Shepard, and Hack (2000) highlight the need for students to learn that their clinical effectiveness will be enhanced by "a nonjudgmental approach to patients" (p. 42). While most professionals understand that they must put aside their personal feelings about people's life choices and treat all patients or clients with the same level of professional respect, judgment in the form of believing one knows what's best for the patient is subtler and therefore more challenging to expose.

Strategy: The "Should" Experiment

To help students better recognize the judgment and subsequent negative effects inherent in this assumption, consider the common clinical frustration of the "noncompliant" patient. Even with their limited experience, most students already have strong emotional feelings about patients who do not comply with home exercise programs or other healthcare recommendations. Frustrated, they press, "How do you make them do their exercises?" "I don't," I say. "I don't consider it my job, nor am I able, to *make* my patients do anything." I can, however, provide information and instruction that I hope is compelling because of its relevance and meaning to the patient. When I suggest that presuming that they know what the patient should do actually implies judgment, I am often met with stout denials. "But we *do* know what they need to do! Why else are we learning all this?"

To bring this point home, I ask students to go 24 hours without saying the word "should" or any of its cousins such as "must," "need to," "have to," and "ought to." When they do find themselves starting to say "should," they are to stop and replace the phrase with information. In their student status, most "should" statements are internal rather than used with actual patients, so reframing often sounds like, instead of "I should study," a statement such as, "If I study this material now for an hour, I'm going to do better on tomorrow's test, which will make me feel good."

Reflection on the "Should" Experiment

The students' written reflections, shared here with permission, typically demonstrate an increased awareness of the judgmental and unhelpful nature of expressing what someone "should" do:

> Adapting my usual speech was an experience I did not believe would have major consequences on my thinking, but changing words made a difference in how I felt about myself and my whole day. I realized how overly critical I am toward both myself and friends. When giving relationship advice to a friend in need, I caught the phrase, "you should have" or "need to" much more than I anticipated, putting a negative spin on guidance meant to be encouraging.

Sometimes students also reveal deeper questioning of assumptions they have held about their anticipated roles as experts:

> The assignment really made me think. I started questioning *why* I wanted to do a particular task. I also started to question who I was and what authority I had to tell other people what they should or should not do. The assignment

really made me reflect upon my own beliefs and how much I have projected them onto other people.

In our discussion of the experiment, students comment on the paradoxical effect "should" statements have on their behavior. I ask them what one word almost always follows "should," and they all agree: "but." That word is inevitably followed by *not* doing the very thing they *should* do. "I should study," becomes "I should study, *but* I really want to see this movie," and the movie wins out.

As a side note, the word "compliance" is no longer considered acceptable in medical literature because of its air of passivity and paternalism, favoring instead the more collaborative term, "adherence." Still, the implication is that the patient will adhere to what the healthcare professional deems appropriate. Until the underlying attitudes and assumptions of superiority change, the effects of wording changes will be limited. True empowerment comes with mutual respect and recognition. Schein (2011) sums it well: "How the helping relationship evolves. . .depends on the degree to which the client grants value to the helper and the degree to which the helper grants value to the client" (p. 14).

Assumption: Helping Is a One-Way Transaction

In one sense, professional helping is obviously unidirectional in that the professional's job is to serve the patient; *we* help *them*. At a more complex level, however, helping is an inherently reciprocal interaction embedded with social status and the related implications and consequences. When they view helping as merely a clinician-to-patient transaction, healthcare practitioners tend to overlook opportunities for the patients to inform the clinical decisions of the provider. Furthermore, there is an unspoken expectation that the patients will, in fact, be willing recipients of the assistance that is being offered to them. Many of our most frustrating experiences both as clients and helpers, Schein (2011) asserts, occur because of our expectation that things should be different from the way they are; when assumptions are violated, negative emotions ensue. When a patient fails to follow through as expected, clinicians' feelings of anxiety, annoyance, and anger are common.

The assumption of unidirectionality makes it easy to conclude that the source of this problem lies with the patient who has not kept up his or her part of the bargain. In so doing, the therapist does not consider his or her own limiting beliefs that may be contributing to the failed interaction. Consequently, the professional also misses a valuable prompt for self-reflection and the opportunity to be on the receiving end of the learning exchange.

Recognizing negative feelings as indicators of deeper conflicts, the therapist can choose to reframe the situation as a "disorienting dilemma," the entry point into transformative learning (Mezirow, 1990). When emotions are strong, however, a systematic, external tool can be useful to support the transformative learning process.

Nowhere do the frustrations and misconceptions of helping become more evident than during difficult patient encounters. Difficult patient encounters are a reality of clinical practice, challenging even seasoned clinicians (Essary & Symington, 2005; Steinmetz & Tabenkin, 2001). Students, too, with their limited exposure to physical therapy practice, already have strong opinions about the types of patients they find difficult to work with in practice settings.

Difficult patient situations can test even strong positive values in the healthcare professional. Working with patients they consider difficult can cause clinicians who are otherwise positive and compassionate to feel discouraged, manipulated, angry, and emotionally drained (Essary & Symington, 2005; McCauley & Tarpley, 2004; Steinmetz & Tabenkin, 2001). Patients themselves also suffer, realizing poorer outcomes despite a higher utilization of the healthcare system (Essary & Symington, 2005; Jackson & Kroenke, 1999).

Numerous articles and books on difficult patient encounters have been written in the nearly 40 years since Groves (1978) published his seminal work on caring for the "hateful patient." Although patient descriptions in subsequent literature vary, it is important to note that, ultimately, "difficult patients" are defined by their ability to elicit negative emotions *in the healthcare provider* (De Marco, Nogueira, & Yazigi, 2005; Groves, 1978; Steinmetz & Tabenkin, 2001). Even as the term "difficult patient" is being replaced by the less judgmental term (though still conveniently ambiguous in its attribution of responsibility) "difficult patient encounter" (De Marco et al., 2005), the advice for dealing with such situations continues to focus on modifying the patient's behaviors. Whether the recommendation is to convey expressions of empathy, practice active listening, or implement behavior modification (De Marco et al., 2005; Essary & Symington, 2005; Haas, Leiser, Magill, & Sanyer, 2005), the goal is to reduce the patient's demanding, irritating, or otherwise difficult behaviors.

Rarely is the health professional urged to look inward, even though reflective insight has been deemed essential to the development of professional expertise and virtuous practice (Jensen & Paschal, 2000; Macdonald, 2002). In addition to the lack of educational guidance toward such inward responses, honest self-assessment is difficult and uncomfortable. Recognizing that attempts at self-reflection in the face of strong emotion usually benefit from the aid of a guided, systematic process, I developed the Mirror

Insight Tool (MIT) to facilitate clinicians' self-examination in response to difficult patient encounters.

Strategy: The Mirror Insight Tool

Rather than attempting to get rid of "problem patient behaviors" or compartmentalize our own responses, the MIT uses the energy created by the tension between what we want to experience (consistent with values such as compassion and tolerance) and what we actually experience (such as anger, resentment, and frustration) to fuel our own development. To implement the MIT, the clinician identifies the patient behavior that is eliciting the negative emotional response and the character trait that behavior represents. For example, if the clinician is irritated by the patient's fearfulness and refusal to attempt even the most basic rehabilitation tasks despite the clinician's confident reassurance, the clinician might identify cowardice as the associated character trait.

Next, the clinician places that character trait on a continuum. Aristotle described ideal traits, or "virtues," as located in the middle between extreme deficiency of that trait on one end and extreme excess of that trait on the other (Bostock, 2000; see Figure 1.1). He labels these extremes of deficiency and excess at each end of the continuum "vices." Using the example above, the clinician would place cowardice at one end of the continuum, representing a deficiency of courage. The virtue courage is placed in the middle, and the excess of courage, foolhardiness, is placed at the far end of the continuum (see Figure 1.2).

With the virtue continuum in place, the clinician uses it to look inward. As I have advised students and clinicians engaged in difficult patient encounters, when someone "pushes your button," remember whose button it is. Rather than attempting to change or fix others, we can focus on what we might be able to alter within ourselves to achieve personal and professional growth. To do this with the MIT, we apply the following axiom: "We

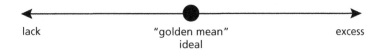

lack   "golden mean"   excess
ideal

Figure 1.1 Character trait plotted on a continuum with the ideal trait in the middle between extreme trait deficiency and extreme trait excess.

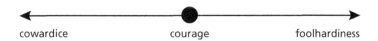

cowardice   courage   foolhardiness

Figure 1.2 The virtue courage plotted on a continuum between lack of courage and an excess of courage.

resist most in others what we fear most in ourselves." For example, the clinician who experiences strong resistance to expressions of cowardice will commonly find that he or she identifies strongly with the other extreme of foolhardiness, perhaps even taking pride in engaging in reckless or daredevil activities.

Reflection on the Use of the Mirror Insight Tool

In my first experience applying this process to my own difficult patient encounter, the trait I found irritating in the patient was an exaggerated expression of helplessness and dependence. Disturbed by my feelings, I tried on the axiom. "I resist most in others what I fear most in myself?" "That's ridiculous," I thought. "I'm not afraid of being dependent; I'm way too independent for that!" It dawned on me, of course, that I was, in fact, so afraid of being dependent that I was living at the other extreme of the continuum, insisting on fierce independence in every endeavor. I then identified the "golden mean" between the extremes of helplessness and extreme independence, that of interdependence (see Figure 1.3).

In another example, a student once confessed that she became internally furious at a 12-year-old patient during her first clinical rotation because he invariably stumbled over the edge of the treatment mat on the floor every time he came to therapy. Aware that her emotions were out of proportion to the patient's behavior, she willingly took part in the MIT. As the process unfolded, I learned that her aversion to being clumsy was so profound that she had spent years learning to control her movements through the precise and formalized practice of ballet. In completing the MIT, the student recognized that she found her patient's clumsiness so objectionable because it represented a characteristic that she was unwilling to accept in herself. Once she recognized where her own emotional reaction originated, however, she was better able to separate her personal fear of being clumsy from her patient's actual situation.

Having plotted both the patient's and clinician's behaviors on the continuum, however, is only the beginning. Transformation in one's own perspectives requires more than mere awareness; newfound understanding must be followed by congruous action. Change is possible, transformative learning authority Jack Mezirow (1990) asserts, only when critical self-reflection results in "reflective action" (p. 7). Having considered that the source of

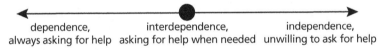

Figure 1.3   The virtue interdependence plotted on a continuum between extreme dependence and extreme independence.

the emotional response to a patient's behavior may lie internally, the next step in the guided process is to explore ways in which the clinician might inch closer to the "golden mean" by engaging in behaviors that represent the trait lying in the middle between the patient's excess and one's own, for it is by practicing a virtue that the clinician moves toward virtuous practice (Pellegrino, 2002). The student who had been irritated by her stumbling patient began exploring improvisational dance and theater. In my case, I began accepting small offers of assistance and, occasionally, even asking for help, even when I could have managed on my own.

A final key to the MIT is understanding that the vice-virtue continuum is, in fact, not a simple horizontal line with the vices at opposite ends. In reality, the shared quality of excess make the extremes more alike than different, depicted visually by bending the continuum into a circle until the two ends of the arrow almost touch. Although the "vices" may *feel* as far apart as possible from each other, it is actually a very short jump from one excess to the other (see Figure 1.4).

This phenomenon is often evident when a patient who has behaved at one extreme for a lifetime suddenly flips to the other extreme when incapacitated by illness or injury. One student told of her grandmother who, before a stroke left her unable to walk, was "the most giving and selfless person you could ever imagine. All of a sudden," the student exclaimed, "she turned into this selfish, demanding person!" The student and I considered the possibility that what had on the surface appeared to be a genuine virtue of selflessness may, in truth, have been an excess. Perhaps she engaged in self-sacrificing behavior to the exclusion of her own self-care which, in Aristotle's view, would have represented a behavioral extreme. It would not be surprising, then, that when a stroke prevented her from continuing at one extreme, she made the small leap to excessive behaviors at the other extreme of selfishness. Had she previously practiced a more

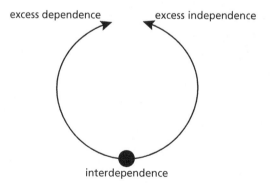

Figure 1.4 The reshaped continuum with the character trait extremes in close proximity to each other and at a maximum distance from the character trait ideal.

balanced approach of sometimes saying "no" to others so that she could care adequately for herself, perhaps her behaviors would not have changed so drastically after her stroke. As illustrated in the MIT diagram, the greatest distance lies not between the two extremes but between the extremes and their corresponding virtue or ideal trait.

Although most of us know better than to use patients to meet our needs, when patient behaviors elicit defensiveness within us as clinicians, we often hold the patient responsible for the negative feelings that result. In this way, we are, in fact, using our patients; they, and the negative feelings we hold about them, become buffers between us and our unconscious, allowing us to maintain the illusion of distance from that which we fear. When we are able to use the MIT successfully, not only do we improve our ability to meet a patient's underlying needs, but we change, expanding our capacity to be therapeutically present for similar patients in the future. Such change holds the potential to be transformative for the therapist. Unexamined assumptions and expectations about how our patients should behave, on the other hand, set healthcare practitioners up for frustration and, ultimately, burnout.

Willingness to share the healing role, whether played out in structured exercises such as the MIT or cultivated as an ongoing attitude, facilitates the uncovering of unconscious assumptions about what it means to help and be helped. In his lessons on mindfulness in medicine, Santorelli (2000) describes this reciprocity:

> Perhaps our real work, whether offering or seeking care, is to recognize that the healing relationship—the field upon which patient and practitioner meet—is, to use the words of the mythologist Joseph Campbell, a "self-mirroring mystery"—the embodiment of a singular human activity that raises essential questions about self, other, and what it means to heal thy self. (p. 12)

Santorelli sums up the potential for those practitioners willing to share in the healing role by looking within: "Being in the presence of others who are suffering and who, in turn, if we allow them to, reflect back to us unwanted or undisclosed elements of our own lives is an enormous opportunity" (p. 167). This openness to another human being, this shared sense of vulnerability that affects us at the deepest levels, can yield the greatest wisdom for healing and growth for both patient and therapist.

Assumption: Giving Help Is More Virtuous Than Receiving Help

A final assumption regarding helping that pervades healthcare professions and threatens the therapist's ongoing well-being is the belief that helping is more virtuous than being helped. While this assertion may at first seem overstated and even offensive to those in helping professions, everyday experiences bear it out. It is no secret in the medical world that healthcare providers often make the worst patients. While commendably dedicated to giving care, many resist asking for or accepting assistance from others. Being in need of help—Schein (2011) explains—creates a temporary loss of status. Our discomfort and even shame at being in this "one down" (p. 31) position betrays the often-unconscious sense of superiority in the role of helper. Until the therapist learns to value the receiving of care as much as the giving of care, the relationship with the patient will continue to be affected by this embedded disparity. Along with anxiety or even guilt, there is a perverse pride in working too hard and not taking time for self-care, even though those within the profession preach the cost of such behaviors to their patients.

Experiences of Burnout and Compassion Fatigue Among Helping Professionals

This devaluing of care receiving takes a toll on the professional helper as well, evidenced by the prevalence of mentally, physically, and emotionally exhausted therapists. Burnout and compassion fatigue are all too common among healthcare professionals. Burnout, characterized by emotional exhaustion, depersonalization, and a decreased sense of personal achievement (Maslach, 1982; Maslach & Jackson, 1976), is prevalent among human service professions in which client interaction revolves around a provider-receiver relationship (Balogun et al., 2002). Several investigators have determined that high stress and burnout in the health professions are more prevalent than in the general population (Anderson, 2015; Balogun et al., 2002; Passalacqua & Segrin, 2012; Shanafelt et al., 2010). In addition to costly organizational effects, high stress and burnout have been found to negatively affect both patient care and the well-being of healthcare providers (Aiken, Clarke, Sloane, Sochalski, & Silber, 2002; Balogun et al., 2002; Cimiotti et al., 2012; Lyndon, 2016).

Investigations into the causes of burnout have typically focused on organizational factors, but Balogun and colleagues' (2002) study of physical therapists found that work-related and sociodemographic factors accounted for only 26% of the burnout experienced. Physical and occupational therapists, they claim, "are prime candidates for burnout because their clinical roles are demanding and require close interaction with clients" (Balogun et al., 2002, p. 132). Campo and colleagues (2009) speculate that a possible burnout mechanism within client interactions is that therapists "experience a conflict between clinical realities and personal ideals" (p. 947). Similarly, Cherniss (1980) hypothesizes that new graduates are especially susceptible to burnout because they tend to have idealized expectations of patient responses to their efforts.

Within the realm of patient interaction, role ambiguity has been identified as a potential cause of burnout (Deckard & Present, 1989; Maslach & Jackson, 1976). What role is more fundamental to the helping professions than that of helping? Embracing the reciprocity of helping reminds us that it is not the impartation of knowledge that "makes" the patient do or be anything; in fact, it is the open, respectful interaction with the patient that can end up making, and remaking, the therapist.

The phenomenon of compassion fatigue—the state of exhaustion and dysfunction that results from exposure, whether intense or prolonged, to clients' traumatic or stressful events—has gained increasing recognition as a significant threat to the welfare of healthcare workers (Craig & Sprang, 2010; Slatten et al., 2011). Novice physical therapists, with their enthusiasm and caring, are particularly susceptible to this affliction. As Klappa, Howayek et al. (2015) state, "New graduate PTs [physical therapists] are ready to assume their professional responsibilities and enter the field with great satisfaction. However, many are not prepared for the challenges of everyday practice, leading to a state of compassion fatigue" (p. 100).

What on the surface seems paradoxical—that our commitment to compassion, one of the seven core values of the physical therapy profession, leads to an ultimate depletion of compassion in the caregiver—is actually revelatory of our lopsided assumption about the value of helping. When people care only for others and not for themselves, they eventually become depleted, one facet of "pathological altruism" (Oakley, Knafo, Madhavan, & Wilson, 2012). In a conversation on compassion fatigue with the host of *On Being*, medical anthropologist Joan Halifax (2013) claims that a lack of self-care among caregivers can lead to "empathic distress," a condition in which people resonate with the suffering of others but are too overwhelmed to respond in any meaningful way. As challenging as this experience is, this crisis is also an opportunity for transformative learning. Halifax describes empathic distress as an "edge state," a condition that calls people to the edges of their capacity and challenges their self-identities. In redefining themselves as caregivers who also attend to self-care, she explains, people gain stability. It is this stability, Halifax declares, that gives people the resilience to respond to the profound needs continually surrounding them. To embrace our role as partners in the healing process, therefore, we must tend to ourselves as well as to our patients, anchoring ourselves with self-compassion.

Strategy: Engaging in Self-Care

Physical therapists and others who are deeply invested in caring for others often have difficulty making self-care a priority in their lives by allowing others to care for them. The evidence is increasingly clear, however, about the relationship between the lack of self-care and the presence of compassion fatigue (Alkema, Linton, & Davies, 2008; Figley, 2002; Klappa, Howayek et al., 2015). Self-care can take many forms: contemplative rituals, exercise, nurturing relationships, true vacations. O'Halloran and Linton (2000) recommend a holistic approach to self-care, addressing emotional, spiritual, social, cognitive, physical, and vocational needs. At its essence, self-care is healing, renewing, and stabilizing. Muller (2000), in his book *Sabbath*, explains:

> Sabbath is more than the absence of work; it is not just a day off, when we catch up on television or errands. It is the presence of something that arises when we consecrate a period of time to listen to what is most deeply beautiful, nourishing, or true. It is time consecrated with our attention, our mindfulness, honoring those quiet forces of grace or spirit that sustain and heal us. (p. 8)

Muller makes the plea for the integration of Sabbath in our lives "in part for ourselves, in part so that when we go forth to heal the wounds of our world, whatever we. . .serve will have the wisdom of rest in it" (p. 10).

Research results corroborate the importance of this approach. In a study of hospice healthcare providers, compassion fatigue was significantly negatively associated with all aspects of self-care except for physical self-care (such as diet and exercise); as compassion fatigue increased, the number of reported self-care activities, other than physical self-care, decreased (Alkema et al., 2008). The authors concluded that while a variety of self-care activities may lessen burnout and compassion fatigue, only emotional and spiritual self-care and personal–professional balance were predictive of higher levels of compassion satisfaction.

This commitment to self-care must begin early. Some scholars suggest that, like burnout (Cherniss, 1980; Kolb, 1994), compassion fatigue among physical therapists begins while therapists are still students (Klappa, Howayek et al., 2015). Indeed, Balogun, Pellegrini, Miller, and Katz (1999) found burnout rates among physical therapy students were even higher than rates among practicing physical therapists. In speaking to the educational needs of physical therapy students, Jensen et al. (2000) urge : "Our novice colleagues need to be supported for exhibiting the virtues of caring, compassion, and commitment" for patients (p. 42). I would add that our novice colleagues should also be equally supported in their behaviors of self-caring and self-compassion.

In many cases, this commitment to self-care may require the redesign of more than course content in professional curricula. A lecture on the topic of mindfulness or stress reduction is not sufficient to promote true self-care. For many years (from 1933 to 1977), the accreditation of physical therapy curricula lay in the hands of the American Medical Association (Moffat, 1996). Thus, entry-level physical therapy education has been strongly influenced by the same entity that is responsible for the education process for physicians. Western medical education, however, is well known for the physical, psychological, and emotional strain it places on its students (Cooke, Irby, & O'Brien, 2010; Dyrbye, Thomas, & Shanafelt, 2005). Rarely do these programs make self-care an overt objective within the structure and implementation of the curriculum, and the effects on these care providers and on their patients are disturbing.

Finally, the practice of setting healthy boundaries and regularly making time for renewal must be embraced by healthcare educators themselves. Jensen et al. (2000) stress the importance of modeling compassionate patient care: Physical therapy students "need to witness practitioners who demonstrate these virtues in practice" (p. 42). Again, I would suggest that Jensen et al.'s declaration be extended to the practice of self-compassion; students in the helping professions need to witness practitioners and educators who overtly demonstrate effective self-care.

MAKING MEANING OUT OF HELPING

Working through these and other assumptions during entry-level training, educators can assist students in discovering who they are as helping professionals. The liminal state of physical therapy students who are committed to a profession that has not yet fully admitted them makes them particularly poised for change. Expert therapists are marked by ongoing transformation throughout their professional lives (Jensen & Paschal, 2000). How students learn transformation informs this journey. By making students aware of transformative learning *in the process of becoming what they are studying*, educators equip graduates for just such a lifetime of transformation and resilience.

Extracting the transformative learning process from the content at hand often begins with recognition of a disorienting dilemma or critical incident and the negative emotions such as confusion, frustration, and anger that often accompany this state. When students are encouraged during the learning process to recognize and appreciate these emotions for the potential transformation they signify, they are more likely to sit with their feelings long enough to mine them for the gold that lies beneath. In the classroom, strategic learning opportunities often intentionally push students out of their comfort zones. If the resulting feelings of anxiety and confusion are not overtly acknowledged and validated, however, students may quickly deflect them. The easiest means of deflection is to assume the anxiety and confusion stem from a poorly constructed or executed learning experience, in other words, by blaming the instructor. When a student attributes the discomfort of a critical incident in education to bad teaching or testing, the moment for critical self-reflection is lost. Just as clinicians frequently have difficulty making a distinction between a difficult encounter with a patient and a patient who is inherently difficult, students have difficulty differentiating between their bad feelings associated with a learning experience and a genuinely flawed teaching activity.

With skilled guidance, on the other hand, the negative feelings of vulnerability and discomfort that emerge from disorienting dilemmas can become welcomed invitations to growth. In her scholarship on healthcare education, Clouder (2005) challenges educators' reluctance to acknowledge the emotional and affective aspects of caring in favor of more rational topics and suggests that more discourse on the complexities of caring be incorporated into the implicit healthcare curriculum. Following students' constructive disruptions, educators can offer repeated and guided opportunities to practice critical self-reflection, safe environments for dialogue, and avenues for affirming actions. Educating students in all components of the transformative learning process positions the emerging professional for a lifetime of continued growth in the face of adversity. Thus, armed with a personal understanding of the transformative learning process, students can choose to cultivate an ongoing internal culture of transformation.

The personal nature of transformation is such that we, as educators, cannot guarantee it (Taylor, 2006). We can, however, make the environment ripe for these deep changes. When we engage in the transformative learning process ourselves, our teaching is made even more powerful (Jensen & Paschal, 2000). What we share as educators is more than knowledge: It is our ability to acknowledge what we do not know, to reveal our vulnerabilities, and to choose to know more deeply. This knowledge is not just about the science of physical therapy, but about ourselves as helping professionals.

Students typically enter the doctoral program believing that physical therapy expertise is achieved by learning about the anatomy, physiology, and, even, the psychology of the patient. They expect to learn about others, but what they often do not expect is that, to achieve their goals of expertise, they must learn about themselves. The best patient care skills are dependent on the therapist's ongoing commitment to self-awareness and transformation.

Students also bring with them previously formed notions of what it means to help and expectations of who they will be as professional helpers. If we allow students to invest so deeply of their time, energy, emotions, and finances while leaving this fundamental concept of helping unexamined, as educators, we pave a road to future exhaustion and professional breakdown. Taking on tightly held assumptions about what it means to help, both as educators and healthcare providers, requires courage. Questioning what we view as successful helping, what we expect in return from those we help, and what it means when we ourselves need help requires that we be vulnerable and dig deep into the reservoir of our own assumptions. It allows eager prospective students leaning forward in their chairs during their interviews to maintain, and even deepen, their enthusiasm. It allows them, years later, to remain bright-eyed rather than burned out, their compassion still fueled rather than fatigued. The seemingly altruistic desire to *make* patients better contains within it a host of assumptions that, left unexplored and unchallenged, jeopardize long-term professional well-being. In fact, it is the continuous remaking of ourselves that allows us to be the most effective therapists. We are all therapists in the making.

AUTHORS' NOTE

Students' reflections on the "should" experiment were submitted as a required part of a course. Permission to share de-identified samples of their reflections was granted through Elon University's Institutional Review Board, protocol #18-185.

REFERENCES

Aiken, L., Clarke, S., Sloane, D., Sochalski, J., & Silber, J. (2002). Hospital nurse staffing and patient mortality, nurse burnout, and job dissatisfaction. *Journal of the American Medical Association, 288*(16), 1987–1993.

Alkema, K., Linton, J., & Davies, R. (2008). A study of the relationship between self-care, compassion satisfaction, compassion fatigue, and burnout among hospice professionals. *Journal of Social Work in End-of-Life & Palliative Care, 4*(2), 101–119.

Anderson, E. Z. (2015). *Stress and burnout in physical therapists* (Doctoral dissertation). Retrieved from Dissertation Abstracts International database. (No. 3717027)

Balogun, J., Pellegrini, E., Miller, T., & Katz, J. (1999). Pattern of physical therapist students' burnout within an academic semester. *Journal of Physical Therapy Education, 13*(1), 12–17.

Balogun, J., Titiloye, V., Balogun, A., Oyeyemi, A., & Katz, J. (2002). Prevalence and determinants of burnout among physical and occupational therapists. *Journal of Allied Health, 31*(3), 131–139.

Bostock, D. (2000). *Aristotle's ethics*. New York, NY: Oxford University Press.

Campo, M., Weiser, S., & Koenig, K. (2009). Job strain in physical therapists. *Physical Therapy, 89*(9), 946–956. https://doi.org/10.2522/ptj.20080322

Cherniss, C. (1980). *Professional burnout in human service organizations*. New York, NY: Praeger Press.

Cimiotti, J., Aiken, L., Sloane, D., & Wu, E. (2012). Nurse staffing, burnout, and health care-associated infection. *American Journal of Infection Control, 40*(6), 486–490. https://doi.org/10.1016/j.ajic.2012.02.029

Clouder, L. (2005). Caring as a 'threshold concept': Transforming students in higher education into health(care) professionals. *Teaching in Higher Education, 10*(4), 505–517. https://doi.org/10.1080/13562510500239141

Cooke, M., Irby, D. M., & O'Brien, B. C. (2010). *Educating physicians: A call for reform of medical school and residency.* San Francisco, CA: Jossey-Bass.

Craig, C., & Sprang, G. (2010). Compassion satisfaction, compassion fatigue, and burnout in a national sample of trauma treatment therapists. *Anxiety, Stress and Coping, 23*(3), 319–339. https://doi.org/10.1080/10615800903085818

Deckard, G., & Present, R. (1989). Impact of role stress on physical therapists' emotional and physical well-being. *Physical Therapy, 69*(9), 713–718.

De Marco, M., Nogueira-Martins, L., & Yazigi, L. (2005). Difficult patients or difficult encounters? *QJM, 98*(7), 542–543. https://doi.org/10.1093/qjmed/hci083

Dyrbye, L. N., Thomas, M. R., Shanafelt, T. D. (2005). Medical student distress: Causes, consequences, and proposed solutions. *Mayo Clinic Proceedings, 80*(12), 1613–1622. https://doi.org/10.4065/80.12.1613

Essary, A. C., & Symington, S. L. (2005). How to make the "difficult" patient encounter less difficult. *Journal of the American Academy of Physician Assistants, 18*(5), 49–55.

Figley, C. (2002). Compassion fatigue: Psychotherapists' chronic lack of self care. *Journal of Clinical Psychology, 58*(11), 1433–1441. https://doi.org/10.1002/jclp.10090

Groves, J. (1978). Taking care of the hateful patient. *New England Journal of Medicine, 298*(16), 883–887.

Haas, L., Leiser, J., Magill, M., & Sanyer, O. (2005). Management of the difficult patient. *American Family Physician, 72*(10), 2063–2068.

Halifax, R. J. (2013, December 26). Compassion edge states: Roshi Joan Halifax on caring better (K. Tippet, Interviewer) [Audio recording transcript]. Retrieved from https://onbeing.org/programs/joan-halifax-compassions-edge-states-and-caring-better/

Jackson, J., & Kroenke, K. (1999). Difficult patient encounters in the ambulatory clinic: Clinical predictors and outcomes. *Archives of Internal Medicine, 159,* 1069–1075.

Jensen, G., Gwyer, J., Shepard, K., & Hack, L. (2000). Expert practice in physical therapy. *Physical Therapy, 80*(1), 28–52.

Jensen, G., & Paschal, K. (2000). Habits of mind: Student transition towards virtuous practice. *Journal of Physical Therapy Education, 14*(3), 42–47.

Johansson, C., & Felten, P. (2014). *Transforming students: Fulfilling the promise of higher education.* Baltimore, MD: Johns Hopkins University Press.

Killian, K. (2008). Helping till it hurts? A multimethod study of compassion fatigue, burnout, and self-care in clinicians working with trauma survivors. *Traumatology, 14*(2), 32–44. https://doi.org/10.1177/1534765608319083

Klappa, S. G., Fulton, L., Cerier, L., Pena, A., Sibenaller, A., & Klappa, S. P. (2015). Compassion fatigue among physiotherapist and physical therapists around the world. *Global Journal of Medical, Physical and Health Education, 3*(5), 124–137.

Klappa, S. G., Howayek, R., Reed, K., Scherbarth, B., & Klappa, S. P. (2015). Compassion fatigue among new graduate physical therapists. *Global Journal of Medical, Physical and Health Education, 3*(4), 100–111.

Kolb, K. (1994). Graduating burnout candidates. *Physical Therapy, 74*(3), 264–265.

Lyndon, A. (2016). Burnout among health professionals and its effect on patient safety. *Patient Safety Network.* Retrieved from https://psnet.ahrq.gov /perspectives/perspective/190/burnout-among-health-professionals-and-its-effect-on-patient-safety

Macdonald, G. (2002). Transformative unlearning: Safety, discernment, and communities of learning. *Nursing Inquiry, 9*(3), 170–178.

Maslach, C. (1982). *The cost of caring.* New York, NY: Prentice-Hall.

Maslach, C., & Jackson, S. (1976). Burned out. *Human Behavior, 5,* 16–23.

McCauley, J., & Tarpley, M. (2004). Irritability (yours and theirs). *Journal of the American Medical Association, 291*(8), 921–923. https://doi.org/10.1001/jama.291.8.921

Mezirow, J. (1990). How critical reflection triggers transformative learning. In J. Mezirow & Associates (Eds.), *Fostering critical reflection in adulthood: A guide to transformative and emancipatory learning critical reflection* (pp. 1–20). San Francisco, CA: Jossey Bass.

Moffat, M. (1996, June). Presidential address presented at the Scientific Meeting and Exposition of the American Physical Therapy Association, Minneapolis, MN. Retrieved on April 14, 2018 from http://www.ncope.org/summit/pdf/ PTEducationTimeLine.pdf

Muller, W. (2000). *Sabbath: Finding rest, renewal, and delight in our busy lives.* New York, NY: Bantam Books.

Najjar, N., Davis, L., Beck-Coon, K., & Carney Doebbeling, C. (2009). Compassion fatigue: A review of the research to date and relevance to cancer-care providers. *Journal of Health Psychology, 14*(2), 267–277. https://doi.org/10.1177 /1359105308100211

Oakley, B. A., Knafo, A., Madhavan, G., & Wilson, D. S. (Eds.). (2012). *Pathological altruism.* New York, NY: Oxford University Press.

O'Halloran, T., & Linton, J. (2000). Stress on the job: Self-care resources for counselors. *Journal of Mental Health Counseling, 22*(4), 354–364.

Passalacqua, S., & Segrin, C. (2012). The effect of resident physician stress, burnout, and empathy on patient-centered communication during the long-call shift. *Health Communication, 27*(5), 449–456. https://doi.org/10.1080/10410236.2 011.606527

Pellegrino, E. (2002). Professionalism, profession and the virtues of the good physician. *The Mount Sinai Journal of Medicine, 69*(6), 378–384.

Potter, P., Deshields, T., Berger, J., Clarke, M., Olsen, S., & Chen, L. (2013). Evaluation of a compassion fatigue resiliency program for oncology nurses. *Oncology Nursing Forum, 40*(2), 180–187. https://doi.org/10.1188/13.ONF.180-187

Santorelli, S. (2000). *Heal thy self: Lessons on mindfulness in medicine.* New York, NY: Random House.

Schein, E. H. (2011). *Helping: How to offer, give, and receive help.* San Francisco, CA: Berrett-Koehler.

Shanafelt, T., Balch, C., Bechamps, G., Russell, T., Dyrbye, L., Satele, D., . . . Freischlag, J. (2010). Burnout and medical errors among American surgeons. *Annals of Surgery, 251*(6), 995–1000. https://doi.org/10.1097/SLA.0b013e3181bfdab3

Slatten, L., Carson K. D., & Carson, P. P. (2011). Compassion fatigue and burnout: What managers should know. *Health Care Manager, 30*(4), 325–333.

Smith, M. (2008). Helping relationships—principles, theory, and practice. *The encyclopaedia of informal education.* Retrieved from www.infed.org/mobi/helping-relationships-principles-theory-and-practice/

Steinmetz, D., & Tabenkin, H. (2001). The 'difficult patient' as perceived by family physicians. *Family Practice, 18*(5), 495–500.

Taylor, E. W. (2006). The challenge of teaching for change. *New Directions for Adult and Continuing Education, 2006*(109), 91–95. https://doi.org/10.1002/ace.211

West, C., Huschka, M. M., Novotny, P. J., Sloan, J. A., Kolars, J. C., Habermann, T. M., & Shanafelt, T. D. (2006). Association of perceived medical errors with resident distress and empathy: A prospective longitudinal study. *Journal of the American Medical Association, 296*(9), 1071–1078. https://doi.org/10.1001/jama.296.9.1071

CHAPTER 2

DEVELOPING PROFESSIONAL IDENTITIES AND FOSTERING RESILIENCE IN MEDICAL STUDENTS AND RESIDENTS

Transformative Learning on the Texas–Mexico Border

Judith E. Livingston
The University of Texas Health Science Center at San Antonio

Marsha R. Griffin
The University of Texas Rio Grande Valley School of Medicine

ABSTRACT

Community for Children (CforC) is a voluntary, 4-week program on the Texas–Mexico border designed to prepare physicians-in-training to provide compassionate, effective leadership to advocate for social justice and the

Transformative Learning in Healthcare and Helping Professions Education, pages 23–45
Copyright © 2019 by Information Age Publishing
All rights of reproduction in any form reserved.

rights of all children. The elective is situated in transformative learning theory, informed by Freire's critical pedagogy, the pedagogy of privilege, and an epistemology of empathy. In this chapter on practice, we begin by examining the ethos of conventional medical education and these theoretical underpinnings which disrupt the status quo. We describe CforC's educative spaces and teaching methods that promote transformative learning, foster resilience, and support professional identity formation. We use direct quotes and examples of learners' work to augment the narrative and highlight ways in which the elective impacted them. We discuss resilience strategies and provide recommendations for professional identity formation and resources for resilience applicable to all healthcare professionals.

After a night of violence in Valle de Juarez, a mother and her four-year-old son fled across the border and were detained by U.S. Customs and Border Protection. As the boy was being separated from his mother, he asked ¿Mama, ya nos van a matar? [Momma, are they going to kill us now?]

—Griffin, Son, & Shapleigh, 2014

We were working in the colonia and invited to visit a family's 10x10 square foot home built of pallets and salvaged wood. The mother offered us two plates of beans and rice. A thin little boy saw us and ran into the house. He pleaded for food. "Why do they get to eat and not me?" Uncontrollable tears came to my eyes. I called to the boy and gave him my food. He ate like he hadn't eaten in days.

—Story from a medical student

Into the milieu of a militarized zone with significant poverty, fourth-year medical students and pediatric residents from across the United States and other countries travel to South Texas' Lower Rio Grande Valley (LRGV) to participate in an elective course, Community for Children (CforC). In this chapter on practice, we describe the characteristics of CforC, a program designed to prepare physicians-in-training to provide compassionate, effective leadership to advocate for social justice and the rights of all children. We examine the theoretical underpinnings, educative spaces, and teaching methods that promote transformative learning, foster resilience, and support the professional identity formation of learners. We discuss resilience strategies and provide recommendations for professional identity development and resources for resilience. These themes are covered in six sections: medical education and the theoretical underpinnings of CforC; geopolitical context; educative spaces and teaching methods; strategies for resilience and healing; transformative learning in CforC; and resources for professional identity formation, followed by a few concluding thoughts.

MEDICAL EDUCATION AND THE THEORETICAL UNDERPINNINGS OF COMMUNITY FOR CHILDREN

The medical students and residents who travel to the LRGV choose to come, bringing a variety of experiences and perspectives. They come for multiple reasons, chiefly related to professional development. Some arrive with idealism about their futures while others are dispirited and longing for respite. What they share in common is immersion in the culture of medicine and medical education involving 4 years of undergraduate medical education and a minimum of 3 years of graduate medical education in residency. Their professional identities are in formation in an adaptive developmental process that happens simultaneously at the individual level, involving the person's psychological development, and at the collective level, involving the person's socialization in appropriate roles and forms of participation in the community's work (Jarvis-Selinger, Pratt, & Regeher, 2012).

Professional Identity Formation and the Ethos of Medical Education

Professional identity formation has been characterized as the "integrative developmental process involving establishment of core values, moral principles, and self-awareness" (Holden, Buck, Clark, Szauter, & Trumble, 2012, p. 246). For physicians-in-training, professional identity formation occurs within a formal curriculum of codified knowledge, an informal curriculum of everyday learning experiences, and a hidden curriculum that shapes values and behaviors. "A great deal of what is taught—and most of what is learned—in medical school takes place not within formal course offerings but within medicine's 'hidden curriculum'" (Hafferty, 1998, p. 403). The hidden curriculum has positive elements, such as role modeling "where a certain level of positive affect between learner and model is a *sine qua non* of occupational socialization" (Shuval & Adler, 1980, p. 6). However, negative elements dominate the literature (Gaufberg, Batalden, Sands, & Bell, 2010; Martimianakis & Hafferty, 2016) where physicians-in-training must learn to navigate in a culture with rigid hierarchies (Dankoski, Bickel, & Gusic, 2014) and where they encounter "a demand for 'right' answers (avoidance of uncertainty), intimidation, public shaming, and humiliation" (Haidet & Stein, 2006, p. S17) that collectively puts them at risk for professional "deformation" (Rabow, Evans, & Remen, 2013, p. 13).

It should not be surprising that there is a reported decline in empathy and humanism as medical students and residents progress through their training (Bellini & Shea, 2005; Hojat et al., 2009; Newton, Barber, Clardy, Cleveland, & O'Sullivan, 2008). This decline has been attributed, in part, to the ethos of dominant medical culture "based on a particular kind of logic that embraces heroism, rationalism, certainty, the intellect, distance, objectification, and explanation before appreciation" (Bleakley, 2013, p. 63), leading to "the well-rehearsed argument that doctors see so much suffering that they must protect themselves, through objectification and distancing" (p. 63). Professional identity formation is also affected, where

> the rapid growth in scientific knowledge and technology, the qualities of predictability, measurability, efficiency, productivity, cost-effectiveness, and objectivity have come to assume a priority equal to, if not exceeding, older professional qualities of compassion, avoiding harm, service, altruism, and a reverence for life. (Rabow, Remen, Parmalee, & Inui, 2010, p. 310)

Theoretical Underpinnings

The status of CforC as an elective course is indicative of the hidden curriculum, with social justice education and the altruism of advocacy for human rights subjects generally relegated to the margins in medical education. Although some medical schools are beginning to make strides in this area, CforC educators and those in other programs have recognized the need for substantive social justice education in the medical curriculum (DasGupta et al., 2006; Schiff & Rieth, 2012) and the need for healing in the culture of medicine (Krugman, Jones, & Lowenstein, 2014; Rabow et al., 2013; Suchman et al., 2004). CforC's purposes are to contribute to the development of reflexive, socially responsible physicians while also providing an opportunity for learners to heal from negative experiences in their medical education to develop resiliency. To do this, CforC draws on four theoretical perspectives to inform its curriculum: critical pedagogy, pedagogy of privilege, an epistemology of empathy, and transformative learning theory.

The critical pedagogy of Freire (1998, 2000), who viewed teaching and learning as political acts, underpins CforC's efforts to foster critical consciousness that emphasizes critique and disruption of oppressive systems to promote social change. Freire identified "the development of a critical consciousness as prerequisite for liberating personal development and social action" (Mezirow, 1978, p. 103) and posited that critical consciousness is brought about through the union of reflection and action—praxis (Freire, 2000). CforC is about helping learners develop their reflective capacity and work with communities for social justice.

Medical students and residents are privileged by their position as future physicians. With this understanding, pedagogy of the privileged also informs the elective. This pedagogy seeks to transform those who are advantaged into allies of those who are not and to build a commitment to engage in practices that promote social justice (Curry-Stevens, 2007). Although CforC participants volunteer for this elective, the meaning of privilege and the power that comes with their profession has been largely unexamined. CforC faculty are reflexive of their own positionality and engage the learners throughout the elective in an ongoing dialogue about the great privilege they have stepping into the powerful physician role and their responsibility to acknowledge and address abuses of privilege and power. CforC faculty and learners discuss their own personal experiences with systemic privilege and oppression and consult the literature in the CforC reference collection. CforC learners are thus challenged to develop a structural competency, attending to power and privilege in language and within the social structures that both privilege and oppress (Angoff, Duncan, Roxas, & Hansen, 2016; Tsevat, Sinha, Gutierrez, & DasGupta, 2015).

CforC draws on an epistemology of empathy (Kasl & Yorks, 2016) derived from Heron (1992) who posited four ways of knowing: experiential, presentational, propositional, and practical. In their epistemology, Kasl and Yorks (2016) apply a working definition from the literature that distinguishes cognitive and emotional empathy. They locate emotional empathy in experiential knowing which Heron's (1992) model positions as the foundation for all others. Kasl and Yorks (2016) assert that cognitive empathy is a flawed concept because it is in the realm of propositional knowing, "a mental model of another's emotional state, simulated from one's personal experience" (p. 6). Cognitive empathy fails to produce an accurate model when two people's experiential worlds are dissimilar. Encountering the dissimilar "other" is an essential feature of CforC which critiques the idea that teaching cognitive empathy alone is sufficient for developing empathy. CforC learners encounter the "other" directly, bearing witness to the effects of social injustice on the people of the LRGV. They work side-by-side with community members, learning from them as they address the very real problems associated with poverty and oppression. CforC learners spend significant time in the field with the "other" where they can develop relationships and sensitivity to others' feelings that foster emotional empathy.

Mezirow (1978) first posited a theory of perspective transformation, "involving a structural change in the way we see ourselves and our relationships" (p. 100) that became known as transformative learning theory. He defined transformative learning as

> the process by which we transform our taken-for-granted frames of reference [meaning perspectives, habits of mind, mind-sets] to make them more inclusive, discriminating, emotionally capable of change, and reflective so that they may generate beliefs and opinions that will prove more true or justified to guide action. (Mezirow, 2012, p. 76)

Over time, transformative learning has been theorized "as cognitive and rational, as imaginative and intuitive, as spiritual, as related to individuation, as relational, and as relating to social change, to name just a few of the most common perspectives" (Cranton & Taylor, 2012, p. 7). Although there is diversity in the understanding of the process of transformation, the outcome involves a deep shift in perspective that leads to more open and better-justified meaning perspectives (Cranton & Taylor, 2012). CforC provides learners with multiple, compelling opportunities for perspective transformation that can lead to transformative learning.

GEOPOLITICAL CONTEXT

Space is not neutral but "plays a significant role in producing power relations in adult education and lifelong learning. Where educational programs are 'located' not only influences their purposes and processes but also helps produce the power that participants in education exercise in society" (Edwards et al., 2002, p. 99). CforC recognizes the significance of space in adult education, the theme of the XI International Conference on Transformative Learning (Nicolaides & Holt, 2014), where preliminary work for this chapter was presented (Livingston, Griffin, Brooks, Son, & Monserrat, 2014). The LRGV, its history, geography, and people are all part of the CforC classroom.

Known locally as El Valle, the four-county region of the LRGV has a population of over 1.3 million of which 90% are Hispanic or Latino (Texas Department of State Health Services, 2017). Children comprise 32% of the population with 45% living in poverty (Annie E. Casey Foundation, 2017). A brief history provides some context for this level of poverty. A little more than a century ago, land developers promoted the region, persuading thousands of Anglos to settle in the area where they practiced irrigated agriculture in a place that quickly developed into a major horticultural region sustained by impoverished and segregated Hispanic workers (Brannstrom & Neuman, 2009). The long-term effects of the exploitation of people and resources are still evident. Prime examples are the colonias, unincorporated communities often lacking basic living necessities such as running water, sewer service, electricity, paved roads, and habitable housing (Escquinca & Jaramillo, 2017). Half a million people reside in the estimated 2,294 Texas colonias where 40% live below poverty (Barton, Perlmeter, & Marquez, 2015). Sixty percent of Texas colonias are in the LRGV's Hidalgo County (Mier et al., 2007).

Many families in the colonias and in the other LRGV communities have members living on both sides of the border, and there are undocumented immigrants in families of mixed immigration status, such as the undocumented mother caring for her U.S. citizen children. In 2014, there were 11.1 million undocumented immigrants living in the United States, with an estimated 1.65 million living in Texas (Pew Research Center, 2018). These numbers do not include the thousands of unaccompanied children and families who have crossed the border, fleeing primarily from gangs and drug-related violence in Central America and Mexico. U.S. Customs and Border Protection reported in fiscal year 2016 that they apprehended 59,692 unaccompanied children and 77,674 family units at the southwest U.S. border (U.S. Customs and Border Protection, 2016). Unaccompanied children who are detained are housed in facilities operated by the U.S. Department of Health and Human Services, Office of Refugee Resettlement until released to parents, other adult family members, or nonfamily individuals throughout the United States while awaiting prosecution of their cases (Linton, Griffin, & Shapiro, 2017).

Entering the LRGV from northern Mexico means crossing harsh terrain and the Rio Grande River, the natural boundary that separates Texas from Mexico. The LRGV is also bordered with stretches of an 18-foot steel fence (Schwartz, 2017). An attempt to build a contiguous barrier between Texas and Mexico beginning a decade ago proved extraordinarily difficult given the river's convolutions and the disputes of private property owners, leaving only 10% of the border fenced (Schwartz, 2017).

Despite these conditions, the LRGV can be a place of healing and restoration. There is great natural beauty with South Padre Island National Seashore, parks, and nature preserves. There is also a vibrant culture, including a dynamic network of community-based advocacy groups working with impoverished communities whose members are themselves resilient and who persevere to improve their lives (Brodner, 2005 Karlin, 2012). The region is burgeoning as it undergoes significant development. In 2013, two universities merged to form a single large, public university (The University of Texas Rio Grande Valley [UTRGV], 2017). It includes a medical school, many years in the making, and is the academic home of CforC.

EDUCATIVE SPACES AND TEACHING METHODS

CforC is directed by a board-certified general pediatrician, who provided indigent care for a decade in a community health center before joining the faculty at UTRGV. CforC is a tuition-free elective offered two to three times annually for cohorts of four to eight learners. Since the 2007 program inception, 105 medical students and residents from 72 U.S. and international medical schools have participated in 23, 4-week rotations (in medical education parlance, a rotation is a specific block of time in upper level training). Learners are between ages 25–35, with 75% female and 35% representing ethnic or racial minority groups.

Educative Spaces

CforC is a nonclinical elective that removes the medical students and residents from the comfort zone of the clinical setting with its power dynamic that privileges doctor over patient. Instead, CforC situates the learners in community settings that create disjuncture in taken-for-granted worldviews. Colonias, federal detention facilities for unaccompanied children, immigration court, and a church-based refugee clinic are the primary settings where learners interact with children, families, and other members of the community on their own turf. CforC also creates protected spaces, where learners can express themselves freely and reflect on their journeys in becoming physicians. These include the home of the CforC director and a spiritual retreat center. In addition, classrooms and office spaces are used for lectures with small group discussion. Most of the training occurs *in situ*, appropriate to the topic. CforC curricular components include children's rights; social determinants of health; cultural humility; the impact of poverty, immigration, and violence; preparing for advocacy; fostering a culture of compassion; and professional development. These themes are addressed primarily through lecture and small group discussion, community-based advocacy work, and individualized developmental counseling.

The first day's orientation begins in the CforC director's home, located less than a mile from the border in a neighborhood where some of her former patients reside. The setting, with its many photographs, books, artwork, and artifacts, reflects passion and commitment to working with the poor and marginalized. The living room is arranged with comfortable chairs and sofa around a low wooden table. In this intimate space, CforC learners are invited, not pressed, to share stories of their journeys in becoming physicians, after the CforC director and other faculty share their own stories and vulnerabilities in professional development.

Teaching Methods

The daylong orientation begins formation of a learning community for collective learning and action (Merriam, 2010). Learners receive information packets with course schedule, syllabus, a bibliography of resources in the CforC library reserve collection, two nonfiction books on immigration and global health, and a blank journal for reflections. Journals are private and not read by faculty. Faculty explain to learners that formal evaluation is based on their professionalism, defined for them in humanistic terms—a way of being as opposed to a way of acting (Jarvis-Selinger et al., 2012) and that they, in turn, have the opportunity to provide formal evaluation about the elective using an instrument with open-ended questions in a process that protects confidentiality. When asked, learners have consented readily to sharing their responses on the CforC website and in this chapter, with some further elaboration on their experiences.

Role Modeling

During the elective, CforC learners meet with 16 volunteer faculty members, comprised of pediatricians, legal aid attorneys, community organizers, and other community leaders who contribute to the education of learners. Pediatric faculty, who teach during the elective, include women and men faculty leaders recognized nationally and internationally for their important contributions in advocating for socially-marginalized people. CforC learners are able to observe physicians as they advocate for social justice and human rights. The importance of role modeling in professional formation has been acknowledged in the medical literature, as well as in other disciplines (Kenny, Mann, & MacLeod, 2003; Shuval & Adler, 1980), with role models critical to professional, character, and career development of the trainee (Passi & Johnson, 2016). CforC faculty interpret role modeling as manifesting positive professional characteristics (Passi et al., 2013) and endeavor to be positive role models for professionalism and resiliency. CforC learners frequently allude to role modeling in their written feedback with comments such as, "she also role-models how you need deep and lasting relationships in order to do good work...It was good to see how community leaders throughout the region support each other in a strong network of love and cohesion."

Advocacy Fieldwork

CforC subscribes to learner-centered teaching precepts that give students choice while also holding them responsible for learning autonomously (Weimer, 2012). In advance of the elective, CforC learners are provided a synopsis of advocacy options from which to choose their advocacy work. Options routinely offered include opportunities to work in community-based organizations embedded in colonias, federal detention centers for unaccompanied children, legal aid organizations focused on child refugees, a midwifery-based birthing center, and a shelter for women and their children fleeing intimate partner violence. Learners spend approximately 80 hours implementing projects to address needs identified in collaboration with these community-based organizations. During the final week of the elective, they present their work to community-based collaborators and to their learning community, as well as summarize it in an abstract for presentation at national conferences.

Examples of projects in the colonias include surveying residents to explore effects of substandard housing on mental health, presenting on topics such as emergency medical care and adolescent pregnancy, making home repairs, and facilitating group discussions on dealing with the toxic stress of living in a militarized zone. Being in the community has a powerful effect on learners who observe the resiliency of the people. One learner commented on what she has learned from the community, "Resilience. Don't give up. Keep on trying. Hope." Another reflected on the nature of change that was possible when the physician is someone who becomes integral to the community:

> This elective has changed me for the better. As a physician, I am capable of doing so much more than just seeing patients and treating them. I can implement change on a larger scale and that begins with learning my community and truly becoming part of it.

Other learners realized the potential to cultivate activism as an aspect of professional identity:

> I am determined to incorporate activism and advocacy into my long-term career plans. I am further encouraged to form successful community partnerships to help serve my patients more effectively. I also hope to become increasingly involved in policy by utilizing my position as a pediatrician to its fullest advantage.

One resident, new to the role of advocate, described the significance of belonging to a community of practitioners, all of whom were striving to improve the lives of children and families in the region:

> This is one of my first experiences conducting any advocacy and it has been the biggest project in my medical career thus far ... It is reassuring to know that you are among an army of advocates who are fighting for the same universal goals ... as we traversed the colonias, we found many others who wanted to help their communities.

At the federal detention facilities, CforC learners listen to the odysseys of unaccompanied children awaiting a decision on their fates. They read stories together with the children, drew, and painted. In consultation with shelter staff, they provide health education classes to children and adolescents at the facilities. CforC learners attend immigration court where they observe young children without legal representation standing alone and confused before a judge who tries to explain that they have violated U.S. immigration laws. CforC learners are deeply troubled by these experiences; many weep. One learner's reflection expresses feelings and thoughts shared by others who bear witness to the proceedings:

The border breaks families every day and, in these children, it tears asunder one of the few things they have—their hope. This, of all things I have seen in the valley, is the most awful. As an American who was saturated with the history of lofty rights our founding fathers established here, I am ashamed to see them so blatantly forgotten. Truly ashamed.

Reflection

During the elective, CforC learners reflect on their experiences with the "other" through various art forms such as poetry, music, and collage in presentational knowing (Heron, 1992). In doing so, CforC learners connect their experiential knowing with their propositional knowing (Kasl & Yorks, 2016) which leads to an understanding of the other's life world, derived from encountering the "Other" rather than from simulations based on one's personal experience. We believe this process supports empathic professional identity formation. Examples of reflections, used with permission, are a sketch by a pediatric resident, Dr. Pearl Tsou (Figure 2.1) and a written reflection on children's rights by a medical student, Sarah Lusk (Figure 2.2).

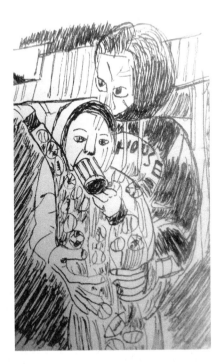

Figure 2.1 Sketch reflection.

You Have the Right....

A Convention on the Rights of the Child in the Rio Grande Valley

You are special; an ever-evolving, learning, loved and growing human being. You were born that way and as a child in the Rio Grande Valley you have the right...

To run and skip and play in a safe, clean environment, where you get your heart rate up because of the sheer joy of all of the energy that comes with your youth

To see a border inspection station and know that it's only purpose is to keep you safe and it is there to keep out those things (guns, invasive plant species, spoiled cheese) that will harm all of *us*...because you are now one of *us*

To proclaim loudly for all to hear where you come from and what you miss about that place, as well as what you have suffered to come here

To know who your parents are and to be with them if you so choose, without having to board trains, swim rivers, survive bandit attacks or go without food and water for long periods of time

To never see a fence or a wall that is meant to be a barrier to human beings and to know that you are welcome and safe while you are here, as long as that may be

To know that the community of which you are now a part welcomes you with open arms and wants you to take the beautiful culture you have brought with you and make it a part of each and every one of us

To contribute to your community by sharing your culture, beliefs and concerns in whatever way you feel best

To share in the same privileges of health care, schooling, college and career as children who were born just a few miles north of you

To know that you are perfect just the way you are and regardless of how or when you came to be a part of this community, you have more to contribute than you will ever know.

So, go forward as the perfect, evolving, loved, learning, growing and dear child that you are, regardless of your age, gender or country of origin. Tell your story to all who will listen, because you have something wonderful to become in this beautiful place known as the Rio Grande Valley.

Sarah Lusk, May 2009
Community for Children

Figure 2.2 Written reflection.

In a culminating event on the final day, learners present their reflections and abstracts to the learning community. It is an emotional time, again in the protected space of the program director's home. Only faculty who have spent time with the learners are present at this intimate exchange which strengthens the bonds of the learning community, indicated by comments such as "I felt like it was an incredible bonding experience to share with the group." Through this collective reflection, learners are able to process their

CforC experiences and depart with beautiful works of art and memories to fortify their resilience. As one learner wrote,

> The reflection component was so meaningful and made the rotation complete for me. It was nice to get to take something home that means something to me, and see what means a lot to the other students... The reflection component definitely set this rotation apart from typical rotations, and allows us to take something huge from the month and apply it in the future.

The bonds formed during the elective, supported through ongoing outreach to CforC alumni, help to sustain a sense of community. As one learner shared 4 years after his CforC experience, "Thanks again for the outstanding experience I had with CfC. It's a global community, and though we may be spread far and wide, we are all connected in heart, soul, and mission."

STRATEGIES FOR RESILIENCE AND HEALING

Resilience has been defined as the ability to respond to stress in a healthy, adaptive way where individuals are able to face and overcome obstacles, experiencing personal transformation and growth in the process (Epstein & Krasner, 2013; Tempski et al., 2015). Physicians-in-training are under chronic stress with significant numbers experiencing burnout and depression with some reporting suicidal ideation (Beresin et al., 2016; Goebert et al., 2009). Researchers suggest developing learners' resilience as a strategy to minimize emotional distress and enhance medical training (Tempski et al., 2015, p. 1). CforC faculty are keenly aware of the need to foster learners' resilience to help them deal with the dehumanization and sheer demands of their training, as well as process experiences of the elective. To do this, CforC employs three primary strategies for healing: mentoring, contemplative retreat, and professional identity formation counseling.

Mentoring

CforC faculty mentor the learners individually and as a learning community over the course of the elective. Mentoring in this context is not the traditional mentor and protégé dynamic but draws on the archetypal concept of mentors who guide us on a journey and who understand they are part of a relationship (Daloz, 2012). Part of this mentoring occurs twice a week when CforC learners and faculty gather in the director's home for dinner and authentic discussion—the reflective discourse central to Mezirow's transformative learning theory (Cranton, 2006). In this protected space, learners can express their emotions genuinely. CforC's learning community is a container for hearing all viewpoints and for critical self-reflection where group work can lead to personal growth, relational empathy, and critical consciousness (Schapiro, Wasserman, & Gallegos, 2012). Mentoring continues beyond the elective as learners become CforC alumni who stay connected through social media, professional meetings, and communications with CforC faculty who nurture relationships with learners as a core practice. As others who have written about professional identity development have noted, a relationship-centered approach to education contributes to resilience (Wald et al., 2015, p. 704).

Contemplative Retreat

There is a growing movement in higher education, including medical education, to incorporate contemplative practices, such as meditation, in the curriculum (Zajonc, 2013). Research on meditation has demonstrated increased concentration and attention, improved mental health and wellbeing, increased creativity and insight, and other benefits (Barbezat & Bush, 2014, p. 23). As a contemplative practice, CforC learners and faculty spend a weekend at a spiritual retreat center located in a remote, rural setting. CforC faculty encourage contemplative practices with the understanding that in the educational setting these must remain separated from ideology or religious belief. Instead, we encourage learners to explore their own spiritual beliefs. They are invited to gather as a group and break silence each afternoon for an hour or so, to share thoughts or contemplations. During this gathering, we often discuss self-care as a way to maintain resiliency while navigating medical education and as practicing physicians. Several self-care strategies that are repeated themes include: (a) staying connected with a supportive professional community, (b) pursuing a life of personal meaning as a defense against burnout, (c) practicing good health habits (i.e., healthy eating, physical exercise, and adequate rest), (d) meditating or maintaining some form of spiritual practice, and (e) keeping a journal or participating in other forms of creative expression regularly. Faculty are available during the retreat for one-on-one time should a learner request it. Participation in the retreat is optional.

Professional Identity Formation Counseling

In the final week, each participant has the opportunity to meet with a clinical psychologist for professional identity formation counseling in the privacy of the CforC director's home. Learners have the opportunity to further process their experiences and discuss their dreams, hopes, and fears. The meeting is non-compulsory, confidential, and typically lasts about 2 hours. We believe this is an essential healing component of the elective that contributes to learners' professional identity formation, helping learners "find out who they are, who they are becoming, and who they wish to become" (Cruess, Cruess, Boudreau, Snell, & Steinert, 2014, p. 1449), as well as prepare them for reentry into their medical education training programs at home. During CforC, the medical students and residents find respite from their harried lives which leave little time for contemplation. As one learner expressed, "Community for Children allowed me time. Time to listen, really listen, to the world around me. Time to consider problems larger than my daily patient load and time to ponder a solution. Time to reflect." Learners need preparation to aid their transition back into the demands of clinical training.

TRANSFORMATIVE LEARNING
IN COMMUNITY FOR CHILDREN

CforC creates conditions Daloz (2000) described as necessary for transformation: presence of the other; reflective discourse; a mentoring community; and opportunities for committed action. Through its elements of meaningful and productive engagement with the community, reflective discourse in a safe space, and ongoing relational mentoring within a learning community, CforC lays the groundwork for learners to experience transformative learning. Most participants experience a perspective change, becoming more critically conscious, aware of their privileged positions and their capacity to be a force for social justice.

Recurrent themes in the feedback and reflections from CforC participants, at the end of the rotation and through subsequent interactions with them as alumni, include a sense of awakening, clarity of vocational mission, and a complete embrace of the social justice advocacy role. Over the course of the 23 elective rotations, we have repeatedly received comments such as, "I have found my mission and I wanted to thank you for exposing me to a world I needed to see and for your continued efforts in the fight..." and "My experience with Community for Children led me to discover my calling in life... I am able to advocate for my patients and learn what their needs are from them."

As a pediatric resident, Dr. Ryan Van Ramshorst penned this feedback, "Community for Children has re-energized and re-affirmed my intense drive to seek justice—unrelenting and uncompromising justice—for the children and families I care for" (Livingston et al., 2014, p. 350). During the CforC elective, he secured a grant and implemented a bicycling fitness program for indigent families in the LRGV. As an academic general pediatrician, he has become a fierce and eloquent advocate for children's health, holding leadership positions in medical organizations and testifying regularly before state and national legislative bodies against policies detrimental to children and families.

Dr. Elizabeth Losada came to us as a pediatric resident in the Fall of 2012. Her reflection, spoken at the culminating event of her CforC rotation, was a poem filled with her observations of the juxtaposition of poverty and wealth and metaphors questioning the positionality of the privileged when contrasted with the oppressed people in the LRGV. Her CforC advocacy work involved researching local perceptions of barriers to optimal health in the colonias, identifying a major problem with stray dogs and dog bites requiring emergency medical care. She and her CforC coresearcher, Dr. Preeti Dave, were influential in effecting policy changes to improve the situation and went on to present their research at the American Pediatric Association's Community, Advocacy, Research, and Education Conference in 2013. In 2017, as a CforC alumnus and a general pediatrician, Dr. Losada shared these thoughts:

> My time on the border solidified my desire to work with Spanish-speaking immigrants, and gave me a very intimate look at the challenges many families face on their journey to the United States. This has influenced my daily practice in pediatrics and has allowed me to better serve this population, especially with regard to trauma and other mental health issues arising from their experiences. Working alongside community activists while on the border was very inspiring and broadened my focus to make community health and activism a part of my daily practice.

As a pediatric resident in the Fall of 2013, Dr. Hilda Loria commented in her CforC evaluation:

> It wasn't until I came home did I realize how much I had changed... Now, apathy toward the challenges of others elicits frustration I never felt before. Some things just don't get better by pulling yourself up by the bootstraps. Not everyone is born on the same starting line.

Dr. Loria has become a staunch advocate for immigrant children as a practicing pediatrician, giving voice to the voiceless through the media:

> We cannot continue creating adversity for our immigrant children or the U.S. citizen children of immigrant parents. They need to feel safe and protected. As their caretakers, neighbors, and community leaders, we need to invest in their health and fight for their rights. They need us to be their voice and their advocate... Learn about the struggles of the immigrant families in your community and get involved! Call, email, or visit your representatives and talk

about ways to ensure the health and well-being of *all* of our children ... Our children need us, and we can't fail them (Loria, 2017, para. 7–8).

In the Spring of 2016, Hannah Palm participated in CforC as a fourth-year medical student. She was so moved by her experience that she had her wrist tattooed with the Spanish word, "Adelante," used to exclaim "Forward!" A year later, Dr. Palm wrote saying,

> I think about my month on the Texas–Mexico border daily . . . I think about it when I scrub into surgeries for sick patients who were unable to come to the doctor earlier because they have no insurance. I think about it when people start talking about "the wall." I think about it every day, as I wash my hands, and see my wrist tattoo saying, "Adelante." It is a simple word that, to me, holds so much power. What my time on the border taught me is that we do not have to look far to see the constant struggle for basic human rights. It is in our backyard, if we choose to see. But that is the key—that we see it. It is easy, in our world, to remain self-centered and have our individual problems and struggles overwhelm our lives. But next door, there is a woman who is sick and has no access to healthcare. There is a child with no way to get to school safely. There is a father struggling to provide for his family. And I am so fortunate, as a doctor, as a member of the middle class, as a U.S. citizen, as a White woman, to have influence, to have my words listened to. So I have started to speak and act for the rights of every human, to treat every patient that walks through the door as an equal, no matter what. And when I get tired, I remember my experience on the border—the stories I heard, the people I met, the tears they shared—and I take a deep breath and continue forward. Adelante. We have so much work to do.

There have been very few learners who did not engage in the elective beyond a superficial level of participation. Some were underdeveloped in professionalism and others behaved in ways that suggested they were in distress. For example, a few learners did not attend didactic presentations as expected of them, made only a token effort in their advocacy work or behaved inappropriately toward other learners and faculty. In these cases, the CforC program director and the clinical psychologist intervened to provide emotional support and guidance. Given the challenges an elective course such as this one pose to learners, it is vital to maintain close mentoring and to have some type of professional psychological services that learners can access.

RESOURCES FOR PROFESSIONAL IDENTITY FORMATION

In a comprehensive report on professional formation in medicine, Rabow et al. (2010), who prefer the more encompassing term professional formation to professional identity formation, state,

The goal of professional formation is to anchor students in foundational principles while helping them navigate the inevitable moral conflicts in medical practice. The consequences of inadequate support for professional formation are profound, impacting individual learners, patients, the profession, and society at large. (p. 310)

They outline the following essential elements for learners' professional formation, synthesized from multiple sources in the literature: mindfulness; reflection (journaling, storytelling, critical incident review, reflection on role modeling); positive role modeling and mentoring; evaluation and feedback about values and choices; and sharing with a professional community (Rabow et al., 2010, p. 315). We concur but suggest this list of elements should also include action for social justice where learners engage with the "Other" on their terms and in creative expression to integrate ways of knowing that engender transformative learning for empathic, moral professional identity formation. We further believe that these elements apply to other health professions learners, as well as medical students.

While the specifics of CforC are unique to the LRGV, every community has its own set of issues and opportunities for transformative learning that contribute to professional identity formation and resiliency. Similar educational experiences can be offered in other settings and for other health professionals through a relationship-centered curriculum, mentoring, positive role-modeling, community-based advocacy, space for contemplation and reflection through discourse and creative expression. The CforC website (http://www.communityforchildren.org) provides details about the elective and a toolkit with resources for program development.

Other resources we suggest related to empathic professional identity formation and resiliency include: (a) Association for Contemplative Mind in Higher Education (http://www.acmhe.org); (b) the Healer's Art course (http://www.rachelremen.com/learn/medical-education-work/the-healers-art/); (c) American Balint Society (ABS), an organization of clinicians and teachers using a group process of exploration and training called the Balint group. The ABS website (http://www.americanbalintsociety.org) explains the focus is on empathic care of others and of physicians' professional selves and development of resiliency and longevity in practice; and (d) a book for medical, nursing, and allied health professionals, *Overcoming Secondary Stress in Medical and Nursing Practice: A Guide to Professional Resilience and Well-being* (Wicks, 2005), which includes a secondary stress self-awareness questionnaire, information on developing a self-care protocol, and recommendations for many other related resources.

In our 10 years implementing CforC, we have observed that learners are able to reconnect to the heart motivations that first called them to become physicians. Reflection on this calling in the context of tremendous need and in dialogue with others who share their vocational aspirations is central to their transformative learning. Participation in CforC also enables learners to recover from the hurts in their medical training and develop a practice to maintain resilience throughout their lives. CforC is an imperfect and ever-evolving attempt at helping learners develop as resilient, empathic healers committed to social justice in their transformation of becoming physicians. Our engagement with the learners continues to astonish, transform, and heal us. They give us hope and remind us of our own purpose.

REFERENCES

Angoff, N., Duncan, L., Roxas, N., & Hansen, H. (2016). Power day: Addressing the use and abuse of power in medical training. *Journal of Bioethical Inquiry, 13*(2), 203–213. https://doi.org/10.1007/s11673-016-9714-4

Annie E. Casey Foundation. (2017). *Kids count data center.* Retrieved from http://datacenter.kidscount.org/data#TX/2/0/char/0

Barbezat, D. P., & Bush, M. (2014). *Contemplative practices in higher education: Powerful methods to transform teaching and learning.* San Francisco, CA: Jossey-Bass.

Barton, J., Perlmeter, E. R., & Marquez, R. R. (2015). *Las colonias in the 21st century: Progress along the Texas-Mexico border.* Dallas, TX: Federal Reserve Bank of Dallas Community Development. Retrieved from https://www.dallasfed.org/~/media/microsites/cd/colonias/index.html

Bellini, L., & Shea, J. (2005). Mood change and empathy decline persist during three years of internal medicine training. *Academic Medicine, 80*(2), 164–167.

Beresin, E., Milligan, T., Balon, R., Coverdale, J., Louie, A., Roberts, L., . . . Roberts, L. W. (2016). Physician wellbeing: A critical deficiency in resilience education and training. *Academic Psychiatry, 40*(1), 9–12. https://doi.org/10.1007/s40596-015-0475-x

Bleakley, A. (2013). Gender matters in medical education. *Medical Education, 47*(1), 59–70. https://doi.org/10.1111/j.1365-2923.2012.04351.x

Brannstrom, C., & Neuman, M. (2009). Inventing the "Magic Valley" of South Texas, 1904–1941. *The Geographical Review, 91*(2), 123–145.

Brodner, S. (2005). In America: Stories of struggle and improbable success from the colonias of South Texas. *Texas Monthly, 33*(5), 156–165.

Cranton, P. (2006). *Understanding and promoting transformative learning: A guide for educators of adults* (2nd ed.). San Francisco, CA: Jossey-Bass.

Cranton, P., & Taylor, E. W. (2012). Transformative learning theory: Seeking a more unified theory. In E. W. Taylor & P. Cranton and Associates (Eds.), *The handbook of transformative learning: Theory, research and practice* (pp. 3–20). San Francisco, CA: Jossey-Bass.

Cruess, R., Cruess, S., Boudreau, J., Snell, L., & Steinert, Y. (2014). Reframing medical education to support professional identity formation. *Academic Medicine, 89*(11), 1446–1451.

Curry-Stevens, A. (2007). New forms of transformative education: Pedagogy for the privileged. *Journal of Transformative Education, 5*(1), 33–58. https://doi.org/10.1177/1541344607299394

Daloz, L. A. (2000). Transformative learning for the common good. In J. Mezirow & Associates (Eds.), *Learning as transformation: Critical perspectives on a theory in progress* (pp. 103–123). San Francisco, CA: Jossey-Bass.

Daloz, L. A. (2012). *Mentor: Guiding the journey of adult learners.* San Francisco, CA: Jossey-Bass.

Dankoski, M., Bickel, J., & Gusic, M. (2014). Discussing the undiscussable with the powerful: Why and how faculty must learn to counteract organizational silence. *Academic Medicine, 89*(12), 1610–1613.

DasGupta, S., Fornari, A., Geer, K., Hahn, L., Kumar, V., Lee, H. J.,...Gold, M. (2006). Medical education for social justice: Paulo Freire revisited. *Journal of Medical Humanities, 27*(4), 245–251. doi:10.1007/s10912-006-9021-x

Edwards, R., Cervero, R., Clarke, J., Morgan-Klein, B., Usher, R., & Wilson, A. (2002). *Cartographical imaginations: Spatiality, adult education and lifelong learning.* Retrieved from the ERIC database. (ED471622)

Epstein, R. M., & Krasner, M. S. (2013). Physician resilience: What it means, why it matters, and how to promote it. *Academic Medicine, 88*(3), 301–303. https://doi.org/10.1097/ACM.0b013e318280cff0

Escquinca, M., & Jaramillo, A. (2017, August 22). Colonias on the border struggle with decades-old water issues. *Texas Tribune.* Retrieved from https://texastribune.org/2017/08/22/colonias-border-struggle-decades-old-water-issues/

Freire, P. (1998). *Pedagogy of freedom: Ethics, democracy, and civic courage.* Lanham, MD: Rowman & Littlefield.

Freire, P. (2000). *Pedagogy of the oppressed* (M. B. Ramos, Trans.; 20th anniversary ed.). New York, NY: Continuum.

Gaufberg, E., Batalden, M., Sands, R., & Bell, S. (2010). The hidden curriculum: What can we learn from third-year medical student narrative reflections? *Academic Medicine, 85*(11), 1709–1716. https://doi.org/10.1097/ACM.0b013e3181f57899

Goebert, D., Thompson, D., Takeshita, J., Beach, C., Bryson, P., Ephgrave, K.,...Tate, J. (2009). Depressive symptoms in medical students and residents: A multischool study. *Academic Medicine, 84*(2), 236–241.

Griffin, M., Son, M., & Shapleigh, E. (2014). Children's lives on the border. *Pediatrics, 133*(5), e1118–e1120. https://doi.org/10.1542/peds.2013-2813

Hafferty, F. W. (1998). Beyond curriculum reform: Confronting medicine's hidden curriculum. *Academic Medicine, 73*(4), 403–407.

Haidet, P., & Stein, H. F. (2006). The role of the student-teacher relationship in the formation of physicians: The hidden curriculum as process. *Journal of General Internal Medicine, 21*(S1), S16–S20. https://doi.org/10.1111/j.1525-1497.2006.00304.x

Heron, J. (1992). *Feeling and personhood: Psychology in another key.* Newbury Park, CA: SAGE.

Hojat, M., Vergare, M. J., Maxwell, K., Brainard, G., Herrine, S. K., Isenberg, G. A.,...Gonnella, J. S. (2009). The devil is in the third year: A longitudinal study of erosion of empathy in medical school. *Academic Medicine, 84*(9), 1182–1191.

Holden, M., Buck, E., Clark, M., Szauter, K., & Trumble, J. (2012). Professional identity formation in medical education: The convergence of multiple domains. *HEC Forum, 24*(4), 245–255. https://doi.org/10.1007/s10730-012-9197-6

Jarvis-Selinger, S., Pratt, D. D., & Regehr, G. (2012). Competency is not enough: Integrating identity formation into the medical education discourse. *Academic Medicine, 87*(9), 1185–1190. https://doi.org/10.1097/ACM.0b013e3182604968

Karlin, M. (2012, April 22). Latina leaders of Texas colonias help remake shantytowns into empowered communities. *Truthout*. Retrieved from http://truthout.org/news/item/8638-empowering-the-texas-colonias-with-an-equal-voice

Kasl, E., & Yorks, L. (2016). Do I really know you? Do you really know me? Empathy amid diversity in differing learning contexts. *Adult Education Quarterly, 66*(1), 3–20. https://doi.org/10.1177/0741713615606965

Kenny, N. P., Mann, K., & MacLeod, H. (2003). Role modeling in physicians' professional formation: Reconsidering an essential but untapped educational strategy. *Academic Medicine, 78*(12), 1203–1210. https://doi.org/10.1097/00001888-200312000-00002

Krugman, R., Jones, M., & Lowenstein, S. (2014). Can we learn civility? Reflections on the challenge of changing culture. *Academic Medicine, 89*(12), 1586–1588.

Linton, J., Griffin, M., & Shapiro, A. (2017, March 13). AAP policy says no child should be in detention centers or separated from parents. *AAP News*. Retrieved from http://www.aappublications.org/news/2017/03/13/Immigration031317

Livingston, J., Griffin, M., Brooks, A., Son, M., & Monserrat, C. (2014). Transforming privilege in marginal spaces: Teaching medical students on the Texas-Mexico Border. In A. Nicolaides & D. Holt (Eds.), *Spaces of transformation and transformation of spaces: Proceedings from the XI International Conference on Transformative Learning* (pp. 347–354). Athens, GA: University of Georgia.

Loria, H. (2017, July 7). We are failing our immigrant children. *TribTalk*. Retrieved from https://www.tribtalk.org/2017/07/07/we-are-failing-our-immigrant-children/

Martimianakis, M. A., & Hafferty, F. W. (2016). Exploring the interstitial space between the ideal and the practised: Humanism and the hidden curriculum of system reform. *Medical Education, 50*(3), 278–280. https://doi.org/10.1111/medu.12982

Merriam, S. B. (2010). Globalization and the role of adult and continuing education. In C. E. Kasworm, A. D. Rose, & J. M. Ross-Gordon (Eds.), *Handbook of adult and continuing education* (pp. 401–409). Los Angeles, CA: SAGE.

Mezirow, J. (1978). Perspective transformation. *Adult Education, 28*(2), 100–110.

Mezirow, J. (2012). Learning to think like an adult: Core concepts of transformation theory. In E. W. Taylor & P. Cranton and Associates (Eds.), *The handbook of transformative learning: Theory, research, and practice* (pp. 73–95). San Francisco, CA: Jossey-Bass.

Mier, N., Millard, A. V., Flores, I., Sánchez, E. R., Medina, B., & Carbajal, E. S. (2007). Community-based participatory research: Lessons learned from practice in South Texas colonias. *Texas Public Health Association Journal, 59*(1), 16–18.

Newton, B. W., Barber, L., Clardy, J., Cleveland, E., & O'Sullivan, P. (2008). Is there hardening of the heart during medical school? *Academic Medicine, 83*(3), 244–249.

Nicolaides, A., & Holt, D. (Eds.). (2014). *Spaces of transformation and transformation of space*. Proceedings of the XI International Transformative Learning Conference. New York, NY: Teachers College.

Passi, V., & Johnson, N. (2016). The impact of positive doctor role modeling. *Medical Teacher, 38*(11), 1139–1145. https://doi.org/10.3109/0142159X.2016.1170780

Passi, V., Johnson, S., Peile, E., Wright, S., Hafferty, F., & Johnson, N. (2013). Doctor role modelling in medical education: BEME Guide No. 27. *Medical Teacher, 35*(9), e1422–e1436. doi:10.3109/0142159X.2013.806982

Pew Research Center. (2018, November 27). *Unauthorized immigrant population trends for states, birth countries, and regions.* Retrieved from http://www.pewhispanic.org/interactives/unauthorized-trends/

Rabow, M., Evans, C., & Remen, R. (2013). Professional formation and deformation: Repression of personal values and qualities in medical education. *Family Medicine, 45*(1), 13–18.

Rabow, M., Remen, R., Parmelee, D., & Inui, T. (2010). Professional formation: Extending medicine's lineage of service into the next century. *Academic Medicine, 85*(2), 310–317. https://doi.org/10.1097/ACM.0b013e3181c887f7

Schapiro, S. A., Wasserman, I. L., & Gallegos, P. V. (2012). Group work and dialogue: Spaces and processes for transformative learning in relationships. In E. W. Taylor & P. Cranton and Associates (pp. 355–372). *The handbook of transformative learning: Theory, research, and practice.* San Francisco, CA: Jossey-Bass.

Schiff, T., & Rieth, K. (2012). Projects in medical education: "Social Justice in Medicine" a rationale for an elective program as part of the medical education curriculum at John A. Burns School of Medicine. *Hawai'i Journal of Medicine & Public Health, 71*(4), 64–67.

Schwartz, J. (2017, March 12). 'It feels like no man's land' The border fence cuts off areas of Texas in places; will extending the existing barrier make it worse? *Austin-American Statesman* (p. A1). Retrieved from https://projects.statesman.com/news/texas-border/noman.html

Shuval, J., & Adler, I. (1980). The role of models in professional socialization. *Social Science and Medicine. Part A: Medical Psychology and Medical Sociology, 14*(1), 5–14.

Suchman, A., Williamson, P., Litzelman, D., Frankel, R., Mossbarger, D., & Inui, T. (2004). Toward an informal curriculum that teaches professionalism: Transforming the social environment of a medical school. *Journal of General Internal Medicine, 19*(5), 501–504.

Tempski, P., Santos, I. S., Mayer, F. B., Enns, S. C., Perotta, B., Paro, H. S.,... Martins, M. A. (2015). Relationship among medical student resilience, educational environment and quality of life. *PloS ONE, 10*(6). https://doi.org/10.1371/journal.pone.0131535

Texas Department of State Health Services. (2017). *Center for health statistics.* Retrieved from https://www.dshs.texas.gov/chs

Tsevat, R. K., Sinha, A. A., Gutierrez, K. J., & DasGupta, S. (2015). Bringing home the health humanities: Narrative humility, structural competency, and engaged pedagogy. *Academic Medicine, 90*(11), 1462–1465.

The University of Texas Rio Grande Valley. (2017). *History of The University of Texas Rio Grande Valley.* Retrieved from http://www.utrgv.edu/en-us/about-utrgv/history/

U.S. Customs and Border Protection. (2016). *United States Border Patrol Southwest Family Unit and unaccompanied alien children apprehensions fiscal year 2016.*

Washington, DC: Author. Retrieved from https://www.cbp.gov/newsroom/stats/southwest-border-unaccompanied-children/fy-2016

Wald, H. S., Anthony, D., Hutchinson, T. A., Liben, S., Smilovitch, M., & Donato, A. A. (2015). Professional identity formation in medical education for humanistic, resilient physicians: Pedagogic strategies for bridging theory to practice. *Academic Medicine, 90*(6), 753–760. https://doi.org/10.1097/ACM.0000000000000725

Weimer, M. (2012). Learner-centered teaching and transformative learning. In E. W. Taylor & P. Cranton and Associates (Eds.), *The handbook of transformative learning: Theory, research, and practice* (pp. 439–454). San Francisco, CA: Jossey-Bass.

Wicks, R. J. (2005). *Overcoming secondary stress in medical and nursing practice: A guide to professional resilience and personal well-being.* New York, NY: Oxford University Press.

Zajonc, A. (2013). Contemplative pedagogy: A quiet revolution in higher education. *New Directions for Teaching & Learning, 2013*(134), 83–94. https://doi.org/10.1002/tl.20057

CHAPTER 3

A TALE OF TWO AFRICAS

Transformative Learning
in Global Health Electives

Scott T. Armistead
Virginia Commonwealth University School of Medicine

with
Teresa J. Carter
Virginia Commonwealth University School of Medicine

ABSTRACT

Two global health electives in Africa during 2017 and 2018 led to the discovery of important factors contributing to or inhibiting transformative learning among U.S. medical and health professions students. Conditions of high moral and ethical dissonance in one group of students situated in the context of a rural hospital in western Africa served to inhibit meaning-making in student learning, while a more relational and affective learning experience in southern Africa appeared highly supportive of instances of transformed perspectives. Multiple contextual variables within the two settings emphasized the significance of professional identities already well-developed among student learners in how they responded to ethical challenges.

Transformative Learning in Healthcare and Helping Professions Education, pages 47–65
Copyright © 2019 by Information Age Publishing
47

When students develop a professional identity as providers of healthcare in the United States, they are privileged to learn and work in one of the most technologically advanced societies in the world. The array of diagnostic tests and treatment options continues to grow with each passing year, providing increased possibilities for what can be done to diagnose and treat illness, prolong life, and ameliorate suffering. What happens when U.S. students, who have been trained in the values, culture, and norms of Western medicine experience the healthcare system of a developing nation? What do they learn about justice, poverty, and the causes of suffering, and what lessons might they find applicable to their own lives and future career plans? Ultimately, are their experiences transformative (Mezirow, 1991; Mezirow & Associates, 2000) according to the theory that describes how adults revise the meaning of experience to encompass perspectives that are more open to alternative viewpoints? These were some of the questions that framed an examination of two global health electives (GHEs) in Africa offered to health professions students at Virginia Commonwealth University in the Spring of 2017 and 2018.

A BRIEF REVIEW OF THE LITERATURE IN GLOBAL HEALTH ELECTIVES

Many students in the health professions have interest and prior experience in global health, and the number of students involved in international "medical mission trips" has burgeoned since the 1970s (Jeffery, Dumont, Kim, & Kuo, 2011; Rahim, Knights, Fyfe, Alagarajah, & Baraitser, 2016; Roche, Ketheeswaran, & Wirtz, 2017). In 2015, around 30% of U.S. medical students completed an elective in global health by the time of their graduation (Gwinn & Frank, 2015). In the United Kingdom, the numbers are even higher, with 90% percent of medical students going abroad for their mandatory elective and four-fifths of these students choosing to spend time in a low- or middle-income country (Bowsher, Parry-Billings, Georgeson, & Baraitser, 2018). Most of these trips are a month in duration, the timeframe for a typical "rotation" in a specialty during the latter, clinical years of medical training. Although some students travel independently, many state and private medical schools and residency programs in the United States have established relationships with healthcare providers in developing countries to host GHEs, and students are often accompanied on these trips by one or more faculty members. In recent years, the extent to which North American medical schools have global health tracks within the curriculum has been considered an asset for students drawn to the humanistic aims of the profession (American Academy of Family Physicians, 2018; Association of

American Medical Colleges, 2018), and the value of this clinical training for students has been considered "profound" (Gwinn & Frank, 2015, p. 2). GHEs have provided advanced learners with exposure to healthcare in the developing world, broadened their experience in dealing with diseases and conditions not typically found in the United States, inspired them as future providers to care for the underserved, and fostered career interests in primary care (Jeffrey et al., 2011; Haq et al., 2000; Sawatsky, Nordhues, Merry, Bashir, & Hafferty, 2018). Medical educators have described these international experiences as offering future healthcare professionals the opportunity to enlarge their perspectives, provide alternative frames of reference about what it means to provide healthcare, and foster the positive development of a professional identity (Dowell & Merrylees, 2009; Sawatsky et al., 2018). In addition, professional schools find that GHEs provide opportunities for learners that are not always adequately addressed within the current curriculum, including lived experience in understanding the social determinants of health (Haq et al., 2000; Lumb & Murdoch-Eaton, 2014). Haq and colleagues (2000) are among those who assert the need for physicians-in-training to gain greater appreciation for the global dimensions of health in an era of heightened international travel and immigration.

Previous research has pointed to the transformative nature of participation in GHEs by describing it as altering students' worldviews (Dowell & Merrylees, 2009; Haq et al., 2000; Sawatsky et al., 2018). The expectation of many educators has been that contexts of severe resource limitations, significant cultural variances, and the complexities and ethical ambiguities encountered in GHEs offer the kind of dissonant milieu and challenging personal experiences that Mezirow's (1991, 2000) transformative learning theory considered necessary for deep and enduring learning. How people make sense of such critical events or "disorienting dilemmas" (Mezirow, 1991) is the essence of this transformative potential.

In one of the more thorough investigations of global service learning, Kiely (2005) conducted a 10-year longitudinal case study using transformative learning theory (Mezirow, 1991, 2000) as the theoretical lens for examining student experiences abroad. While the students in this study were undergraduates and not healthcare professionals in training, the intensity and thoroughness of analysis into both reflective and nonreflective learning in a global context has much to offer healthcare educators when analyzing the potential for transformative learning in GHEs. The students in Kiely's study worked and conducted research on health and social problems in an impoverished area of Nicaragua. As co-instructor of the Nicaragua program from 1994–2001, Kiely was able to observe participation in service-learning activities and gain an in-depth perspective on the specific events described by students. Data analysis included extensive field notes and video footage, as well as interview and focus group data that were analyzed yearly.

Kiely's (2005) analysis discovered five categories that described how students experienced transformative learning in service learning contexts. He labeled these: (a) *contextual border-crossing*, (b) *personalizing*, (c) *dissonance* (both high-level dissonance and low-level dissonance), (d) p*rocessing*, and (e*) connecting*. The category of contextual border crossing included four important elements of context that affected students' transformative learning before, during, and after participation in the program. These consisted of personal, structural, historical, and programmatic elements that interacted to either enhance or hinder possibilities for transformative learning. Personal elements were composed of students' personality traits, social roles, professional background, knowledge, skills, beliefs, values, interests, needs, learning styles, expectations, motivations, desires, fears, and sense of efficacy (p. 9). Since these are all highly individualistic attributes, Kiely felt that they created a foundation of "biographical baggage" (p. 9) that influenced how students made sense of the experiences they encountered and influenced the assumptions they held.

Kiely (2005) discovered that many of the students in his study held established assumptions and beliefs that included an uncritical acceptance of their own cultural competence based upon prior international travel or study experiences; a Western view of health that asserted the superiority of medical knowledge as prescribed by expert doctors, based upon scientific knowledge; and individualistic explanations of social problems, among others. The service learning experience led many of his students to reevaluate these assumptions, returning home with an entirely different perspective about their identity and the world (p. 9). Kiely also offers a specific critique on the emphasis that Mezirow (1991, 2000) makes on reflection and dialogue in processing dissonant experiences without adequate attention to the visceral, emotional, and affective reactions that occurred. Among the critiques of Mezirow's theory has been lack of emphasis on the emotion-laden and affective nature of experiences that influence transformative learning (Taylor, 2007; Kiely, 2005; Sawatsky et al., 2018).

I approached my study of the potential for transformative learning among U.S. medical students with my interest in leading GHEs for a large, urban, state-supported medical school. Based upon my own highly rewarding experience of living and working as a medical doctor in a resource-poor nation in south Asia, I began to think about the learning potential for health professions students who would accompany me on my first GHE elective in the Spring of 2017. I thought that accompanying students on a month-long elective at a hospital in the developing world would provide a context in which we could work together in a GHE, process the deeper meaning of the experience, and explore its implications for students' futures.

MY PERSONAL EXPERIENCE
OF WORKING IN GLOBAL HEALTHCARE

As someone who practiced medicine for 16 years in a radically different context than that in which I was trained, my goal was to share the joy of this life-changing experience with students. During those years, I worked in a village mission hospital in Pakistan. I practiced medicine in another language, wore non-Western clothes, and was immersed in a premodern culture quite different from the postmodernism of the United States. I learned how to treat diseases I had never seen before, about the interaction of the local culture and health, how communal cultures differ from individualistic ones like the United States, and how an honor–shame orientation to understanding human behavior and relationships plays itself out. Over the course of these years, a handful of medical students from Western countries completed GHEs under my supervision, but these students were predominantly Europeans, not North Americans. Our rural hospital also accepted primary care residents from a wealthy, urban area within Pakistan for a month at a time. My teaching experience was with these medical students and residents, and not with Westerners.

After this extensive time abroad, when family needs necessitated a return to the United States for a season, I was happy to find a practice among the underserved in a university teaching setting in which I could mentor students, particularly those with a similar sense of calling and beliefs as my own. In the United States, I found an eagerness for knowledge of and experience in global health among students, much more so than I remembered as a student 25 years earlier. I found that faculty and students viewed their role in addressing the vast needs of global health predominantly within the framework of short-term service abroad. What I did *not* find were other voices of physicians within the medical school who had served internationally on a long-term basis who could share experiences with students about medical care abroad.

Because of my desire to encourage and influence students with global health interests to consider career service in the developing world, I began hosting student meetings in my home. We discussed possible careers and some of the challenges a doctor might face, such as family considerations, appropriate training, what to look for in a sending organization, risk and suffering, children's educational options, dependency issues, and more. I also created an international medical mission elective for approval within the school's curriculum for final-year medical and health professions students at the university.

LEADING A GLOBAL HEALTH ELECTIVE ABROAD

Accompanying a group of students abroad for a GHE was an undertaking requiring greater preparation than anticipated. Our trip was originally intended to be in a rural hospital within a remote part of south Asia, with many similarities to my previous service abroad. Problems obtaining the necessary visas for myself and the students made that trip impossible, and locating an alternative site required research into many different medical mission possibilities. We finally settled on a country in western Africa for our GHE placement in a religious-affiliated healthcare system. There was also extensive educational preparation required of the students, as well as myself, before engaging in the global health experience, which we completed during the month before our departure.

Three learning objectives framed the GHE experience for students who aimed to (a) participate as active members of a clinical team to assess and treat patients in a resource-poor context under the supervision of both U.S.-trained and local physicians; (b) participate in group reflective discussions both during and after the rotation, with a written reflective paper to be submitted upon completion of the elective; and (c) gain exposure to an international, cross-cultural medical mission experience among an underserved population as part of an overall emphasis on thinking about the role of service in their lives and career paths. Before our trip, I worked with a faculty colleague (Carter) to design a qualitative research study to explore the learning outcomes of this elective. We obtained institutional review board approval for the study of human subjects and the study was carried out soon after our return from western Africa with the assistance of my colleague as the focus group facilitator.

Case Study of the Experience in Western Africa

As the course director, it was essential that a third-party facilitator explore student experiences so that there would be no coercion to participate for any of the small number of students involved. It was also important that I was not involved in any consent process or in the data gathering since I was responsible for determining students' final grades. In the Spring of 2017, four senior medical students and one senior nursing student, all in their mid-to late 20s and just months away from graduation, accompanied me on our journey. There were three women among the students and two men. We traveled with another physician colleague; three of the students worked with her in one hospital setting, and I worked with the other two students in another rural hospital that was approximately 150 kilometers away.

I had interviewed and selected students for this elective to ensure we had a team with a shared vision and goals. All had prior short-term, cross-cultural experience, although none had ever worked in Africa. We met together two times before our trip, and the students were given a workbook about a short-term mission experience to encourage reflection during the month. They were also provided digital recorders for recording personal reflections and they brought laptop computers should they want to keep written journal reflections. Other than the final, required reflective essay to be graded by me upon their return to the United States, any written or recorded reflections were primarily for personal benefit, although they were given the option to share these as part of the study. There was no requirement to do so, and many did not. While we were in west Africa, one group met together daily in the morning to reflect on their experiences as a group in open dialogue and pray, and the other met more sporadically and informally, with students primarily engaged in individual journaling according to their choice. The hospitals we visited had been founded by European medical missionaries, but had been entirely nationalized for several decades so that both medical providers and staff were local.

Since there were only five possible study participants bounded by the context of a single institutional elective of one month, the study was ideally suited to a single case (Creswell, 1998; Merriam, 1988). A focus group discussion was the main data source, with questions framed by the goals and objectives of the GHE, and any voluntarily-submitted student journal reflections. My colleague who assisted with the study took care to preserve the confidentiality of their written and audio-recorded reflections, requesting that they only share content they were comfortable in contributing to the study. The graded, reflective essay due at the end of the course for each student was not included as study data to preserve the confidentiality of study participants who would receive a pass or fail grade from me as the course director.

All students voluntarily participated in the 90-minute focus group session. We used Glaser and Strauss's (1967) method of constant comparison in an inductive analysis of themes that emerged from de-identified data that had been professionally transcribed. My colleague and I each reviewed the data independently, then discussed it together during multiple sessions to ensure that we had captured the nuances and meaning associated with student learning experiences.

Evidence of Transformative Learning?

Early analysis of data left us wanting greater understanding of student experiences than we gleaned from the focus group and journal entries alone. Where was the evidence of transformative learning that we expected? Surely, their emphasis on what was wrong about medical care in this rural part of a western African country was not all there was to discover. We were distracted by conversations of having to buy drinking water that was sold in plastic bags and purchase computer access by the gigabyte. Most of all, we wondered, why did these students seem to be so *offended* by their experiences in this healthcare context?

It was only after thinking about these data for an extended period of time that my colleague and I came to a better understanding of what was occurring, and, even now, we suspect our understanding is still incomplete. We realize that our window into the potential for transformative learning in a GHE was just that—a window in time within an experience that these young doctors and nurse are still making sense of as part of their professional lives. Mezirow (2000), Taylor (2008), Baumgartner (2012), and others have described the sometimes slow, gradual changes that take place over time to transform the meaning made of experience. Our glimpse into their accounts was only the first leg of a potential transformative journey—we wondered how future training and practice would affect perspectives as they acquired greater experience in medical and nursing care.

Students' Experiences in Western Africa

We found four major themes emerging from these data about what they experienced in the rural hospital setting in western Africa. These were contrasted with what the students had come to think of as the *right way* to practice medicine: (a) acceptance of the current situation; (b) standards of timeliness, urgency, and responsiveness to patient situations; (c) moral stances about healthcare; and (d) expectations for patient privacy and family support. Only in the area of family support was there an admiration for differences present in a communal culture that they perceived as superior to their experiences in the United States.

Their stories were events to be commented upon, disapproved of, or, in a few cases, appalled or shocked by in their discrepancies with U.S. medical care. My colleague found their conversation in the focus group animated, marked by a strong emotional tenor and often interspersed with laughter or a sense of disbelief. They were also thoughtful, sad, and regretful, and sometimes indignant, especially when describing many of the patient situations they encountered but were unable to influence. Clearly, the meaning they made of these experiences was still in transition, and the pain of them was evident.

Acceptance of the Current Situation

Several students commented upon the culture of this country as one of acceptance and contentment with the present situation, whatever it was. This made a strong impression in light of how little material goods, health status, or wealth the people of this nation had. They were amazed by it, while also dismayed by its effects in a healthcare context. In this example, the student was working in obstetrics and gynecology in the hospital with a pregnant patient who had lost one of her twins before birth:

> They [local doctors] were trying to keep the pregnancy going for a certain amount of time before doing a C-section. What struck me the most was this patient was not really downtrodden. The patient was still smiling at me, like glad to see me, like welcoming me, asking questions . . . I was just taken aback by it . . . just contentment, regardless of the situation.

While this willingness to accept the present situation without complaining about her loss was somewhat amazing to one student, others perceived acceptance as passivity in the local healthcare staff's willingness to intervene on behalf of a patient. An example of this which greatly distressed them was that of a young girl with Down's syndrome who had been sexually assaulted. There seemed to be no system in place to address the violation, either legally or with a view to protection in the future:

> So we had a little girl come in, she's the age of one of my younger sisters . . . she had fingernail marks in her neck, she had a fractured arm, and nobody really seemed upset about it, except us. Even the grandmother was, well, I think the grandmother had . . . seemed bothered by it. But the rest of the medical staff, they're like, "Oh, yeah, it's sad." But they weren't visibly disturbed by it.

Differing expectations and the willingness to be accepting of situations that had no obvious system in place to remedy them were troubling to these U.S. students. They were especially upset by situations over which they had no control, ones that they perceived did not embody professional care. One student recounted an incident in which a patient, who had been beaten by her husband, was treated and then sent home with her abuser:

> I feel like there's a wrong and a right, and there is, but who am I to make that call in this situation because I'm not the [medical care] provider and I have no authority here. Yet I feel in my gut that there's something wrong about this . . . and yet [hospital staff] are not doing anything about it. So, those were some of the things that I think challenged me.

While students recognized that this lack of effort to influence some of life's tragic circumstances probably reflected a cultural sense of acceptance of situations beyond their control, it caused them much frustration, especially when it meant that patient care was less than optimal by their standards.

Standards of Timeliness, Urgency, and Responsiveness to Patient Situations

It became apparent during the analysis of the focus group discussion that the students felt emotional and professional distress at the ethos and standards of care they encountered. One student recalled seeing the operating theatre chief of nursing pick up a fallen surgical instrument off the floor and place it on the sterile collection of instruments. Another student told the story of a profoundly short of breath patient with what they suspected to be a collapsed lung. The patient was seen by the students during morning rounds, a chest x-ray was ordered, and the patient was handed off to the national staff for follow-up. At the end of the workday, the students returned to find out that no intervention had been made:

> The chest x-ray wasn't done by the time we were doing afternoon rounds... eventually we encouraged them to roll him into the x-ray department to have the x-ray done. He had a very obvious pneumothorax and so, immediately, my gut reaction having done trauma rotation, I realize, "like, oh, man, we really need to put a chest tube in this person." And they were like, "You want to put in a chest tube? We haven't seen one of those things in months."

Many of the students' concerns were for the seriousness of the patient's situation if quick action was not taken:

> We need to do something right now, this person could die secondary to heart strain, and I just felt very helpless in that moment, but wanting to be a patient advocate, so at the end of the day, the orthopedic surgeon helped us place this MacGyvered [improvised] chest tube in this gentleman and he improved a lot the day after.

The student sums up the experience upon reflecting on it: "We talked a lot about how the medical system there works very differently where they're much more passive... there's not really a sense of urgency when things are done a lot of times."

Students were also dismayed with diagnoses and treatments that failed to consider all of the possibilities, as they had been taught to do in clinical care, so that antibiotics were overly prescribed for many of the situations that presented in the hospital:

There were several situations I can think of where, the little girl we were treating on that last day with the knee... I remember talking to one of the doctors and they were treating her with antibiotics like they treat everybody with antibiotics, and I brought up the idea, "Well, maybe this is something different, like maybe autoimmune or something else?" and the doctor's like "Well, no, probably not, it's probably just infectious cellulitis or it could be a septic joint but we'll just treat that with antibiotics." And I'm like... in the United States, we wouldn't just treat a septic joint, but that's an emergency, like you deal with that. I don't know... just different ways of thinking about things.

During the focus group discussion, the students reflected upon the nature of cultural assumptions, and how different they can be in different parts of the world. While they were acutely aware that much of what they experienced was embedded within the norms and values held by institutions as well as individuals, reconciling these differences was difficult when providing healthcare:

I think I learned how much of the way I look at the world is shaped by culture... it's something you kind of know, like intuitively, but I don't think you really get an understanding for it until you're immersed in a different culture and you're surrounded by people who do things very differently.

Moral Responsibilities As Healthcare Professionals

Already deeply instilled within these students were the moral values inherent in their roles as professional healthcare providers. When they observed an instance of medical practice that they deemed reprehensible in their moral judgment, it was offensive, no matter what rationale had been provided for the situation. One student recounted the conversation with a doctor in the rural hospital who performed surgery to "tie women's tubes" without permission among those who had previous Cesarean sections:

He said... "sometimes I do it without them knowing because if I don't then they may continue to have babies and they won't come back [to the hospital] for C-sections and they think that they can deliver at home and they will die"... and so he was making this judgment call... he wasn't telling anyone, he wasn't getting their permission, and yet his reasons for doing it were very much heartfelt and sincere.

The students were disturbed by instances that violated their sense of duty. They were at a loss to reconcile their sense of what was right with the moral stances of others who were also healthcare providers.

Expectations for Patient Privacy and Family Support

Among the many differences experienced in this country in western Africa, students were both surprised and complementary of how extended families often provided support for a person who was sick, even those with psychiatric illnesses. This student describes her experience by contrasting it with what she had seen at home:

> Something that stands out for me... I was in an outpatient clinic a lot and a psych clinic and so often patients were brought in by family almost 100% of the time and families were never asked to leave the room, it was always a very collaborative environment... the patient's family would get handed the medication. They would talk about... how they are going to provide housing and food for this patient... it *did* feel like invasion of patient privacy, but the patients that I saw were very comfortable with having everyone involved.

With the tremendous attention given to patient privacy in the United States, the communal culture of this country was a very positive contrast to what she had experienced in her training, one that left the student feeling that it was a superior situation for patient care.

Making Sense of the Experience in Western Africa

We began to believe that the dissonance between students' lived experiences in western Africa and what they had internalized from their healthcare training in the United States was too great. From the stories they shared, these students appeared to be in cultural and professional shock. They found what they experienced to be irreconcilable with what they had learned in their professional training. Some of their experiences were described as violations of everything they held as sacred; others were merely frustrating because they had no control over the situation.

In his observations of U.S. students in global contexts, Kiely (2005) had described high intensity dissonance as catalyzing ongoing learning. The high level of dissonance that we heard in student stories had another effect altogether; it was acting as a *barrier* to inhibit their meaning-making. It appeared as though the assault they experienced on their basic values resulted in a defensive posture as they asserted their own professional norms in contrast to what they had experienced. Though they were able to identify aspects of the culture they appreciated and areas in which their diagnostic acumen and medical knowledge improved, when broached with questions of deeper lessons learned or worldview assumptions challenged as indicators of transformative learning, there was awkward silence. The meaning of these experiences was yet to emerge, and they were unsure as to where it would lead them.

It was also evident that the socialization process by which healthcare professionals internalize the values, acceptable practices, and beliefs upon which their professions depend was already well-developed in these students. They were well on their way in the formation of a professional identity and the assimilation of its ideals. They knew how healthcare was *supposed* to work, and what they experienced contrasted strongly with their expectations. Although they had all traveled internationally, these students lacked previous exposure to severely dissonant contexts in the practice of medicine, so that what they experienced violated practices they perceived as the right way to do things. They were caught in the perplexing dilemma of uncertainty. With their own standards intact, they had the difficult task of making sense of what was acceptable elsewhere.

Though certainly many of the things they (and I) experienced *were* unacceptable, could it be that these students lacked the broader perspective of cultural understanding that comes from time and reflection developed within the context of relationships? Would experience gained over time have put them in a better position to deal constructively with the extreme dissonance they experienced? I wondered what might have led them to greater appreciation of the complexity of cultural and professional differences, and not simply disdain. Was it simply a bad placement for the GHE? Though I made an attempt to process some of the difficult experiences with the students, I also acknowledge what I might have done differently as their attending physician and mentor to help them deal with the angst they felt. I had to consider whether my own experience of cultural and ethical dissonance influenced theirs, as well.

A GLOBAL HEALTH ELECTIVE
EXPERIENCE IN SOUTHERN AFRICA

The following year, in the Spring of 2018, I took another group of five students to a mission hospital in southern Africa. I chose not to pursue returning to the western Africa sites because of the complexity and extreme dissonance experienced by the students, reflected in the focus group data we had analyzed. Like the elective in western Africa the year before, I interviewed and selected students to accompany me so as to have a team with shared vision and goals. All had prior short-term, cross-cultural experiences; two had worked for several months in Africa during their undergraduate years. We met together prior to the trip and met each evening while there for processing the day's events, as well as reflection and prayer, using the same workbook I had used in the west African country.

Both sites, the national-run hospitals in western Africa and the Western-run mission hospital in southern Africa, were limited resource sites.

Apart from location, there are major differences in the economic status of these two countries. The southern Africa country's gross domestic product (GDP) per capita in 2017 was $1,079 compared to that of the western Africa country's GDP of $1,641 per capita (The World Bank Group, 2017). The western Africa country's infrastructure and health care system, though certainly not without problems, is more advanced than that of the southern Africa country. This disparity was reflected in the severity of the diseases we encountered in which the pathology of disease was more advanced, the goiters larger, the cancers more commonly Stage 4, and the distances patients traveled to receive healthcare were significantly longer. It was not uncommon to see patients who traveled several hours from the capital to our rural mission hospital in southern Africa because of the inaccessibility, lack of affordability, or perceived poorer quality of care in the capital. The HIV and AIDS burden in the two African countries also differed significantly. In the southern Africa country, according to the statistics website Index Mundi (2017a, 2017b), 13.5% of the adult population between the ages of 15 and 49 was living with HIV or AIDS at the end of 2016, while the prevalence in the western Africa country was 1.6% for the same year.

After arriving in our host country in southern Africa, and prior to arriving at the hospital, we were able to visit villages in which an American missionary nurse from our home city (a personal friend of mine) had been working for many years. These rural villagers greeted us with dancing and singing and graciously gave us their huts for sleeping while they slept outside. We participated in church services with them, watched their choirs sing and dance, and held simple clinics under their thatched-hut church structures. Though brief, the students gained a contextual understanding in these village encounters of the world of their future hospital patients by sleeping in typical village huts, eating at their tables, worshipping in their churches, and bathing in open, thatched structures under the sky. Despite language barriers, friendships began to develop quickly between the students and villagers.

Unlike the hospitals in our western Africa host site, the mission hospital in southern Africa was run by North American missionary staff. This hospital operated under the same mission oversight organization for which I had worked for 16 years in Pakistan. Though there was a national doctor on site and nearly all the nurses and ancillary staff members were nationals, most of those in leadership positions were Westerners. Reflecting the economic situation of the southern African country, the hospital seemed to have lower resources for patient care, including laboratory services, than that of the country in western Africa. Despite this, the students and I felt as if the standard of care was as congruous as possible with that in a Western context, considering the resources available.

As the faculty member with them for the entire month, I had extensive time with the students during the workday and intentional time for group reflection in the evenings. Each evening when we shared a "high" and a "low" of the day, the topics were about the courage and fortitude of a patient with an advanced cancer, the severity of illnesses encountered, and the tragedy of illnesses which could have been prevented. Students commented upon the difficulty of working without usual laboratory services and the horror of childhood AIDS. They also mentioned the positive relationships developed with host country staff and many of the local children, and they expressed admiration for those who had been in long-term service at the hospital.

Their overall experience was positive; none of them felt as though the standards of care at the hospital violated their own. This was in sharp contrast to the experience I had with the students a year earlier in the country in western Africa. The dissonance these students in southern Africa expressed was that of economic disparity, resource deprivation, and the severity of diseases of poverty. After the students returned to the United States, one wrote to me, confirming her sense of calling to a career in global surgery in Africa. Another wrote of his admiration for the long-term Western mission workers in this southern Africa country, his continued wrestling with the implications of disparities in living standards, and his desire to return for future service. Though a formal study of the students who traveled to south Africa with me was not held, it appeared to me that they were making meaning out of the challenging, but overall, positive experience of their work in a way that fostered transformed perspectives. Their worldviews had been challenged by the disparities they had encountered in this developing country. The experiences affected them deeply, emotionally and spiritually, but none of them seemed to be offended by how patients were treated or by the lack of infrastructure to provide the best possible care with the limited resources in place. The affective response brought about by the village visits and the many relationships they developed while in southern Africa seemed to be central to their meaning-making. These relational experiences allowed students to enter into the affective processes of personalizing and connecting, two of the five categories Kiely (2005) identified when describing how students experience transformative learning through service learning.

Student Experiences in Learning and Reflection

The overall experience of our U.S. health professions students—their ability to learn from and engage in reflection—and their resulting desire for future service, was in striking contrast within the two different GHE contexts. One left our students, at least at the time of the focus group, offended by much of what they experienced, seemingly closing their minds to further reflection. None of them mentioned a desire to return, whereas the experience in southern Africa left students admiring the healthcare provided. They seemed open to broadening their perspectives of what it means to deliver healthcare in the developing world, and several expressed a desire to return for further service. Why was this so? These differences appeared to be more than individual differences alone among the two groups. What factors contributed to flourishing reflective learning in one context and the stifling of learning in another?

Potential for Transformative Learning

Kiely's (2005) research looked at different types and intensities of dissonance and the effects of this dissonance on the potential for transformative learning. Types of dissonance he mentioned were political, economic, historical, and social, asserting that these led students to "rethink their political assumptions, spending habits, loyalties, and global position on the map of power and wealth" (p. 12). Kiely also found that service learning in conditions of poverty and suffering causes powerful emotional reactions that necessitate a response that cannot be ignored: "Students express 'moral outrage' and 'feel compassion for poor people's struggle.' They experience a variety of emotions including shame, guilt, anger, confusion, compassion, denial, and sadness" (p. 12). He does not, however, mention the type of dissonance the medical and health professions students in western Africa experienced, that of *ethical* or *moral* dissonance, a clash of values between their own professional identities and those found within the host site. The moral outrage of students participating in the west African GHE was directed at the healthcare system and those within it who did not exemplify all that these students had been taught as professional standards and codes of conduct. This violation of ethical and professional standards appeared to stifle further inquiry and exploration.

This "closing of the mind" was also found in research on the experiences of UK medical students in GHEs by Bowsher and colleagues (2018). In an intensive look at students' responses to difficult ethical situations, these scholars found similar results to those I encountered among students in our GHE in western Africa. Among the five themes that emerged in Bowsher et al.'s analysis of ethically dissonant experiences, three were similar, including adopting a position on ethical issues without overt analysis, presenting issues in terms of their effects on students' ability to complete medical tasks, and describing local contexts and colleagues as "other" (pp. 5–6). When looking for evidence of transformative learning in such disturbing, ethically dissonant contexts, the conclusions reached in this research study were that there *was* no evidence that transformative learning had occurred. The same can be said for the students who accompanied me to west Africa, although it is difficult to know if the passage of time and lessons learned in future practice settings will change this outcome.

One can only imagine what factors might have prevented these barriers to transformative learning in our students in western Africa. Perhaps, if the students had a more intensive orientation to the local culture or an immersion experience in a nonmedical setting prior to arrival at the hospitals, like we had the following year in southern Africa, they would have approached the dissonance differently. In a study of African providers hosting GHEs, advance preparation that included cultural awareness training with an emphasis upon cultural bias and cultural humility was strongly advocated by Fotheringham, Craig, and Tor (2018). Had the students stayed longer in the culture, perhaps they would have gained a deeper understanding which could have tempered such a strong critique. If they had been earlier in their professional training, with less well-developed professional identities, they might have been less deeply offended at differences in the standards of care.

The students who accompanied me to western Africa were also of very strong moral and religious conviction; this also may have influenced entrenched notions of what was right or wrong. Had they been more accepting of modern notions of pluralism, perhaps they would have taken less offense. What was clear is that the full story of how these students might incorporate this GHE experience into their personal and professional lives in the future has not yet been told. Their experience of severe dissonance seems *not* to have been conducive to transformative learning. Each of the two GHEs in Africa reflected the cultural context in which it was embedded, and each institution was the product of its broader organizational culture and the ethics of its leadership. These aspects of experience appeared to have been significant to the learning experience for students.

CONCLUSION

The potential for transformative learning within GHEs for students in the health professions is complex and worthy of further exploration. That GHEs are a highlight of clinical training for many medical and health professions students is not in doubt. That GHEs have the potential to present Western students with opportunities for dissonant learning experiences, including difficult ethical challenges not faced in their home countries, is indisputable. What is worthy of further consideration is the variety of contexts that might be conducive to or detrimental to transformative learning and the fostering of a professional identity that includes a global health perspective. Selection of GHE sites requires careful attention to the cultural context as well as the environment of specific institutions. Affective and relational possibilities within a GHE context and the necessity of mentoring students before, during, and after their GHEs are important factors for faculty and students to consider. Leading a GHE and mentoring the students involved is no small or simple task, and, as I have discovered, is worthy of considerable preparation and reflective exploration by the educator.

REFERENCES

American Academy of Family Physicians. (2018). *Global health education for medical students and residents.* Retrieved from https://www.aafp.org/patient-care/global-health/education.html

Association of American Medical Colleges. (2018). *Students in the U.S. pursuing electives abroad.* Retrieved from https://students-residents.aamc.org/attending-medical-school/article/students-us-pursuing-electives-abroad/

Baumgartner, L. M. (2012). Mezirow's theory of transformative learning from 1975 to present. In E. W. Taylor, P. Cranton, & Associates, *The handbook of transformative learning: Theory, research, and practice* (pp. 99–115). San Francisco, CA: Jossey-Bass.

Bowsher, G., Parry-Billings, L., Georgeson, A., & Baraitser, P. (2018, April 11). Ethical learning on international medical electives: A case-based analysis of medical student learning experiences. *BMC Medical Education, 18*(78), 1–9. Retrieved from https://doi.org/10.1186/s12909-018-1181-7

Creswell, J. W. (1998). *Qualitative inquiry and research designs: Choosing among five traditions.* Thousand Oaks, CA: SAGE.

Dowell, J., & Merrylees, N. (2009). Electives: Isn't it time for a change? *Medical Education, 43*(2), 121–126. https://doi.org/10.1111/j.1365-2923.2008.03253.x

Fotheringham, E., Craig, P., & Tor, E. (2018, May 23). International medical electives in selected African countries: A phenomenological study on host experience. *International Journal of Medical Education, 9*, 137–144. https://doi.org/10.5116/ijme.5aed.682f

Glaser, B. G., & Strauss, A. L. (1967). *The discovery of grounded theory: Strategies for qualitative research.* New York, NY: Adline de Gruyter.

Gwinn, L. A., & Frank, I. M. (2015, August). Medical schools offering international elective courses: Average number of medical students in international elective courses. *Association of American Medical Colleges (AAMC) Curriculum Inventory in Context, 2*(8), 1–4. Retrieved from https://www.aamc.org/download/464774/data/ciic02-8aug2015.pdf

Haq, C., Rothenberg, D., Gjerde, C., Bobula, J., Wilson, C., Bickley, L., . . . & Joseph, A. (2000, September). New world views: Preparing physicians in training for global health work. *Family Medicine, 32*(8), 566–572.

Index Mundi. (2017a). *HIV/AIDS—Adult prevalence rate in Ghana* [Table]. Retrieved from https://www.indexmundi.com/g/g.aspx?v=32&c=gh&l=en

Index Mundi. (2017b). *HIV/AIDS—Adult prevalence rate in Zimbabwe* [Table]. Retrieved from https://www.indexmundi.com/g/g.aspx?v=32&c=zi&l=en

Jeffrey, J., Dumont, R. A., Kim, G. Y., & Kuo, T. (2011, January). Effects of international health electives on medical student learning and career choice: Results of a systematic literature review. *Family Medicine, 43*(1), 21–28.

Kiely, R. (2005, Fall). A transformative learning model for service-learning: A longitudinal case study. *Michigan Journal of Community Service Learning, 12*(1), 5–22.

Lumb, A., & Murdoch-Eaton, D. (2014). Electives in undergraduate medical education: AMEE Guide No. 88, *Medical Teacher, 36*(7), 557–572. https://doi.org/10.3109/0142159X.2014.907887

Merriam, S. B. (1988). *Case study research in education: A qualitative approach.* San Francisco, CA: Jossey-Bass.

Mezirow, J. (1991). *Transformative dimensions of adult learning.* San Francisco, CA: Jossey-Bass.

Mezirow, J., & Associates. (2000). *Learning as transformation: Critical perspectives on a theory in progress.* San Francisco, CA: Jossey-Bass.

Rahim, A., Knights, F. (neé Jones), Fyfe, M., Alagarajah, J., & Baraitser, P. (2016). Preparing students for the ethical challenges on international health electives: A systematic review of the literature on educational interventions. *Medical Teacher, 38*(9), 911–920. https://doi.org/10.3109/0142159X.2015.1132832

Roche, S. D., Ketheeswaran, P., & Wirtz, V. J. (2017, January). International short-term medical missions: A systematic review of recommended practices. *International Journal of Public Health, 62*(1), 31–42. https://doi.org/10.1007/s00038-016-0889-6

Sawatsky, A. P., Nordhues, H. C., Merry, S. P., Bashir, M. U., & Hafferty, F. W. (2018, September). Transformative learning and professional identity formation during international health electives: A qualitative study using grounded theory. *Academic Medicine, 93*(9), 1381–1389. https://doi.org/10.1097/ACM.0000000000002230

Taylor, E. W. (2007). An update of transformative learning theory: A critical review of the empirical research (1999–2005). *International Journal of Lifelong Education, 26*(2), 173–191. https://doi.org/10.1080/02601370701219475

Taylor, E. W. (2008, Fall). Transformative learning theory. *New Directions for Adult and Continuing Education, 2008*(119), 5–15. https://doi.org/10.1002/ace.301

The World Bank Group. (2017). GDP per capita (Current US$). *The World Bank Data.* Retrieved from https://data.worldbank.org/indicator/NY.GDP.PCAP.CD

CHAPTER 4

A LONG TRADITION WITH IMPLICATIONS FOR PROFESSIONAL LEARNING

Situated Learning in a Community of Practice

Teresa J. Carter
Virginia Commonwealth University School of Medicine

Bryan Adkins
Denison Consulting

ABSTRACT

This chapter examines the theoretical roots and practical application of learning that is socially constructed and situated in a community of practice, with implications for the professional preparation of learners in healthcare and the helping professions. Situated learning theorists define learning as

---

Transformative Learning in Healthcare and Helping Professions Education, pages 67–89

a form of social co-participation in which members of a community are not only engaged in common work practices, but also create knowledge and shared ways of knowing. Situated learning theory in a community of practice developed from anthropological studies in the 1970s and 1980s to describe a radically different view of learning than that of transmission or assimilation. This chapter provides historical context for the social construction of knowledge through communities of practice since the seminal writings of Lave and Wenger, and includes early anthropological accounts that led to the theory's creation. While communities of practice are often intentionally created in organizations today, they continue to be defined by membership that is engaged in shared work practices within a domain of knowledge.

* * *

= problem

Our institutions, to the extent that they address issues of learning explicitly, are largely based on the assumption that learning is an individual process, that it has a beginning and an end, that it is best separated from the rest of our activities, and that it is the result of teaching. Hence we arrange classrooms where students—free from the distractions of their participation in the outside world, can pay attention to a teacher or focus on exercises... To assess learning we use tests with which students struggle in one-on-one combat, where knowledge must be demonstrated out of context, and where collaborating is considered cheating. As a result, much of our institutionalized teaching and training is perceived by would-be learners as irrelevant, and most of us come out of this treatment feeling that learning is boring and arduous, and that we are not really cut out for it. (Wenger, 1998, p. 3)

Perhaps the study of learning that is socially constructed in a community of practice would not be so fascinating if we knew for certain how knowledge is produced and shared among learners. The question of how learning occurs and whether what is learned in one situation can be transferred to another has long been of interest to learning theorists. In the workplace and in in our professional schools, the issue of transfer of learning is key to what educators attempt to do in healthcare and the helping professions. How successful are they? If students learn in the classroom, are they sufficiently prepared to apply that knowledge in the workplace? If they fail in the classroom, are they likely to fail in the learning necessary for practice environments?

This chapter examines the theoretical roots and practical application of learning that is socially constructed and acquired in practice by a community of learners, called a community of practice (CoP). Situated learning theorists define learning as a form of social co-participation in which members of the community are not only engaged in common work practices, but they also create knowledge and shared ways of knowing through their actions. These actions are not necessarily the ones officially prescribed in job descriptions or in manuals that outline routine procedures. Instead, they are noncanonical, meaning that they arise from communal under-standings, shared stories and practices, negotiated meanings, and a common way of viewing the world within the context of practice environments (Brown, Collins, & Duguid, 1989; Brown & Duguid, 1991, 1993; Lave, 1985; Lave & Wenger, 1991; Orr, 1990; Wenger, 1998).

Who becomes a part of this "community," and how does one gain access to it? What does it have to do with learning in healthcare and the help-ing professions? The answers lie within the concept of professional identity formation—the socialization process through which novices within a pro-fessional field of study acquire the skills, knowledge, beliefs, values, and mores associated with their discipline (Cruess, Cruess, Bordreau, Snell, & Steinert, 2015). Situated learning in a CoP is the *means* by which learners in professional studies come to embody all that it means to be a doctor, nurse, therapist, or social worker, and more. It is the pathway, the route traveled through years of arduous study, rites of passage, and skill acquisition that enables learners to perform competently, while also displaying the values and beliefs associated with the profession. In short, it is how lay members of the population become professionals (Wald, 2015).

Early scholars who explored the nature of situated learning in a CoP conceived of knowledge and the learning process as a communal en-deavor, existing in the relationships between individuals and their envi-ronment as they sought to solve ill-defined problems of practice (Lave & Wenger, 1991). In this view, the unit of analysis for studying learning within a CoP is collective, rather than the individual learning of its members. Ac-cording to Lave and Wenger (1991), it is the community, rather than the person, who learns. Learning is distributed among co-participants accord-ing to the role of each within the community. Thus, original definitions of a CoP were distinct from traditional views of a group or team unified by common goals or by learning perspectives that asserted the importance of context. These early conceptions of a CoP, rooted in cognitive psychology and cultural anthropology, described a radically different view of learning than that defined by cognitive theories of knowledge acquisition. "Rather than asking what kinds of cognitive processes and conceptual structures are involved, they [Lave and Wenger] ask what kinds of social engagements provide the proper context for learning to take place" (Hanks, as cited in Lave & Wenger, 1991, p. 14).

Even though this view of learning as socially constructed within a CoP has received considerable attention during the past 28 years, the idea of a CoP still remains a relatively underappreciated construct. Much of its original meaning as a naturally-occurring and informally-organized group of learners who share common work practices has evolved to meet the needs of organizations for achieving productive workplaces (Wenger,

McDermott, & Snyder, 2002). In the context of higher education, the term is sometimes now used to include intentionally organized groups of either faculty or students who come together for a defined period of time to explore a topic and learn from each other in a learning community (Cox, 2004; Cross, 1998; Richlin & Essington, 2004). However, the theoretical underpinnings of this concept were quite different from either of these more recent perspectives.

While more recent views of a CoP diverge from the informal, naturally occurring and self-organizing entity in support of learning and innovation that was described by early scholars (Lave & Wenger, 1991; Wenger, 1998), they have nonetheless proven useful as strategies cultivated by organizations and institutions to advance team productivity, develop novice teachers, and advance skills and knowledge of educators and students alike (Cox, 2004; Newman, 2010; Young & MacPhail, 2015). Scholars have found CoPs to be a useful lens for examining the nature of learning and identity development in medicine, nursing, and other domains of professional practice (Andrew, Ferguson, Wilkie, Corcoran, & Simpson, 2009; Cruess et al., 2015; Kubiak et al., 2015; Sprouse, 1998).

Original notions of learning as socially constructed within a CoP arise from anthropological and sociocultural studies conducted in the 1970s to contradict notions of learning as an assimilation or transmission process in acquiring knowledge. In a situated learning perspective, learning does not involve absorbing the "body of knowledge" associated with a discipline (Wenger-Trayner & Wenger-Trayner, 2015b). This perspective differs from views of knowledge as something passed from expert to novice through observation and imitation, or that which is discovered experientially. Rather, the origins of a CoP assert learning occurs through the situationally-specific actions of members *acting in concert*, shaped by what the community pays attention to and what is does not, and realized in the negotiated meanings given to practice situations. These meanings, in turn, come to define what it means to become a skilled and knowledgeable professional practitioner. According to Lave and Wenger (1991), a situated perspective on learning within a CoP is characterized by mutual engagement of practitioners of different levels of experience and expertise. The learning that occurs is usually dilemma-driven and is often associated with skillful manipulation of a tool, such as a surgeon's scalpel (Lave & Wenger, 1991). Such knowledge is neither static nor stable, but continuously shifting in response to the changing nature of practice situations as they emerge (Wenger-Trayner, Fenton-O'Creevy, Hutchinson, Kubiak, & Wenger-Trayner, 2015). It is highly characteristic of the messy, gray, and indeterminate areas of professional practice that were described years ago by Schön (1987):

Through countless acts of attention and inattention, naming, sensemaking, boundary setting, and control, they make and maintain the world matched to their professional knowledge and know-how. They are in transaction with their practice worlds, framing the problems that arise in practice situations and shaping the situations to fit the frames, framing their roles and constructing practice situations to make their role-frames operational. (p. 36)

Even before Schön (1983, 1987) explored the world of professional practice, Oakeshott (1962) described a community of practice as apprentice-style learning carried out within the context of work, with knowing and action intimately related to the social context. Oakeshott referred to an "idiom of activity" as the tacit knowledge of how to behave appropriately and of how and when to apply the rules that related to a profession or craft. He believed that knowledge was either technical or practical, and considered practical knowledge as that which could neither be taught nor learned, but only imparted and acquired.

The concept of a collective memory, sustained by the social practices of members of a community and passed on to newcomers, can be traced to Soviet writers; in particular, the psychologist Lev Vygotsky, who lived between 1896 and 1934. Bakhurst (1990) describes the Vygotskian model as one in which the human child enters the world endowed by nature with certain elementary mental functions. As a child grows and develops, the higher mental functions arise from an internalized set of external social practices of the community into which the child is born. In Vygotskian thinking, only as these social practices are mastered does the child become a conscious being capable of thought and experience.

In this chapter, we provide examples of this socially constructed learning theory as it was described in early anthropological and sociocultural studies. It was these early investigations that led scholars, including Jean Lave (1985, 1988), Etienne Wenger (1998), Lave and Wenger (1991), Julian Orr (1990), and Sylvia Scribner (1984), among others, to describe CoPs as naturally occurring, practice-based learning environments. Theirs is a learning theory distinct from traditional behavioral, cognitive, or social cognitive theories that continues to challenge many established ideas about how we acquire knowledge and share it with others.

Next, we describe the evolution of this concept over the last 15 years, explore how it differs from perspectives on informal and incidental learning, and describe its relationship to the many intentionally cultivated CoPs that exist within workplaces and educational institutions today. We use italics to introduce the terminology associated with early theoretical concepts that undergird the idea of learning situated within a CoP. In this chapter, we explore the unique meanings these terms have for a social learning theory that continues to receive attention for its distinctive view on knowledge creation among learners engaged in work practice.

EARLY DISCOVERIES THAT LED TO THE DEVELOPMENT
OF A SITUATED THEORY OF LEARNING

The first linking of the term communities of practice and situated learning in the literature does not appear until Jean Lave, a cognitive anthropologist, began to examine the connections between cognitive theory, educational forms, and everyday practice (Lave, 1985, 1988). Beginning with her ethnographic studies of the learning and use of mathematics among Vai and Gola apprentice tailors in Liberia between 1973 and 1978, she sought to better understand the distinction between formal and informal educational environments. Lave had expected that the arithmetic skills of Liberian tailor apprentices used on the job would exemplify the kind of concrete, situation-specific learning that would transfer to unfamiliar problems, but she found that the mathematical calculations of tailor apprentices rarely transferred to novel situations.

Further ethnographic research among Vai tailors provided Lave (1985, 1988) with strong evidence that routine calculations in the tailor shops were quite different from those evoked in experiments designed to measure arithmetic knowledge, regardless of whether the tailors had any formal education. For example, she discovered that novice tailors began their work in a manner that enabled them to depict the construction of a whole garment from beginning to end. Rather than stitching or cutting fabric segments, they began to learn their trade by ironing individual pieces that would later be stitched into a whole by more experienced tailors. In so doing, proportions and the relationships among sizes became apparent. The novice tailors appeared to be at the periphery of a practice, learning to appreciate the steps of garment construction in a holistic fashion as they came to appreciate the way the garment was constructed by ironing and assembling pieces for others to sew.

Lave's Liberian research project of the 1970s was significant in that it challenged the importance of learning transfer as a source of knowledge and skill across situations. For Lave, the Liberian tailor studies paved the way for future work to investigate an alternative analytic framework for studying learning in everyday practice (Lave, 1988). Because she perceived issues of learning transfer at the core of cognitive anthropology and psychology, Lave thought it was important to pursue the discoveries of the Liberian Project in a comparable study of everyday mathematics in the United States. The goal of the American Math Project was to find a theoretical framework that would account for "specifically situated structuring of cognitive activity, including mathematical activity, in different contexts" (Lave, 1988, p. xiv).

The California Grocery Shoppers in the American Math Project

Lave, Murtaugh, and de la Rocha (1984) hypothesized that research in cognitive development was overly concerned with describing mental changes attributable to an individual independent of contextual influences. Instead, they sought to study the thinking associated with practical activity, believing that such activity was likely to be adjusted to meet the demands of the situation. In a study of California grocery shoppers, these researchers compared the arithmetic skills of shoppers with their performance on identical mathematical calculations using traditional paper and pencil tests.

They selected grocery shopping as the focus of their study because it is an activity that occurs in a specialized setting to support it, the supermarket. The research of Lave et al. (1984) focused on three questions: (a) What is it about grocery shopping in a supermarket that might create the effective context for what is construed by shoppers as problem-solving activity? (b) What are the general characteristics of problem-solving when something happens in the course of shopping that appears problematic to the shopper? (c) How does the character of problem-solving within grocery shopping specifically affect the nature of authentic activity? The American Math Skills Project was designed to answer these questions.

The grocery shoppers study involved extensive interviewing, observation, and experimental work with 25 adult, expert grocery shoppers in Orange County, California, 22 of whom were female. Shoppers' ages ranged from 21 to 80. At the time of the study, their annual incomes ranged from $8,000 to $100,000 per family, with educational levels that ranged from eighth grade to master's degree attainment. All of the shoppers were native English speakers whose educational histories included U.S. public school systems. The researchers collected data through participant observation by asking shoppers to "think out loud" as they made purchase decisions and calculations. Two anthropologists accompanied each shopper, asking questions and recording the shopper's responses and actions.

Lave and her colleagues (1984) found that typical supermarkets keep a constant stock of about 7,000 items in a relatively stationary setting with items arranged by suppliers and store management. They envisioned the setting as being shaped by the layout of the store and the activity of the shopper who navigates through it. Although arithmetic problem-solving plays various roles in grocery shopping, its most common use is for price comparison. The activity of choosing a best buy can require a series of calculations to achieve appropriate comparisons. Of the 803 grocery items purchased by the shoppers in the study, 312 involved explicit problem-solving as shoppers considered alternate brands and sizes, and 125 of these involved actual arithmetic calculations. Of these, 77 involved price comparisons among different brands within a similar class of product. In only four of the 77 situations did the shopper proceed to purchase the more expensive brand. These same shoppers were given an authentic, pencil-and-paper test that addressed calculations similar to those that had been made *in situ* within the grocery store. Shoppers' scores averaged 59% correct responses on the arithmetic test as compared to 98% correct calculations in the supermarket setting. While variables such as number of years of schooling and years since completion of schooling did influence test scores in the pencil-and-paper tests, they had no impact whatsoever on arithmetic calculations conducted in the context of the supermarket.

Lave and her colleagues (1984) described supermarket calculations as *dialectically constituted* as the grocery store setting and the practice-based activity of shopping jointly contributed to accurate calculations. While shopping, problems generated by the activity of price comparison were resolved by considering several factors: where the item was located on the shelf or within a particular section of the store, whether the item was a generic brand or a specialty product, signage that indicated which items were on sale, and even the size and shape of packages and containers. They found that the correct solution to the problem of a "best buy" is embedded in the context, discovered through a process of internal dialogue and reasoning that they requested the shopper conduct "out loud." It appeared that the activity of shopping for best buys is dialectically constituted in relationship to the grocery store setting, which enabled shoppers to be highly accurate in their situated calculations. In the view of the researchers, the grocery store setting and the activity of shopping jointly create the situated environment; each exists in a realized form only in relationship to the other (Lave, 1988; Lave et al., 1984). They described the engagement of shoppers as *cognition in practice*, thinking that was embedded in a specialized context.

Learning as Legitimate Peripheral Participation

Research in West Africa with tailor apprentices, the American Math Project, and similar studies led Lave and fellow anthropologists (1984, 1988) to view learning as not merely influenced by its social context, a view now widely accepted by many learning theorists, but shaped by the extent of participant engagement in practice. Lave first presented the idea that learning was integral and inseparable from social practice in 1988 while she was working for the Institute for Research on Learning in Palo Alto, California:

> In the concept of situated activity we were developing, however, the situatedness of activity appeared to be anything but a simple empirical attribute of everyday activity or a corrective to conventional pessimism about informal,

experience-based learning. Instead, it took on the proportions of a general theoretical perspective, the basis of claims about the relational character of knowledge and learning, about the negotiated character of meaning, and about the concerned (engaged, dilemma-driven) nature of learning activity for the people involved. That perspective meant that there is *no activity* that is not situated [italics added]. It implied emphasis on comprehensive understanding involving the whole person rather than "receiving" a body of factual knowledge about the world; on activity in and with the world; and on the view that agent, activity, and the world mutually constitute each other. (Lave & Wenger, 1991, p. 33)

A defining characteristic of this engagement is what Lave and Wenger (1991) called *legitimate peripheral participation* (LPP). By LPP, they meant that learners inevitably participate in a community of fellow practitioners. To master knowledge and skill, newcomers are required to move toward full participation in the sociocultural practices of the community in which they belong:

Legitimate peripheral participation provides a way to speak about the relations between newcomers and old-timers, and about activities, identities, artifacts, and communities of knowledge...A person's intentions to learn are engaged and the meaning of learning is configured through the process of becoming a full participant in a sociocultural practice (Lave & Wenger, 1991, p. 29).

Lave and Wenger (1991) saw LPP as a complex notion which included ever-changing relationships as individuals experienced changes in membership related to learning and identity development. They were careful to point out that there is no such place as "the periphery" and no center in a community of practice. LPP can lead to full participation as the learner gains expertise in the knowledge-producing aspects of the community. They viewed peripheral membership as empowering as one moves toward more intensive participation and disempowering when one is kept from participating fully. The power aspect of LPP is influenced by cycles of social reproduction as old timers are replaced by newly developing practitioners. Lave and Wenger (1991) describe the contradictions and power struggles inherent in LPP within a community of practice:

One implication of the inherently problematic character of the social reproduction of communities of practice is that the sustained participation of newcomers, becoming old-timers, must involve conflict between the forces that support processes of learning and those that work against them. Another related implication is that learning is never simply a process of transfer or assimilation: Learning, transformation, and change are always implicated in one another. (p. 58)

In later writings, Wenger-Trayner and colleagues (Wenger-Trayner, Fenton-O'Creevy, Hutchinson, Kubiak, & Wenger-Trayner, 2015) describe competence as a way of knowing that is negotiated and defined within a CoP, asserting that professional expertise is characterized by experience, personal characteristics, and actions that reflect the community's determination of what it means to be competent in a domain of practice. They also note that competence is a quality that is both shifting and stable, shaped by the experiences of individual members who also have the ability to redefine what it means to be a competent practitioner. "Members of a community have their own experience of practice, which may reflect, ignore, or challenge the community's current definition of competence" (Wenger-Trayner & Wenger-Trayner, 2015b, p. 14). They are also careful to note that a claim to competence may be refused by the community, citing the examples of a newcomer who may be marginalized, a dissertation that may be refused, or a new idea that may be dismissed as irrelevant. "Acceptance or resistance may be well founded, groundless, or even politically motivated. However derived, it remains potentially contestable. The power to define competence is at stake. Learning as a social process always involves these issues of power" (Wenger-Trayner & Wenger-Trayner, 2015b, p. 15).

In an exploration of five case studies of apprenticeship-type learning, in addition to the Vai and Gola tailors of West Africa, Lave and Wenger (1991) examined the community-shaped practices of Yucatec midwives, quartermasters in the U.S. Navy, butchers as meat cutters in a supermarket, and nondrinking alcoholics who were members of Alcoholics Anonymous. Within each of these CoPs, common themes emerged, with implications for the nature of LPP. Increasing knowledge and skill development contributed to increased status and standing within the community. New members learned along a trajectory from peripheral membership with lesser standing toward full membership based on skill and problem-solving abilities that garnered respect and decision-making authority. The practice was an ever-changing dynamic that responded to challenges and novel situations, generating new knowledge and redefining membership as the CoP evolved.

Wenger-Trayner and Wenger-Trayner (2015a) define a CoP as a shared domain of human endeavor formed by people who come together to engage in a process of collective learning. This more recent definition makes room for deliberately-cultivated CoPs, in addition to those that are naturally-occurring phenomena of practice situations. They remind us that "this definition allows for, but does not assume, intentionality: learning can be the reason the community comes together or an incidental outcome of members' interactions. Not everything called a community is a community of practice" (p. 2). As they note, a CoP is not merely a club of friends or a network of connections. The most important criteria for defining a CoP is the nature of its members as practitioners who engage in sharing stories, solving problems, negotiating meanings, and developing a collective repertoire of experience that includes the use of tools and specialized terminology. Regardless of allegiance to earlier or later definitions of a CoP, the characteristics of shifting membership trajectories, from newcomers to old timers, and the ability of the collective to generate problem-solving capacities and thereby learn as an entity, remain defining criteria of a CoP.

Lave and Wenger (1991) assert that moving toward full participation in a practice confers a sense of belonging. Such membership not only requires a greater investment of time, greater responsibilities, intensified effort, and more difficult or risky tasks, but also provides an increasing sense of identity formation as a master practitioner (Lave & Wenger, 1991, p. 111). While being a newcomer to a practice entails less responsibility for work than full participation, Lave and Wenger also assert that the newcomer must have full access to areas of mature practice to be able to participate in a peripheral manner. They note that to the extent the CoP isolates newcomers, either directly by denying them access to parts of the practice, or by substituting didactic instruction for participation, newcomers are hindered in their ability to talk about the practice. "For newcomers then the purpose is not to learn *from* talk as a substitute for legitimate peripheral participation; it is to learn *to* talk as a key to legitimate peripheral participation" (Lave & Wenger, 1991, p. 109). They note that when educators assume responsibility for motivating learners by structuring pedagogical content as didactic caretakers, they rob individuals from participating in practice and, instead, attempt to act upon them as objects of change.

War Stories, Narration, and Enculturation in Practice

As people adopt the behaviors and belief systems of people or cultures of which they are a part, they become enculturated into the CoP in the manner in which they engage in practice (Brown & Duguid, 1989, 1991; Lave & Wenger, 1991). A newcomer soon adopts the norms, jargon, and appropriate behavior of those who are more experienced in the community, given opportunities for increasing levels of engagement. A primary characteristic of CoPs becomes the stories that are constructed and held in common by members of the community, stories that often supply needed insight into the workings of the practice as it really happens rather than the more formal, authorized accounts of how work should occur.

In 1979, Julian Orr was a doctoral student who was granted access to Xerox Corporation to complete an ethnographic study of copier repair technicians with the goal of also helping to improve the Xerox technician training program. Orr (1990) viewed the technicians as a culture with unique training needs, and the machines as an important aspect of the technician's social setting. He subscribed to the idea that machines take on a social function in modern society by representing design and function to meet unique needs of a particular community. In analyzing the social relationship between machine and user, Orr described service calls as multi-dimensional, complex situations for the service technician.

Orr (1990) noted that a key element of the technicians' culture within the CoP was their fondness for "war stories," told in conversations that took place during meals and in the evenings after work. Tales of strange and unique machine failures were commonplace, and although none of them related directly to the training course, all of them were examples of real life malfunctions encountered on the job. A senior technician and a technical specialist from the organization served as study participants in a session observed by Orr. During the field work, he observed one prolonged troubleshooting session that offered multiple examples of war stories and the functions they served. The focus of one particular account was a recently installed machine that had never performed reliably. It suffered from repeated, intermittent crashes of its controlling logic system.

The two technicians involved were faced with a failing machine that displayed unreliable diagnostic information (Orr, 1990). Training manuals did not provide a complete representation of the machine, and prescriptions for repair in technical manuals assumed that all malfunctions were likely to be known and understood. The senior technician and the technical specialist begin telling each other about previous machines they had worked on where false error messages were displayed. The stories told created an exchange that illustrated their considerable experience with machine repair and provided a context to determine the applicability of the stories for this particular problem. When the technicians returned from lunch, they discovered that the machine had crashed again. A would-be user of the copier stopped by during these extensive discussions and commented that the machine had crashed more frequently when selecting the size reduction button, which eventually proved significant to the successful repair of shorted wires associated with the reduction feature drivers.

By repeating to each other the process of discovery in which they had participated, the technicians were preparing themselves to tell the whole story to others. Orr (1990) discovered that new problems, as opposed to routine maintenance, were always interesting discussions to others in the community. From the perspective of collective memory, talking about problems preserved and circulated knowledge of how to solve them. War stories themselves became artifacts in possession of the community to be recalled and used as needed. Orr also discovered that another use of war stories was as a claim to status as a member. One technician told Orr that no one was really a member of the team until the member had broken something in a "flagrant and glorious fashion" (Orr, 1990, p. 135). This technician had burned up a power supply in the presence of a customer in a situation of gross oversight and in so doing gained full membership status within the community.

Orr (1990) determined that the use of stories as a vehicle for sharing information was a communal response to an unmet need. Considerable shared history among repair technicians indicated that neither training nor official documentation was able to address the serious problems technicians were required to solve. Orr concluded that participation of the community in remembering and using these stories provided flexibility to adapt to unanticipated situations within the practice setting.

Orr (1990), as well as Brown and Duguid (1991), asserted that divergence between the espoused practice contained in official manuals (canonical practice) and actual, or noncanonical, practice is an important distinction for a CoP that contributes to organizational learning by the collective. This distortion between employee actions specified in procedural manuals and what is actually required in practice can result in the deskilling of positions on the assumption that complex tasks can be outlined as a series of steps without requiring expertise (Brown & Duguid, 1991). The reality of learning within a CoP in an organizational context, according to Brown and Duguid, requires "upskilling" from the usual descriptions contained in procedural manuals to be able to improvise in the face of the many unique problems of practice. This is undoubtedly true for many of the problems encountered today by healthcare and helping professionals.

Brown and Duguid (1991) found several features central to Orr's (1990) study of actual work practice among the Xerox repair technicians: narration (story-telling), collaboration, and social construction of knowledge. All of these they found essential to the work of a technician, but none of these existed within the organization's accounts of what was required to do the job. The technicians' stories became essential in learning to become a skilled practitioner. In Orr's example of the Xerox machine repair, technicians constructed a shared diagnosis of the machine out of conflicting and confusing data. This account illustrates that an important aspect of their skills, though not recognized by the organization, was "the ability to create, to trade, and to understand highly elliptical, highly referential, and to the initiated, highly informative, war stories" (Brown & Duguid, 1991, p. 45).

The Use of Tools: Inert Versus Robust Knowledge

One of the distinguishing characteristics of situated learning involves the learner's involvement with tools or artifacts that are naturally embedded in the context of the environment. Schön (1987) wrote "to become skillful in the use of a tool is to learn to appreciate, directly and without intermediate reasoning, the qualities of the materials that we apprehend *through* the tacit sensations of the tool in our hand" (p. 23). Schön was describing the tools of an architect, but most practice situations make use of specific technologies or tools that are unique to the profession. The feel of the tool in hand enables it to become an extension of the user who has been trained to use it well. Brown and Duguid (1989, 1991, 1993) thought that what is learned cannot be separated from *how* it is learned. In this manner, situations co-produce knowledge through activity which often involves the use of a tool.

Professional practice often involves teaching newcomers how to use a tool appropriately, whether it is a doctor's stethoscope, an engineer's caliper, or a financial analyst's spreadsheet. The study of grocery shoppers by Lave et al. (1984) gave evidence of this when problems situated in the grocery store were solved correctly 98% of the time. The tools of the grocery store setting existed in the packaging displays and containers, along with their location on the shelf in reference to other items of similar kind, package labels, and shelf tags. Brown et al. (1989) noted that concepts can also be considered tools. Research in what was once called the Cognition and Technology Group at Vanderbilt University found that without tools, knowledge is inert, acquired in decontexualized form. It can be recalled on tests, but is not readily used in problem-solving (Choi & Hannafin, 1995). Robust knowledge, by contrast, is full, richly contextual, and completely situated. It is constructed out of whatever tools are at hand and often involves the ability to take something apart and put it back together in a new way. Brown et al. (1991) referred to this reconstruction process adopted by members of a CoP as *bricolage*.

THE NATURE OF SCHOOL ENVIRONMENTS AS SITUATED IN PRACTICE

Some scholars, including Choi and Hannafin (1995), describe school environments as cultures in which students learn to conform. In conceiving of school as a communal endeavor, they assert that students develop test-taking strategies and standard methods for applying the tools of the culture. In her investigations of cognition within everyday practice, Lave (1988) found that "just plain folks," the individuals who were her research study participants, developed general strategies for reasoning intuitively, resolving issues, and negotiating meaning. By contrast, school settings usually involve precise, well-defined problems, formal definitions, and symbol manipulation (Choi & Hannafin, 1995). Choi and Hannafin believed that students tend to accept as valid the knowledge that is provided by a teacher or a textbook as the correct way of thinking or solving problems. These scholars perceived the social context for students as existing within the classroom, but it is a context which promotes uniformity rather than deep understanding or critical thinking.

Choi and Hannafin (1995) address the problems students experience in formal learning environments in contrast with everyday contexts by claiming that decontextualized skills and knowledge are operationalized very differently from the ways that experts and practitioners use these same skills in real life. Therefore, students who can convincingly pass exams may still be unable to apply that same knowledge to everyday situations. This has implications for the high-stakes testing required of many professional students in the early years of their training. When a learner succeeds as a test-taker, it does not necessarily mean that individual will also be as successful in the actual practice setting. Likewise, when a learner fails as a test-taker, that learner is often "remediated" before professional advancement into the practice setting. For these reasons, recent reforms in many healthcare professions emphasize the importance of an integrated curriculum, one that attempts to combine classroom instruction with authentic situations of practice. The most successful remediation efforts are often those that enable the learner to apply skills and knowledge in authentic tasks involved in actual practice.

Perkins and Salomon (1989) proposed two different mechanisms by which transfer of specific skill and knowledge take place within school settings. The first of these they called the "low road" to transfer. This method depends on extensive and varied practice of a skill to near automaticity. In this case, a skill becomes so practiced that it can be applied to perceptually similar situations almost as a response or stimulus generalization. The other method, the "high road" to transfer, depends on a learner's "deliberate, mindful abstraction of a principle" (p. 22). In their view, the learning task has to be decontexualized by the learner, and then stored as a general rule or abstract principle to be recalled from memory. While Perkins and Salomon do not dispute that transfer involves learning in a socially-situated context, they believe that an additional step, decontextualizing the experience and creating an abstract principle which functions as a heuristic, is necessary to enable transfer to occur. This may be the skill involved in clinical reasoning, which is challenging for many learners who have yet to learn how to decontextualize the general diagnostic principles to be able to apply these general principles to other situations.

Cognitive Apprenticeships

Scholars and researchers who have explored the nature of situated learning and CoPs include those who coined the term *cognitive apprenticeships* to describe actions that enable learners to progress along a trajectory of increasing engagement and knowledge acquisition (Brown et al., 1989;

Collins, Brown, & Newman, 1989). In a cognitive apprenticeship, the traditional activities for development of psychomotor knowledge and skills also include conceptual and factual knowledge. Cognitive apprenticeships emphasize the relationship between the thought processes and the content knowledge that experts use to perform complex tasks.

Brown and his colleagues (1989) believed that it was in making thought processes overt that a cognitive apprenticeship creates shared knowledge in the community. Only when the experienced member's thinking was made visible to the novice, and the novice's thinking was also evident to the more experienced member, was it is possible to improve learning (Brown et al., 1989; Collins et al., 1989). In a cognitive apprenticeship, the junior learner acquires the skills of the more experienced individual by imitating or "stealing moves" (Brown & Duguid, 1993).

There are several primary distinctions between Lave and Wenger's (1991) view of LPP and the concept of cognitive apprenticeships as proposed by Brown and his colleagues (1989, 1991). Both are described as the means by which learners become participants in a CoP. However, the term cognitive apprenticeships (Brown et al., 1989; Collins, Brown, & Holum, 1991) is used by many scholars to provide a general framework for designing learning environments. LPP, as Lave and Wenger originally conceived the term, has less to do with instruction and more to do with learning. As such, it focuses solely on the relationship between learning and the social situations in which it occurs. Learning is mediated by the differences in perspective among co-participants. For Lave and Wenger, learning is distributed according to the role of each person in the community. Experts as well as community members change as a result of the learning process and the skill being mastered also evolves through adaptations in novel situations.

ORGANIZATIONS AS COMMUNITIES OF COMMUNITIES: BOUNDARY-SPANNING PRACTICES

The distinction between CoPs and work groups was expressed by Brown and Duguid (1991) as one of boundaries and sanctioned practices. In group theory, groups are usually considered "canonical, bounded entities that lie within an organization and that are organized or at least sanctioned by that organization and its view of tasks" (p. 49). Naturally-occurring CoPs, by contrast, were often considered to be noncanonical, existing without a formal structure. As such, they were part of the informal organization, crossing over otherwise traditional boundaries. These scholars envision organizations as complex systems that consist of overlapping and nested communities within communities.

Another feature which defined CoPs in the early literature and distinguished them from groups was the naturally-occurring fluidity of membership. Brown and Duguid (1991) found that "their shape and membership emerges in the process of activity, as opposed to being created to carry out a task" (p. 49). This was an important distinction in defining a CoP. Brown and Duguid conceptualized CoPs as situated within the organization, but also not limited to it, believing that their membership could include others outside of the formal organizational boundaries. As such, they conceptualized CoPs as nested within other, larger CoPs, much as a community of specialized surgeons exists within the larger community of medical practitioners in a hospital setting. Araujo (1996) extended Brown and Duguid's lens by viewing organizations as multiple, overlapping CoPs and hypothesized interorganizational CoPs that would link organizations to their clients, patients, suppliers, research and development laboratories, university research centers, and other external entities.

Twenty-first century descriptions of CoPs by Wenger and colleagues (2002) and Wenger-Trayner et al. (2015) have no longer insisted on their emergent, naturally occurring and informally organized structure, asserting that value can accrue to both individuals and organizations when CoPs are deliberately cultivated and developed to enhance knowledge sharing and provide strategic knowledge management in organizations. They are careful to state that this does not preclude the existence of CoPs that emerge as a natural evolution of practice situations to involve the legitimate participation of newcomers becoming old timers, but it does indicate an attempt to formalize the structure of a CoP to harness its knowledge-generating capacity in organizational contexts. Much of the recent literature on situated learning in a CoP focuses on this broader definition and explores LPP within deliberately-cultivated contexts, including businesses and institutions of higher education (Burgess & Nestel, 2014; Cambridge, Kaplan, & Suter, 2005; Cuddapah & Clayton, 2011; Wenger-Trayner et al., 2015; Wenger-Trayner & Wenger-Trayner, 2015a).

With this expanded view of the usefulness of CoPs for strategic knowledge sharing and management has come a blurring of the terminology between "learning communities" and "communities of practice." In reconceptualizing CoPs to include those that are intentionally cultivated there is a subtle shift in support needed by a skilled facilitator to realize their full potential for organizational advantage. In 2000, Wenger and Synder attempted to clarify their distinction within traditional learning environments, asserting that learning communities differ from CoPs in several important ways: (a) they need to be continuously fostered to be effective; (b) they depend upon the personal energies and relationships among members to thrive; (c) their success depends upon members' passion for the topic, since passion drives people to share and advance their collective knowledge; and (d) it is the role of institutions to leverage the strategic role of communities.

This newer view of CoPs has been defined more broadly by Wenger-Trayner and Wenger-Trayner (2015a): "Communities of practice are groups of people who share a concern or a passion for something they do and learn how to do it better as they interact regularly" (p. 1). They describe a CoP as involving people who engage in a process of collective learning in a shared domain of human endeavor. Most importantly, "this definition allows for, but does not assume intentionality: learning can be the reason the community comes together or an incidental outcome of a member's interactions" (p. 2). They assert three criteria that are essential in determining whether a community is actually a community of practice: the *domain*, the *community*, and the *practice*. A CoP can be distinguished from a club, a group of friends, or a network of connections by viewing it as an entity with an identity shaped by a shared domain of knowledge interests. By engaging with others who share their interests, members create community, engaging in joint activities and discussions, helping each other, and sharing information. Most importantly, members of a CoP are practitioners. "They develop a shared repertoire of resources: experiences, stories, tools, ways of addressing recurring problems—in short a shared practice. This takes time and sustained interaction" (p. 2). It is these three criteria—a domain of shared knowledge and interests, an involved community, and engagement in situations of practice that create the environment for situated learning and the social construction of knowledge to make the learning community distinctive from other examples of informal or incidental learning.

LANDSCAPES OF PRACTICE

In professional occupations, the Wenger-Trayners (2015b) argue that the social body of knowledge is never a single CoP. Instead, they claim that the body of knowledge of a profession is better understood as a *landscape of practice*. This landscape includes multiple communities of practice and the boundaries between them that professionals must navigate on a regular basis. They refer to competence as a way of knowing that is negotiated and defined within a CoP, and use the term "knowledgeability" to refer to a person's relationship to multiple domains of practice. For Wenger-Trayner and colleagues (2015), this notion of landscape is different from the network of practice that Brown and Duguid (2001) proposed to distinguish close-knit communities from looser networks. The concept proposed by Wenger-Trayner et al. (2015) emphasizes the multiplicity of practices involved, the boundaries between them, the issues of professional identity that must be continuously negotiated as one crosses boundaries, as well as what counts for knowledge as a person works within multiple CoPs. Rather than obstacles to overcome, however, the boundaries of a practice are seen as learning assets. They assert that while no one individual can be competent in all the practices of a landscape, they can still be knowledgeable about them. Becoming knowledgeable about multiple practices requires that learners engage with the perspectives of others and become reflective about them. For these scholars, intentional moments of boundary crossing foster understanding and opportunities for innovation. In navigating boundaries across practice situations, learners are continuously renegotiating meaning and professional identity.

IMPLICATIONS OF A SITUATED
THEORY OF LEARNING FOR PROFESSIONALS

Interestingly, while the concept of LPP in a CoP has garnered much interest as an explanatory model, learning by the collective has been described very rarely. Instead, much of the literature we reviewed uses an individual unit of analysis to examine what seminal writers in this field of study assert is a collective learning process. Consistently, the individual learning trajectories of teachers, students, medical students, and nurses have been explored through individual interviews and then combined to create a collective analysis. This methodological shortcoming limits the value of knowledge-producing research activity into the nature of learning as a communal endeavor. Future scholars will need to consider how to examine the processes of collective learning in a manner that treats the CoP as the unit of activity, with implications for individual learning and professional identity formation as outcomes of participation within the community. Scholarship into the nature of boundaries of practice, and what it means to navigate them in a landscape composed of multiple CoPs, presents an even larger challenge for research, one that could enlighten our understanding of this intriguing concept.

Virtual communities are also emerging as a distinct niche within the medical profession to provide healthcare in areas of isolated or rural practice by sharing knowledge, particularly among general practitioners. These hold potential to bridge disparities between rural and urban emergency providers (Barnett, Jones, Bennett, Iverson, & Booney, 2012; Curran, Murphy, Abidi, Sinclair, & McGrath, 2009). Access to clinical specialists through telemedicine is becoming increasingly common, and online communities comprised of rural and urban emergency physicians create opportunities to seek and share clinical information to address the knowledge gap of many rural practices (Curran et al., 2009).

There are considerable changes involved for educators of professional students and trainees when adopting a situated learning perspective in the structured curricular environment. Discussions of transfer of learning become moot. When learning is completely situated in practice, there is no need for transfer. When an educator is guided by situated learning theory, this perspective can be in direct contrast to other learning theories that view learning as a transmission or assimilation process. It can also be difficult for newer educators to hold a situated learning perspective and adopt its tenets fully in practice situations when senior educators hold different perspectives of teaching and learning in the professions.

We believe that the perspective of situated learning theory presents us with endless opportunities for revisiting the world of professional preparation. In viewing the nature of work and learning through a community of practice lens, there is the potential for better collaboration among learners, greater sharing of knowledge and resources, and enhanced meaning and understanding of how professional identities are shaped by work and learning as simultaneous processes. Such an approach can be transformative (Mezirow, 1991, 2012) for professional educators, as well as learners, as they revise their assumptions about how learning occurs.

AUTHORS' NOTE

The original version of this chapter, entitled "Situated Learning, Communities of Practice and the Social Construction of Knowledge," appeared in *Theory and Practice of Adult and Higher Education* (2017), edited by Victor C. X. Wang, and published by Information Age Publishing, Inc. It has been revised for inclusion in this book with permission from the publisher.

REFERENCES

Andrew, N., Ferguson, D., Wilkie, G., Corcoran, T., & Simpson, L. (2009). Developing professional identity in nursing academics: The role of communities of practice. *Nurse Education Today, 29*(6), 607–611.

Araujo, L. (1996, September). *Knowing and learning as collective work.* Paper presented at the Symposium on Organisational Learning, Lancaster, England.

Bakhurst, D. (1990). Social memory in Soviet thought. In D. Middleton and D. Edwards (Eds.), *Collective remembering* (pp. 203–226). Newbury Park, CA: SAGE.

Barnett, S., Jones, S. C., Bennett, S., Iverson, D., & Booney, A. (2012). General practice training and virtual communities of practice—A review of the literature. *BMC Family Practice, 13*(87), 1–12. https://doi.org/10.1186/1471-2296-13-87

Brown, J., Collins, A., & Duguid, P. (1989). Situated cognition and the culture of learning. *Educational Researcher, 18*(1), 32–42.

Brown, J. S., & Duguid, P. (1991). Organizational learning and communities of practice: Toward a unified view of working, learning, and innovation. *Organizational Science, 2*(1), 40–57.

Brown, J. S., & Duguid, P. (1993). Stolen knowledge. *Educational Technology, 33*(3), 10–15.

Brown, J. S., & Duguid, P. (2001). *The social life of information*. Cambridge, MA: Harvard Business School Press.

Burgess, A., & Nestel, D. (2014, October 30). Development of professional identity through peer-assisted learning in medical education. *Advances in Medical Education and Practice, 4*(5), 403–406.

Cambridge, D., Kaplan, S., & Suter, V. (2005). Community of practice design guide: A step-by-step guide for designing and cultivating communities of practice in higher education. *National Learning Infrastructure Initiative at EDUCAUSE* and the *American Association for Higher Education Bridging VCOP Project*. Washington, DC. Retrieved from https://www.scribd.com/document/235513406/EDUCAUSE-Communities-of-Practice-Design-Guide

Choi, J., & Hannafin, M. (1995). Situated cognition and learning environments: Roles, structures, and implications for design. *Educational Technology Research and Development, 43*(2), 53–69.

Collins, A. S., Brown, J. S., & Holum, A. (1991). Cognitive apprenticeship: Making thinking visible. *American Educator, 15*(3), 6–11, 38–46.

Collins, A., Brown, J. S., & Newman, S. E. (1989). Cognitive apprenticeship: Teaching the craft of reading, writing, and mathematics. In L. B. Resnick (Ed.), *Knowing, learning, and instruction: Essays in honor of Robert Glaser* (pp. 453–494). Hillsdale, NJ: Erlbaum.

Cox, M. D. (2004, Spring). Introduction to faculty learning communities. *New directions for teaching and learning, 2004*(97), 5–23.

Cross, K. P. (1998, July 1). Why learning communities? Why now? *About campus, 3*(3), 4–11. https://doi.org/10.1177/108648229800300303

Cruess, R. L., Cruess, S. R., Boudreau, J. D., Snell, L., & Steinert, Y. (2015). A schematic representation of the professional identity formation and socialization of medical students and residents: a guide for medical educators. *Academic Medicine, 90*(6), 718–725. doi:10.1097/ACM.0000000000000700

Cuddapah, J. L., & Clayton, C. D. (2011). Using Wenger's communities of practice to explore a new teacher cohort. *Journal of Teacher Education, 62*(1), 62–75.

Curran, J. A., Murphy, A. L., Abidi, S. S. R., Sinclair, D., & McGrath, P. J. (2009, September). Bridging the gap: Knowledge seeking and sharing in a virtual community of emergency practice. *Evaluation & the Health Professions, 32*(3), 314–327.

Fenton-O'Creevy, M., Brigham, L., Jones, S., & Smith, A. (2015). Students at the academic-workplace boundary. In E. Wenger-Trayner, M. Fenton-O'Creevy, S. Hutchinson, C. Kubiak, & B. Wenger-Trayner (Eds.), *Learning in landscapes of practice* (pp. 43–63). New York, NY: Routledge.

Hanks, W. F. (1991). Forward. In J. Lave & E. Wenger, *Situated learning: Legitimate peripheral participation* (pp. 13–24). New York, NY: Cambridge University Press.

Kubiak, C., Cameron, S., Conole, G., Fenton-O'Creevy, M., Mylrea, P., Rees, E., & Shreeve, A. (2015). Multimembership and identification. In E. Wenger-Trayner, M. Fenton-O'Creevy, S. Hutchinson, C. Kubiak, & B. Wenger-Trayner (Eds.), *Learning in landscapes of practice* (pp. 64–80). New York, NY: Routledge.

Lave, J. (1985). Introduction: Situationally specific practice. *Anthropology & Education Quarterly, 16*(3), 171–176.

Lave, J. (1988). *Cognition in practice: Mind, mathematics, and culture in everyday life*. New York, NY: Cambridge University Press.

Lave, J., Murtaugh, M., & de la Rocha, O. (1984). The dialectic of arithmetic in grocery shopping. In B. Rogoff & J. Lave (Eds.), *Everyday cognition: Its development in social context* (pp. 67–94). Cambridge, MA: Harvard University Press.

Lave, J., & Wenger, E. (1991). *Situated learning: Legitimate peripheral participation.* New York, NY: Cambridge University Press.

Mezirow, J. (1991). *Transformative dimensions of adult learning.* San Francisco, CA: Jossey-Bass.

Mezirow, J. (2012). Learning to think like an adult: Core concepts of transformation theory. In E. Taylor, P. Cranton, & Associates (Eds.), *The handbook of transformative learning: Theory, research, and practice* (pp. 73–95). San Francisco, CA: Jossey-Bass.

Newman, E. (2010). "I'm being measured as an NQT, that isn't who I am": An exploration of the experiences of career changer primary teachers in their first year of teaching. *Teachers and Teaching, 16*(4), 461–475.

Oakeshott, M. (1962). *Rationalism in politics.* London, England: Methuen.

Orr, J. (1990). Sharing knowledge, celebrating identity: Community memory in a service culture. In D. Middleton & D. Edwards (Eds.), *Collective remembering* (pp. 169–189). Newbury Park, CA: SAGE.

Perkins, D. N., & Salomon, G. (1989). Are cognitive skills context bound? *Educational Researcher, 18*(1), 16–25.

Richlin, L., & Essington, A. (2004). Overview of faculty learning communities. *New Directions for Teaching and Learning, Spring*(97), 25–39.

Schön, D. A. (1983). *The reflective practitioner: How professionals think in action.* New York, NY: Basic Books.

Schön, D. A. (1987). *Educating the reflective practitioner: Toward a new design for teaching and learning in the professions.* San Francisco, CA: Jossey-Bass.

Scribner, S. (1984). Studying working intelligence. In B. Rogoff & J. Lave (Eds.), *Everyday cognition: Its development in social context* (pp. 9–40). Cambridge, MA: Harvard University Press.

Sprouse, J. (1998). Learning nursing through legitimate peripheral participation. *Nurse Education Today, 18*(5), 345–351.

Wald, H. S. (2015). Professional identity (trans)formation in medical education: Reflection, relationship, resilience. *Academic Medicine, 90*(6), 701–705. doi:10.1097/ACM.0000000000000731

Wenger, E. (1998). *Communities of practice: Learning, meaning, and identity.* New York, NY: Cambridge University Press.

Wenger, E., McDermott, R., & Snyder, W. M. (2002). *Cultivating communities of practice.* Boston, MA: Harvard Business School Press.

Wenger, E., & Snyder, W. (2000). Communities of practice: The organizational frontier. *Harvard Business Review,* January–February, 139–145.

Wenger-Trayner, E., Fenton-O'Creevy, M., Hutchinson, S., Kubiak, C., & Wenger-Trayner, B. (2015). *Learning in landscapes of practice.* New York, NY: Routledge.

Wenger-Trayner, E., & Wenger-Trayner, B. (2015a, April 15). Communities of practice: A brief introduction. [Web log post]. Retrieved from http://wenger-trayner.com/wp-content/uploads/2015/04/07-Brief-introduction-to-communities-of-practice.pdf

Wenger-Trayner, E., & Wenger-Trayner, B. (2015b). Learning in a landscape of practice: A framework. In E. Wenger-Trayner, M. Fenton-O'Creevy, S. Hutchinson, C. Kubiak, & Wenger-Trayner, B. (Eds.), *Learning in landscapes of practice* (pp. 13–29). New York, NY: Routledge.

Young, A., & MacPhail, A. (2015). 'Standing on the periphery': Cooperating teachers' perceptions and responses to the role of supervision. *European Physical Education Review, 21*(2), 222–237.

PART II

DEVELOPING A PROFESSIONAL IDENTITY

CHAPTER 5

THE PHYSICIAN ARCHETYPE

Fitting the Pattern,
or Breaking the Mold?

Doug Franzen
University of Washington

ABSTRACT

Medical students, like many others in the health professions who must choose a career path or specialty choice fairly early in their training, are often faced with the dilemmas of career decision-making when they have little to guide them and much is at stake. In this chapter, I introduce the concept of the physician archetype as the internalized ideals that an aspiring physician holds about what a physician is or does that the student draws upon to make important decisions about specialty choice. Advisors have an obligation to challenge students to think deeply and reflectively about these internalized images by questioning the source of their beliefs, which often contain many misperceptions about what it will be like to practice in a particular specialty. In doing so, they can help to facilitate learning that is transformative, with the potential for developing a professional identity that best matches the individual's true career aspirations and proves resilient over time.

Transformative Learning in Healthcare and Helping Professions Education, pages 93–110

The question, "What am I going to be when I grow up?" is one that can recur throughout life. For some, the answer comes early and remains constant; others change jobs every few years, always looking for something new and different. Career aspirations also vary in medical trainees. There is an initial period of certainty when a student is first accepted into medical school and then begins classes, proving it is not just a dream—"I'm going to be a *doctor*!" That certainty can fade as the question of specialty choice comes up when applying for residency training: "What *kind* of doctor?" While some students come to medical school knowing in which area of medicine they ultimately want to practice, it is not uncommon to hear medical students ask one another, "What do you want to be when you grow up?" Even students who are certain of initial specialty choice may face some uncertainty about whether or not to subspecialize or how to choose among subspecialties. These career decisions are not unique to medicine; others in the health professions often face a similar dilemma when there are options for specialization.

In medical education, the road to becoming a practicing physician is very long. An acceptance into medical school may add years to a student's career timeline. Typically, students take the Medical College Admission Test and apply to medical schools in their junior year of college. Most medical schools have prerequisite requirements which students usually take as undergraduates, often with Biology as a popular major. Students who earn a degree without taking the prerequisite courses may do so as part of special postbaccalaureate programs designed to provide them with sufficient background in the sciences to meet admission criteria and prepare them to take the Medical College Admission Test. Some students go through multiple application cycles before they are finally accepted into a medical school, even earning extra degrees to bolster the strength of their applications, since the number of applicants vastly exceeds the number of students accepted into an accredited program.

Medical school is typically 4 years, although some students choose to add a fifth. The medical school curriculum is fairly standard across institutions in the United States, with most curricula divided into two phases. First, there is a classroom-based preclinical phase (usually 2 years), followed by 2 years of clinical education. The clinical phase is also split into two parts. In the third year of medical school, students rotate through the core specialties in a hospital setting: internal medicine, surgery, obstetrics-gynecology, pediatrics, psychiatry, and family medicine. During these rotations, students work alongside practicing physicians, help take care of patients, and learn more about a particular specialty. In the fall of their final year, students apply and interview for positions with residency programs in their specialty of choice. This period of residency training (also known as graduate medical education) can last from 3 to 7 years in a single specialty (internal medicine or surgery, for example). Some amount of residency training is required for state licensure in all states, and board certification requires successful completion of a residency program. After completing residency training, a graduate can go through further subspecialty training ("fellowship") which adds even more years of training but is not required.

Thus, training in medical education requires a minimum of 7 years after completion of an undergraduate degree and can last considerably longer. For example, after 4 years of medical school, a student might decide to complete a residency in internal medicine (3 years) and enter into practice as a general internist. A classmate might do the same 3-year medicine residency, followed by a fellowship in cardiology (an additional 3 years) for a total of 10 years from the start of medical school to becoming a cardiologist. Even more training would be required if the resident wanted to become a pediatric or interventional cardiologist. The debt accrued during this time can be staggering. In 2017, the median debt reported by graduating medical students was $195,000 (Association of American Medical Colleges [AAMC], 2017, p. 3), and that does not include the interest that accrues on the loans while completing residency and fellowship training during which time doctors earn a modest salary. In addition to the time required for training, the AAMC reports that debt is one of many factors affecting career choice, since some physician specialties earn more than others.

This chapter will describe some of my observations as a student adviser and a residency program director from talking with hundreds of students and reviewing thousands of applications for residency training in emergency medicine programs. I discuss the "physician archetype" which I describe as personal images that students have for what a doctor is, does, or should be, based on earlier experiences in life; how these images change during the course of their medical education; and how they influence a student's professional identity formation. I draw on my experiences in mentoring and advising medical students to explore how they might revise their previously held beliefs and assumptions about their "physician archetype" to make career choices and decisions about a practice specialty that is congruent with their developing identity as a medical professional. Finally, I discuss how students can benefit from the type of questioning that leads them to examine previously unexamined assumptions about their future medical career, leading to the potential for transformative learning (Mezirow, 1991).

THE COMPLEX DECISION OF CHOOSING A SPECIALTY

Medical career decision-making is a complex, dynamic, and multifactorial process that is not yet fully understood (Borges, Navarro, Grover, & Hoban, 2010; Querido et al., 2016). Much of the literature tends to focus on why students choose a particular specialty, such as which students are most likely to become surgeons (Kozar, Anderson, Escobar-Chavez, Thiel, & Brundage, 2004). Some scholars have explored various factors affecting career choice, including debt, availability of positions, work–life balance, controllable lifestyle, and more (Boyd, Clyne, Reinert, & Zink, 2009; Scott, Wright, Brenneis, & Gowans, 2009), while others examine the more general process of how students choose one from the wide variety of possible specialties (Cleland, Johnston, French, & Needham, 2012). I have counseled many students and have found that a good percentage of them struggle with the decision of career choice.

This observation is consistent with research on specialty selection (Boyd et al., 2009; Cleland et al., 2012). In 2006, Sinclair, Ritchie, and Lee found that, after initially selecting a specialty, nearly 50% of students changed their specialty choice, some more than once. In another study comparing students' choice of primary care versus non-primary care careers, 22% of those who reported moderate to certain initial preferences switched to another set of preferred specialties (Burack et al., 1997). This lack of clarity about career choice in a specialty or subspecialty is stressful for students, especially when some classmates seem certain of their future. Students are also keenly aware that indecision can be costly in terms of both time and mounting debt. Students appear to welcome any guidance that helps them come to a decision about future careers, even if the advice includes mistaken impressions about specialty choice from classmates, which contributes to the problem.

Learning About Career Choices During Medical School

Most medical schools have programs to introduce students to the different specialties in their preclinical years. These include participation in panel discussions, shadowing programs, or clinical precepting experiences as learners. Many advisers recommend that students suspend a choice of specialty until after their core clinical rotations so that students can rotate through a wide variety of specialties and choose based upon their experiences. However, due to a fairly rigid curriculum, some students may only have a month or two to explore noncore specialties before they have to commit to a career path. Students may be considering a specialty before they complete a rotation experience in it, or be interested in one in which they have had only marginal exposure. For example, students may have been to the emergency department to consult on patients as part of their core rotations, but they may not get an opportunity to actually work along-side emergency medicine physicians until early in the fourth year, with residency application deadlines looming. In less competitive specialties, a late decision may not be problematic, but in very competitive specialties, students may need to demonstrate commitment to the specialty very early in the selection process by performing research, getting early clinical expo-sure, or completing educational projects in that specialty. The result is that sometimes students move toward matching in a specialty with only limited knowledge of the type of work that a doctor in that specialty does. Fortu-nately, many schools have become aware of this problem and are adding career development time to their curricula.

Curricular hurdles aside, firsthand clinical experience would seem to be an ideal way to help provide students a better idea of what a career in a given specialty would be like. In some cases, this holds true. I have worked with students who spent their preclinical years working towards a career in a competitive specialty, only to realize that it was no longer their first choice once they had firsthand experience. However, the value of practical experi-ence in helping students with career decisions is not entirely clear.

While it seems to make sense that practical experience could help a stu-dent decide if a specialty is a good fit, Borges (2007) demonstrated that clinical experiences sometimes resulted in more uncertainty about spe-cialty choice, and often left students unclear about how to make a career decision. Other research suggests that students' knowledge about a profes-sion may not be changed by third-year clerkship rotations (Soethout, ten Cate, & van der Wal, 2008). Additionally, practical experiences have been shown to help cement career choices through reinforcing either positive or negative *preconceptions* students have about a specialty (Sinclair et al., 2006; Soethout et al., 2008). Rather than help students understand clinical work within a specialty, sometimes the experience simply reinforces a preexisting (and possibly incorrect) negative perception. This suggests that something more than experience alone is needed to help students make successful ca-reer choices in medicine, and, most likely, in other fields of practice as well.

Examining Perceptions
and Misperceptions About Career Choices

Students are often unaware of the preconceptions and misconceptions they hold about different specialties. Soethout et al. (2008) demonstrated that students' subjective knowledge about a specialty did not correlate well with objective knowledge of the specialty: "The amount of knowledge the student said they had about the profession had no relationship with the reality at all" (p. 3). However, these unexamined preconceptions carry a lot of weight in specialty decision-making. The same study demonstrated that subjective knowledge correlated with preference for that specialty, but objective knowledge did not. That is, those who stated that they had knowledge about a specialty more often expressed a preference for a career in that specialty, even if their knowledge was incorrect.

Perhaps, then, physicians who advise students, and other advisors in the healthcare professions, should explore the ideas students have about various specialties *prior* to their clinical experiences and work to correct any misconceptions before they are cemented in place. A study by Boyd et al. (2009) suggests that even early preclinical career planning talks may not change fixed ideas about specialty choice. Nieuwhof and his colleagues (2005) demonstrated that students can have coherent and complex beliefs about a specialty, even if they are only casually acquainted with that specialty. Correcting misperceptions, therefore, becomes especially important in the preclinical years of a medical student's career since this is when they encounter others whose misconceptions may influence them through peer interaction and discussion. Even the decision to become a doctor may be seriously questioned after investing heavily in the long journey of a medical career and incurring substantial debt. According to the 2017 AAMC Graduation Questionnaire, when asked, "If you could revisit your career choice, would you choose to attend medical school again?" (p. 29), many would not. Across the nation, 2.1% of student respondents answered "no" and an additional 5.5% answered "probably not" (p. 29). This is disturbing, given the time spent and expense incurred to reach graduation from medical school, which is only halfway along the road to independent practice. It is even more disturbing from the perspective of a patient that more than 7% of the resident physicians that they may encounter in an academic center wish that they had not chosen this career path.

Trying on Possible Selves

Burack et al. (1997) suggested that as they are choosing a specialty, students are "trying on possible selves" (p. 534). They proposed that the specialty choice process is a complex, constructed decision, something much more complicated than just ranking preferences and choosing the best option. Burack and colleagues found that the decision is "constructed through a process sensitive to one's starting point, biases, framing, time pressures, and a range of other factors" (p. 535) as students consider such factors as the technical nature of the work, interpersonal content, and even the social milieu in which the "possible self" would need to function. Similarly, Bland,

Meurer, and Maldonado (1995) proposed that a student's career needs are determined by those things the student values, which are determined by life experiences, demographic characteristics, and personality, all factors determined well before entry into professional education. The student's values are then further shaped by medical school experiences, institutional values, and culture. Bland and colleagues (1995) found that while considering career paths, students often try to match the perceived characteristics of a specialty with their own personal and career needs.

THE PHYSICIAN ARCHETYPE

In my own work with students and residents, I have recognized the weight that life experiences can sometimes have on students' images of what a physician is or does, how they see themselves fitting into that role, and the powerful influence these "possible selves" exert as students consider their future careers. Over time, I developed the idea of a physician archetype as the mental model that a student has of him- or herself as a practicing physician. Unlike a Jungian archetype as described by Cranton (2016), this concept of a physician archetype is not a universal representation, nor does it reside in the collective unconscious. Rather, this concept of physician archetype is deeply individualized—each student's archetype is unique, arising from one or a variety of sources. These can include personal experiences, shared experiences, discussions with physicians, friends, or family members, or experiences that include working in healthcare settings as emergency medical personnel, through shadowing experiences, or in previous roles as a nurse or volunteer.

Physician archetypes may be based on a particular specialty, on practice characteristics, or the perceived personalities of those within a specialty. A student's archetype may even have been influenced by books, stories, or television shows. These experiences and images shape a student's idea of what a physician is and does—the professional identity of what it means to be a doctor—and affect how a student envisions future practice activities and interactions with patients and even colleagues. In my experience, the physician archetype can exert a powerful influence on medical student career choice, similar to the unconscious energies Dirkx discussed as a driving force for transformation (Dirkx, Mezirow, & Cranton, 2006). This archetype can form at any time, in the early years of one's life, or much later in adulthood.

With permission, I am drawing upon the thoughts that these medical students and trainees, as well as some physicians who are already in practice, have shared with me, primarily through personal discussions, email correspondence, blog posts, or in their residency applications. For example, one fairly new physician who was the third generation of doctors in her family to practice medicine, wrote about the influences that affected her career choice, having grown up in a small town where her father, aunt, uncles, and grandfather were all doctors:

> I reflected back on what I knew of what it meant to be a physician from growing up in the family of many: It meant waking up in the middle of the night to answer pages and even going into the hospital, it meant celebrating holidays on a different schedule, and it meant many years of education and training. I remember those experiences, but what I remember more are the people I met who told me, "Your grandfather delivered me!" and the suffering that was alleviated for the patient who came to my father's [practice] for an urgent visit.

In another example, an emergency medicine residency applicant to my program described riding in a taxi in New York City when traffic came to a standstill. She asked the driver what the problem was and the driver said, "It looks like a man is bleeding in the street. I think he got hit by a car." The applicant, who had a successful career in finance at the time this incident occurred, jumped out of the taxi, wanting to help. As she knelt beside the injured man, she realized she didn't know what to do, so she just called 911 and talked to the patient until emergency medical personnel arrived. She told me that as a result of this experience, she changed her life course and went to medical school. She ultimately chose a career in emergency medicine because she decided that she wanted to know what to do should she ever incur a similar situation. As illustrated by this example, the physician archetype can form at any point along the way toward becoming a doctor, and, more importantly, as discussed by Bland et al. (1995), experiences in medical school can help change it.

In another story shared in the context of professional development for faculty in academic medicine, one of the physician participants described his wife's illness several years ago as a shaping influence that changed the trajectory of his career choice. Dr. S (a pseudonym) gave permission for me to share his real life story. During his final year of medical school, Dr. S's wife developed cirrhosis due to a congenital abnormality. Dr. S had already matched into a residency program, and it was during his first year of residency training, known as internship, that his wife became severely ill. She fell into a coma and was in the intensive care unit. Dr. S left his residency position so that he could care for his wife. Ultimately, she became so ill that she required a liver transplant. He described his wife's recovery after the transplant as a "road to Damascus" moment:

> My wife was incredibly sick when she was transplanted . . . In layman's terms, she was rapidly dying of multi-organ failure. Then she got transplanted. She was off [medication to keep her blood pressure normal] by the end of sur-

gery, woke up the same day, and her kidneys started working a couple days later. I simply could not believe she survived. All of that multi-organ catastrophe was caused by the failure of one organ, the liver. As I reflected on that experience over the following weeks and months, it became clear to me that I wanted to be in involved in that [type of care as a physician]. I wanted to know everything about that organ. I wanted to be able to help people get this amazing miraculous [transplant] procedure. I became slightly obsessed...and that obsession continues today [in my work caring for patients with liver disease]...This experience caused a complete and total frame shift for me.

The experience described by this physician, reflecting on a critical juncture in his career, was brought on by what Mezirow (1991) would call a disorienting dilemma, the near-death experience of his young wife. It called into question his intended career path and forever changed how he wanted to spend the rest of his life as a physician. Such a dramatic frame shift, as he expressed it, was clear evidence of transformative learning, reshaping the formative expectations of a physician archetype in favor of a new image that developed upon her miraculous recovery after transplant surgery. In some ways, it was fortunate that Dr. S's revelation came when it did. He was able to change course before he spent a lot of time training in his initial specialty. Now, years later, he works with patients with many different types of liver diseases, many of them needing life-saving transplant procedures. In 2017, about 3% of the 30,478 available residency positions in the United States were filled by applicants who were changing specialties (National Residency Matching Program, 2017). Many represent students who had difficulty with career choice or changed their minds due to a variety of life circumstances. Any number of them may have been transformative for the individuals involved.

In my work advising students and residents, I have noticed some patterns among those who struggled with specialty choice or ended up changing direction after an initial decision had been made. One common theme is that as they begin to gain experience in a specialty, students (or interns, as first-year residents) sometimes decide that practicing in that specialty is not what they anticipated it would be. One student with whom I spoke was interested in switching from family medicine into emergency medicine. She realized that the impression she had gotten from her family medicine rotation as a student was very different from the reality she was now experiencing as a resident. She had completed her student rotation in a very rural location in which her preceptor performed minor surgical procedures out of necessity. She was now in residency training in a large city where surgeons were plentiful, and she had come to realize that a career in family medicine would not offer her the opportunity to do surgical procedures if she wanted to live in a large city. This dissonance between her archetype and the reality of her residency practice led to her decision to change specialties. She realized that a career in emergency medicine would allow her to practice as she wanted to, seeing patients with a wide spectrum of illness and performing minor procedures while living in a large city.

As proposed by Bland and his colleagues (1995), the perception of specialty characteristics is significant in such a situation. A student tries to match her career needs with the characteristics of a specialty as perceived; however, if the student's perception of the specialty is incorrect, this can create dissonance for the student who now has to rethink her choices. Therefore, it is important to explore students' perceptions of the specialty and perceptions of themselves practicing in that specialty since the costs of changing directions mid-career in medical education are significant, and often psychologically daunting. When helping students to discover the true nature of the physician archetype they hold, and the perceptions from which it arises, the opportunity always exists for learning that revises the meaning of previous experience; that is, learning that is transformative (Cranton, 2016; Mezirow, 1991).

A ROLE FOR TRANSFORMATIVE LEARNING

Erin, a pseudonym for a student with whom I worked, is a good example to illustrate the influence of career decision-making factors discussed by Burack et al. (1997) and Bland et al. (1995). While their research was more than 20 years ago, it still has currency today. Erin had a college roommate who worked as an emergency medical technician (EMT) with a local rescue squad. Through her roommate, Erin became interested in emergency medical services, went through training, and began working as a paramedic. She quickly realized that she wanted to do more, admiring her medical director and the emergency physicians who came to teach her paramedic classes and who assumed care for the patients she brought to the emergency department for treatment. Erin realized this was ultimately what she wanted to do in her career.

She enrolled in a postbaccalaureate program designed to prepare premedical students in the sciences, and was accepted to medical school afterwards. She was the first in her family to work in medicine, and, as a result, she felt she had a very open mind about her future career plans. As she described her process of choosing a specialty, Erin told me she went through her core rotations with an open mind, but none of them "felt right." She only felt "at home" when she was in the emergency department to admit a new patient or participate in a consultation. Additionally, she felt defensive when she would hear negative talk about the emergency department and its physicians while she was on other rotations. When we talked about other specialties she had considered, and how they compared to emergency medicine, she said she always returned to her "home" in emergency medicine. Erin successfully matched into the emergency medicine residency program where I was on faculty and it was a pleasure to watch her grow into an excellent physician.

As I met more students like Erin, I realized that the problem is less about *when* to discuss career choices with students but rather more about *how* we discuss career choices with students. The concept of a physician archetype is similar to Mezirow's (2012) concept of a habit of mind: "a set of assumptions—broad, generalized, orienting predispositions that at as a filter for interpreting the meaning of experience" (p. 83). The archetype of a health professional trainee, like Erin, contains many unexamined values, beliefs, and assumptions that are part of the professional identity she associates with being a physician. Many of these have been adopted uncritically from earlier life experiences. Erin's example demonstrates that students may be unaware of the composition of the physician archetype that they hold as a mental image. Although she said she was open-minded about her career choice, the use of words like "return" or "come back" or when she spoke of feeling "at home" in the emergency department suggests that Erin envisioned herself there as she thought about her future career. Comments such as Erin's are opportunities that invite questions to challenge students to consider not only *what* they know, but also *how* they know it, and *why* the knowledge they perceive is important to them.

Questioning Career Choices

Most medical schools hold career talks and encourage interest groups that may help students broaden their ideas about which careers are attainable given class rank and which are needed in a particular part of the country or in a certain area of practice, or even what a physician in a particular specialty can do. However, career planning activities were noted by Boyd et al. (2009) to have minimal influence on medical student decision-making, who hypothesized that these panels may do little to change a student's already fixed perception of a specialty. The purpose of these panel discussions is to provide a broad overview of what a specialty is and is not, what day-to-day practice might look like in that specialty, and to dispel the common rumors that surround practice within the specialty. Commonly, panel participants talk about how much they enjoy the specialty and often mention how they chose it.

Taking into account studies like that of Boyd et al. (2009), a more important function may be to get students to critically examine their perceptions of a specialty and their mental models of a future career within it. Keeping this in mind, one exercise I try to do during these sessions is something I call the "double-edged sword." I ask students to list what they see as advantages and disadvantages of working in emergency medicine. Then I discuss that how what might be considered advantages by some are considered disadvantages by other students. In a different approach to this activity, I ask students to list what they consider the downsides of what they have listed as a positive attribute. For example, many students list "control of schedule" as a positive for emergency medicine since those in this practice work on a shift schedule. While it is true that doctors in emergency medicine have some degree of control over scheduling in their shifts, this irregularity of working hours also comes at the cost of having to cover nights, weekends, and holidays—the emergency department is open 24 hours a day, 7 days a week, 365 days a year, and someone has to be there every hour of every day. Such discussions encourage students to reflect more deeply about what a career in emergency medicine might entail, both the good and the not-so-good.

Feeling "Right"—A Cautionary Tale

As students begin to explore their career paths, some notice that a particular specialty feels "right" for them, just as Erin had described when I spoke with her. This subjective decision-making is an interesting reversal of the dominant biomedical model of scientific questioning they have internalized during medical school with its emphasis on objectivity. Other specialties may be interesting to visit, even becoming leading contenders for a brief period, but as students move out of the immediate experience, they sometimes realize that a specialty holds little to no appeal as a long-term career. As an adviser, it is important to help students recognize that such gut-feelings may be the result of an archetype, one that they may not be aware of, and something that should be explored. It is also important to explore what was appealing about the temporary attraction of the other specialty to get students to reflect deeply on a specialty choice.

In another example, Jamal had always been interested in pediatrics. He had completed his core rotations as a third year medical student, and felt confident in his choice of specialty. He had submitted applications and had already been invited to some early residency interviews in pediatrics prior to starting his rotation in emergency medicine. A few weeks into the rotation, he came to me, somewhat distraught. "I think I chose the wrong specialty! I really enjoy emergency medicine, and I think it's the career for me." We met several times to discuss the difficulty of trying to change specialty choices this late in the process, but Jamal was convinced emergency medicine was the right specialty for him. After a second elective experience rotation in emergency medicine at another medical school, which he did not like as much, Jamal finally realized that the appeal of emergency medicine was not so much the specialty itself, the patients, the environment, or the people, but rather the clinical responsibilities students were given on the emergency medicine rotation in our medical school, which were much greater than the responsibility he had been given on his pediatric rotations. Once he became aware of this aspect of his experience, and realized that he would get this same level of increased responsibility as a resident, he felt much more comfortable leaving emergency medicine behind to continue to pursue a career in pediatrics.

Alternatively, trying on the experience of a specialty may feel "wrong" to a student sometimes. Ted was the child of two physicians. His father was a surgeon and his mother, an oncologist. From an early age, Ted knew he would be going to medical school. He was glad to find how much he enjoyed his coursework as a premed student, and he was overjoyed to get into his first choice medical school. As classes began, he buried himself in his preclinical courses. As he listened to classmates discuss specialty choices, Ted knew he wanted to be a surgeon like his father. He structured his clinical rotations in his third year of medical school, selecting surgery near the end with the thought that the prior rotations that were less important to him would help prepare him to shine on his surgical rotation. A few weeks into his surgery rotation, however, Ted came to my office, nearly in tears. When I asked him what was wrong, he said he was very upset because over the past few weeks on his surgery rotation, he had realized that he was not interested in this specialty as a career. "I hate the operating room!" he said. He was fully aware that his desire to be a surgeon stemmed from his father being a surgeon. However, he had not realized that his experiences with his father were with the loving, caring father who talked with him, read him bedtime stories when he was young, and was there for him while he was growing up. These were experiences of the man as his father, and not of the surgeon who had to make difficult decisions, focus solely on the surgery, and who could not interact with his anesthetized patients.

Ted told me that opportunities in surgery to talk with his patients, such as clinic appointments or postoperative checks, felt rushed and were unfulfilling. He realized that he enjoyed talking with patients, sitting with them, helping them through their illnesses, and watching their progress. As we talked, it occurred to me that his physician archetype was intertwined with his memories of his father as a parent, and he could not make his experience on this surgical rotation or his developing idea of a practicing surgeon fit this archetype. I met with him a few more times during the course of his rotation and we discussed what he had liked from his other rotations and what other specialties might interest him. He ultimately matched into a residency in internal medicine and went on to do a fellowship in oncology. Had Ted explored his career perceptions earlier in his training, he might have benefited more from his other clinical experiences by focusing on finding a specialty better aligned with what he envisioned himself doing as a physician.

Encouraging students to critically examine their unexplored ideas about a specialty can be very eye-opening for them. Over the years, I have had a number of residents express interest in a new subspecialty pathway in our field, emergency medicine-critical care. This emerging field requires a fellowship, additional training completed after residency, that allows them to become board certified in critical care medicine. For some, the decision to pursue subspecialty training can be as difficult a decision as choosing an initial specialty. Mustafa came to my office towards the end of his intern year to discuss his career interests. He mentioned that he was very interested in pursuing a critical care fellowship. I gave him some initial "homework" of talking to two members of our faculty who had completed critical care fellowships, one of whom splits her time between the emergency department and intensive care. Mustafa came to our next meeting several months later even more excited about critical care. "I love taking care of the really sick patients! They [critical care physicians] get to do so many procedures!"

As we spoke, it occurred to me that Mustafa's impression of critical care was very "front-loaded" and that he had not considered all the aspects of a career in this demanding field of practice. I asked him how he felt about weaning patients from the ventilator and managing parenteral nutrition, two tasks that are common in critical care but not in emergency medicine. "Uh, okay, I guess. Why?" he replied. As we spoke further, I encouraged him to look into *all* the aspects of providing critical care. I tasked him with rounding (a term that describes daily inpatient visits with the care team) with Dr. M and really focusing on those patients who had been in the intensive care unit for more than 72 hours. At our next meeting, Mustafa admitted that perhaps a career in critical care medicine was not right for him. He had not considered everything that was part of long-term care of the critically ill and had only focused on the initial resuscitation efforts to save a life, an aspect of providing critical care most like emergency medicine. We discussed how he could focus on this without needing to do a critical care fellowship. Ultimately, he did not pursue fellowship training, but now does research in resuscitation and critical care in the emergency medicine department.

ADVICE FOR ADVISERS

In medical education, the concept of professional identity formation describes the largely tacit processes of socialization of individuals as they begin to assume the values, beliefs, and mores that define what it means to be a physician in our society. However, most individuals do not arrive at the doorstep of a medical career without preconceived, internalized images of what it means to be a doctor, the physician archetype that each one carries within. Unearthing these usually buried images becomes essential in helping students and junior doctors make career decisions that are right for them. Advisors, mentors, and role models can have a tremendous impact on the long-term viability of career specialty choice when they help their junior colleagues in this challenging undertaking. So, how does an advisor help a student explore this internalized physician archetype when making career decisions?

Dirkx (2000), who writes about transformative pedagogy from a mythopoetic perspective, believes in the importance of giving voice to the emotions and internalized images that usually remain hidden from conscious awareness, regardless of subject matter. These, he says, can include stories, myths, poetry, music, drawing, art, journaling, or performance rituals (p. 4). How students express themselves through these alternative strategies can reveal aspects of the psyche that usually remain outside of conscious awareness. When openly expressed, they hold potential to promote self-understanding, and perhaps enable students to identify for themselves aspects of the physician archetype that they seek to honor in personal career choices.

Within a small group of students, what images of a doctor interacting with a patient does each student select as personally resonating from those that can be printed and shared from the many available online? Why does the image hold appeal? What does it say about the type of doctor he or she wants to become?

Other strategies include thoughtful reviews of personal statements in the residency application: What clues are openly hidden there? Was there a particular person or experience that influenced the decision to go into medicine? Why does the student think that person or experience was so significant? What does it say about what is important to achieve in a medical career? When meeting with students, advisors can ask questions that aim to uncover the physician archetype:

- When you first became interested in medicine, what was your mental image of an "ideal" doctor?
- Imagine you are already in practice. What activities are most engaging for you? How do you foresee yourself interacting with patients?
- Imagine you are being honored by your alumni association for the accomplishments of your career as a physician. What did you do over a lifetime to win such an award?

Occasionally, students find themselves heading in the wrong direction, career-wise, by the passion of another person, or by a charismatic mentor or physician. When this happens, the student sometimes mistakenly assumes the other's passion for a particular specialty as his or her own. However, if the student cannot align what this person does with the student's internalized archetype, the "fit" will likely be a poor one and lead to future difficulty. A similar dilemma occurs in the personal anguish that comes with changing specialty after an initial career decision has been made. It becomes important not only to ask "What did you think this specialty would be like?" but also "*Why* did you think it would be like this?" Exploring these previously unquestioned habits of mind becomes a way of unearthing what has been overlooked or misperceived in specialty decision-making.

Some students who appear to have an unexamined archetype may actually lack an internalized image of what they would do as a doctor. These students are usually the ones who have entered medical school and progressed through their studies without really thinking about why they are there or what specialty they will choose. For some, it may be the family's choice of career ("everyone in my family is a doctor"), without any personal exploration of whether or not this expectation is of the individual's choosing. For others, it appears as an overly romanticized image, lacking in any specificity: "I've always wanted to be a doctor. . .I enjoyed all my preclinical courses. . .I loved all of my rotations. . .I loved the excitement of the emergency department, and that's why I want to go into emergency medicine." For me as a residency program director, this red flag merits a serious discussion of whether or not the student understands my field of practice, with its marginalized patients, lack of resources, and social issues. Managing trauma patients and attending to emergency resuscitative efforts are only a small part of what we do.

As advisors, if we are serious about the issue of physician burnout, we have an obligation to help our students make career decisions that promote resilience and serve them well over time. In this way, the rewards of practice in a particular specialty will prove invigorating, rather than draining. In doing so, not only is the individual well served, but all of us benefit from a physician workforce that finds job satisfaction and brings genuine commitment to their work as healers.

AUTHOR NOTE

With appreciation, I wish to thank the physicians, students, and resident trainees whose words are quoted in this chapter. I am grateful for their permission to use the stories that they willingly shared with me as part of their own career decision-making.

REFERENCES

Association of American Medical Colleges. (2017). *AAMC medical school graduation questionnaire 2017 all schools summary report.* Washington, DC: Author.

Bland, C. J., Meurer, L. N., & Maldonado, G. (1995, July). Determinants of primary care specialty choice: A non-statistical meta-analysis of the literature. *Academic Medicine, 70*(7), 620–641.

Borges, N. J. (2007). Behavioral exploration of career and specialty choice in medical students. *The Career Development Quarterly, 55*(4), 351–358. https://doi.org/ 10.1002/j.2161-0045.2007.tb00089.x

Borges, N. J., Navarro, A., Grover, A., & Hoban, J. D. (2010, April). How, when and why do physicians choose careers in academic medicine? A literature reviews. *Academic Medicine, 85*(4), 680–686. https://doi.org/10.1097/ACM. 0b013e3181d29cb9

Boyd, J. S., Clyne, B., Reinert, S. E., & Zink, B. J. (2009). Emergency medicine career choice: A profile of factors and influences from the Association of American Medical Colleges (AAMC) graduation questionnaires. *Academic Emergency Medicine, 16*(6), 544–549. https://doi.org/10.1111/j.1553-2712.2009.00385.x

Burack, J. H., Irby, D. M., Carline, J. D., Ambrozy, D. M., Ellsbury, K. E., & Stritter, F. T. (1997). A study of medical students' specialty-choice pathways: Trying on possible selves. *Academic Medicine, 72*(6), 534–541.

Cleland, J., Johnston, P. W., French, F. H., & Needham, G. (2012). Associations between medical students and career preferences in Year 1 medical students in Scotland. *Medical Education, 46*(5), 473–484. https://doi.org/10.1111/ j.1365-2923.2012.04218.x

Cranton, P. (2016). *Understanding and promoting transformative learning* (3rd ed.). San Francisco, CA: Jossey-Bass.

Dirkx, J. M. (2000). *Transformative learning and the journey of individuation.* Columbus, OH: ERIC Clearing House on Adult, Career, and Vocational Education. (ED448305)

Dirkx, J. M., Mezirow, J., & Cranton, P. (2006). Musings and reflections on the meaning, context, and process of transformative learning: A dialogue between John M. Dirkx and Jack Mezirow. *Journal of Transformative Education, 4*(2), 123–139. https://doi.org/10.1177/1541344606287503

Kozar, R. A., Anderson, K. D., Escobar-Chaves, S. L., Thiel, M. A., & Brundage, S. I. (2004). Preclinical students: Who are surgeons? *Journal of Surgical Residency, 119*(2), 113–116.

Mezirow, J. (1991). *Transformative dimensions of adult learning.* San Francisco, CA: Jossey-Bass.

Mezirow, J. (2012). Learning to think like an adult: Core concepts of transformative learning. In E. W. Taylor, P. Cranton, & Associates (Eds.), *The handbook of transformative learning: Theory, research, and practice* (pp. 73–95). San Francisco, CA: Jossey-Bass.

National Residency Matching Program. (2017). Table 2. In *Results and data: 2017 main residency match* (pp. 8–9). Washington, DC: Author. Retrieved from http://www.nrmp.org/wp-content/uploads/2017/06/Main-Match-Results-and-Data-2017.pdf

Nieuwhof, M. G., Rademakers, J. J., Kuyvenhoven, M. M., Soethout, M. B., & ten Cate, T. J. (2005). Students' conceptions of the medical profession: An interview study. *Medical Teacher, 27*(8), 709–714. https://doi.org/10.1080/01421590500271159

Querido, S. J., Vergouw, D., Wigersma, L., Batenburg, R. S., DeRond, M. E. J., & ten Cate, O. T. (2016). Dynamics of career choice among students in undergraduate medical courses. A BEME systemic review: BEME Guide No 33. *Medical Teacher, 38*(1), 18–29. https://doi.org/10.3109/0142159X.2015.1074990

Scott, I. M., Wright, B. J., Brenneis, F. R., & Gowans, M. C. (2009). Whether or wither some specialties. A survey of Canadian medical student career interest. *BMC Medical Education, 9*(57). https://doi.org/10.1186/1472-6920-9-57

Sinclair, H. K., Ritchie, L. D., & Lee, A. J. (2006). A future career in general practice? A longitudinal study of medical students and pre-registration house officers. *European Journal of General Practice, 12*(3), 120–127. https://doi.org/10.1080/13814780600780833

Soethout, M. B., ten Cate, O. T., & van der Wal, G. (2008). Correlations of knowledge and preference of medical students for a specialty career: A case study of youth health care. *BMC Public Health, 8*(14). https://doi.org/10.1186/1471-2458-8-14

CHAPTER 6

BUILDING PROFESSIONAL IDENTITIES BY LEARNING FROM MENTORS AND ROLE MODELS

Teresa J. Carter, Ellen L. Brock, Frank A. Fulco, and Adam M. Garber
Virginia Commonwealth University School of Medicine

Reena H. Hemrajani
Emory University School of Medicine

Bennett B. Lee and Scott C. Matherly
Virginia Commonwealth University School of Medicine

Emily R. Miller
Michigan State University/Helen Devos Children's Hospital

John G. Pierce Jr.
Liberty University College of Osteopathic Medicine

Transformative Learning in Healthcare and Helping Professions Education, pages 111–127
Copyright © 2019 by Information Age Publishing
All rights of reproduction in any form reserved.

ABSTRACT

Within the literature on mentoring research and practice, which has grown in complexity and depth over the past 30 years, role modeling remains an underrepresented and under-studied psychosocial function of developmental relationships. Yet, scholarship in medical education emphasizes the significance of role modeling for professional identity formation of physicians-in-training and is well-developed in its treatment of both positive and negative role models and their significance for medical education. In this chapter, physician-educators illustrate major themes in the literature with examples of the influence of role models and mentors in determining choice of medical specialty and decisions to teach, as well as the lessons learned from role models that influence how they teach medical students and residents today.

What inspires physicians to want to teach, mentor, and serve as role models for the next generation of doctors? For many faculty members in academic medicine, the opportunity to mentor and model professional behaviors and attitudes serves as a powerful motivator for teaching. All doctors seek to educate their patients about disease, treatments, and prevention of illness. In academic medicine, the teaching role of physicians and surgeons extends beyond the realm of patient care to the education of medical students and residents. These responsibilities are undertaken while also providing quality patient care and leadership for an interdisciplinary team of healthcare providers in the high-intensity environment of a teaching hospital, where many of the most severely ill patients in the healthcare system are treated today.

In academic medicine, mentoring and role modeling have been identified as crucial roles for clinician-educators (Heflin, Pinheiro, Kaminetzky, & McNeill, 2009), with effective role modeling considered an essential skill to enable professional development of learners in the clinical setting (Cruess, Cruess, Boudreau, Snell, & Steinert, 2015; Goldie, 2012; Kenny, Mann, & MacLeod, 2003). A review of literature on role modeling in medical education identified three major attributes imparted by positive role models: demonstration of high standards of clinical competence, excellence in clinical teaching skills, and humanistic personal qualities (Passi et al., 2013).

However, lack of effective, positive role models has been identified as a significant issue within the hidden curriculum of medical education in which learners observe negative behaviors that contradict the desirable professional qualities explicitly taught (Hafferty, 1998; Hafferty & Franks, 1994). For new learners entering the clinical setting as third-year medical students, the hidden curriculum poses a significant threat to the development of professional behaviors (Wear, Aultman, Zarconi, & Varley, 2009). Bandura's (1986) seminal work on social learning theory and his concept of vicarious learning provide a sound basis for examining role modeling in medical education (Jochemsen-van der Leeuw, van Diijk, van Etten-Jamaludin, & Woeromga-de Waard, 2013). In general, the study of role modeling as an important aspect of the mentoring relationship has been underdeveloped and under-researched within mentoring literature (Lankau & Scandura, 2007). One exception has been the work of Gibson (1995) and Gibson and Cordova (1999) who studied the importance of role models as exemplars in organizations.

In academic medicine, those who are mentored include medical students and residents, physicians-in-training who hone their skills and knowledge in the hospital setting where they work under the supervision of faculty members as attending physicians. Medical students, as well as junior residents, called interns, are often taught by senior residents and fellows in addition to the supervision provided by attending physicians in the hospital. The norm for licensure as a physician in most medical specialties within the United States is 7 to 10 years, 4 years of medical school followed by 3 to 5 years of residency training. However, subspecialty or advanced fellowship training can extend the time to practice independently. These years of medical training are demanding on the physical and mental stamina required of those who enter an accredited medical school through a highly competitive selection process. As Cruess et al. (2015) note, acceptance into medical school is symbolically significant in that it begins the process of socialization into the medical profession. Within this profession, mentors and role models increase the sense of belonging, since they are members of the community of practice (Lave & Wenger, 1991) that students wish to join.

During their medical school education, students focus primarily on mastering an extensive domain of content knowledge related to human health and disease before entering the clinical setting in the third and fourth years. After 4 years, medical students earn the MD degree and they become residents in a teaching hospital. This learning environment is known for an apprenticeship-like training method often described as "see one, do one, teach one," in which each level of trainee assists with the education of juniors (Kenny, Mann, Wrixon, MacLeod, & Coles, 2002). Within professional education contexts, the training required of a physician is among the most demanding of disciplines. In recent years, residents have been limited to an 80-hour work week in an effort to increase patient safety and reduce burnout and stress (Walen & Walsh, 2011). Passing on knowledge, skills, attitudes, and values is an integral part of what it means to develop the professional identity of a doctor (Cruess et al., 2015; Kenny et al., 2003).

Even the word, "doctor" has its origins in the Latin *docere*, which means "to teach" (Whitman & Schwenk, 1987). Professional identity formation in medical education has been described as a transformative learning experience that fosters personal and professional development through mentoring and self-reflection, with the goal of affirming best practices, traditions, and ethics of the profession (Holden et al., 2015; Wald, 2015).

This chapter explores mentoring and role modeling in medical education through the words of eight coauthors who are physician-educators in academic medicine. They have reflected upon why they teach as part of their own continuing professional development in a course taught by the primary chapter author. Their words illuminate some of the major themes within current research on mentoring theory and place them in the context of practice within medical education. By drawing on the experience of physicians for whom teaching is a major responsibility, our chapter examines the complex phenomena of mentoring and role modeling within the specialized context of teaching the next generation of doctors.

DEFINING MENTORING AND ROLE MODELING IN THE LITERATURE

Kram's (1985) pioneering research on mentoring dyads discovered two major roles of developmental relationships. These include career-enhancing functions of sponsorship, coaching, protection, exposure and visibility, and the ability to provide opportunities for challenging work, and psychosocial functions. The psychosocial aspects she identified enhance a mentee's sense of competence by shaping a professional identity, and include role modeling, acceptance and confirmation, counseling, and friendship. Of these psychosocial functions, role modeling appears prominently in the medical education literature, including international journals devoted to medical education (Mirhaghi, Moonaghi, Sharafi, & Zeydi, 2015).

Among scholars who have studied mentoring, McCauley and Douglas (1998) adopted a framework for classifying developmental relationships according to their propensity to provide assessment, challenge, or support for the mentee. In the early research on workplace mentoring, McCauley and Douglas, as well as Fletcher (1996), Kram and Hall (1996), and Schor (1997) recognized that the traditional concept of a longstanding dyadic mentor–mentee relationship was far more likely to be replaced in today's work environment by a network constellation of relationships, with multiple individuals fulfilling different roles. Certainly, a network view of the mentoring relationship appears relevant in medical education since the physician-in-training rotates through various clinical services in the hospital with exposure to many potential mentors and role models. In recent years, the concept of a "mentoring episode" (Fletcher & Ragins, 2007; Kram & Ragins, 2007) has addressed the growth potential of short interactions with influential others to provide brief encounters associated with intense meaning. These brief mentoring encounters appear prominently in the narratives of physician-educators in this chapter.

Lankau and Scandura (2007) elaborate upon the distinct qualities of role modeling that enable personal learning within developmental relationships, building upon Kram's (1985) findings that role modeling is a process in which the mentee adopts attitudes, approaches, and values to develop a professional identity. While Kram's (1985) schema highlights role modeling as one of many psychosocial functions of the mentoring relationship, other scholars (Gibson, 1995; Gibson & Cordova, 1999) differentiate the constructs of mentor, role model, and sponsor based on the nature of identification present for the mentee, or protégé. They draw on identification theory to assert that mentoring and sponsorship activities both depend upon interaction with and active intervention by a senior person on behalf of a mentee, whereas role modeling assumes only identification on the part of the observer. Gibson and Cordova (1999) draw upon the scholarship of Bell (1970), Kelman (1961), and Kohlberg, (1963), to associate role modeling with the desire to enhance perceived similarity to another person and to assimilate aspects of the role model's attitudes, behaviors, and values into the self. In this view, the function of role modeling is to emulate by occupying the role model's life situation (Gibson & Cordova, 1999). It is this definition of role modeling that appears in the medical education literature and will be illustrated by our examples.

IDENTIFYING WITH MENTORS AND ROLE MODELS

How do physicians go about identifying with role models or finding a mentor within their specialties? Doctors-in-training seem to look to those whom they admire: the teachers who inspired them, who energetically and enthusiastically shared their love for patients as well as those who demonstrated passion for their choice of medical specialty (Wright, Kern, Kolodner, Howard, & Brancati, 1998; Passi et al., 2013). In our examples, role models appear to be discovered by the learner through specifically remembered incidents. The learner observes the teacher in action and takes notice of his or her commitment to learners and to the profession. The trainee also notices that the teacher stands out from others as exceptional in some way, and this leads the learner to assimilate characteristics of the role model. Dr. Miller's narrative illustrates both the surprise of the discovery and the effect that it had on her choice to become a pediatric endocrinologist in an academic medical center:

You hear throughout medical school and internship that being a physician means you are a "life-long learner," but no one eludes that you will also be a life-long teacher or mentor. That was a stunning insight that occurred in the second year of my residency training, when it was now my responsibility to foster interns or a team of medical students. In medical school and during most of my residency training, I aspired to be an adolescent medicine physician; however, a new pediatric endocrinology faculty member joined our team and derailed my plans. *She embodied everything I wanted to be as a doctor.* She cultivated great relationships with patients and could teach them about their diagnoses in a way that matched their background and level of education. In a lecture setting, she delivered enthusiastic, comprehensive presentations that were understandable at multiple learning stages. Most dramatically, while on [hospital] service, she required residents to read about patients and come up with their own plan rather than dictate the [management] plan herself; impressively, she would let us institute a reasonable, well-thought out plan [of care], even if it was not her exact way of practicing, as long as it did not harm the patient in any way and fit within the management scope. She was relatively fresh out of fellowship and by no means the world's expert on endocrinology, yet she was a remarkable teacher. She became a mentor and an inspiration for me. When I became a fellow, I knew I wanted to bring the skills she demonstrated with me and pass on the knowledge and passion she exemplifies.... It was during that year that I fell in love with teaching myself and knew it is what I want to do as a major part of my career.

The ability to be influenced by an engaging teacher to choose a similar medical specialty has been cited as one of the benefits of a role model in medical education (Wright, Wong, & Newell, 1997). Wright and his colleagues found that exposure to role models in a particular specialty was strongly associated with medical students' choice of clinical field for residency training.

As an example of this phenomenon, Dr. Matherly studied internal medicine with an interest in the subspecialty of gastroenterology. However, he readily admits the influence of his teachers in other specialties whose enthusiastic approach to their work was inspirational during his years of medical education. Matherly describes how he patterned himself after an extraordinary teacher by choosing the same residency training program to develop his specialty in hepatology. For both Drs. Miller and Matherly, the identification was so complete that their professional identities were significantly shaped by role models who were positive influences in choosing the type of medicine they would practice. Additionally, both Miller and Matherly were inspired to become better teachers as a result. Dr. Matherly explains the desire he now has to pass on to trainees what he experienced as a result of an influential mentor and role model:

A variety of teaching techniques and mentors have shaped my teaching style over the years. There was an otolaryngologist who taught me head and neck anatomy who was a huge influence on me. His enthusiasm was so infectious that it made me want to learn more about something I didn't even think I was interested in. Later in my medical school career, I was deeply influenced by one of my Internal Medicine professors. He was fairly young, but his bedside approach to the patient was phenomenal and his physical exam skill was amazing. I patterned my approach to the patient after him even to the point of going to the same residency [program] so that I could be trained in a similar manner. So why do I teach? *My admiration for the teachers who have guided me in the past makes me want to emulate them.* I hope to leave my mark on the world by affecting the lives and practice of a handful of physicians. I hope that in 10 years someone will tell an anecdote about the nutty hepatologist who taught portal hypertension in such a compelling way that he inspired them to want to learn more about it. I hope somewhere, someday, a physician will choose the right thing to do for a patient rather than the easy thing to do because they remember me doing it that way. I am lucky to have a job where I can take care of the patients I love while at the same time influencing the next generation of physicians.

This desire to replicate the quality of education they experienced as learners was universal with the physician-educators who contributed perspectives in this chapter. While all medical educators are well aware that expertise does not develop in a single encounter, the spirit of "see one, do one, teach one" is deeply embedded within this community of practice as the method for transferring knowledge and skills from one generation to the next (Kenny et al., 2002). Newcomers are legitimately peripheral participants (Lave & Wenger, 1991) in the provision of medical care as beginning learners, but with developing expertise, young doctors gradually progress toward full participation as they gain experience. The community of practice that exists within the medical community thus reproduces itself through time-honored traditions of teaching at bedside and in clinical encounters with patients.

In this manner, the medical community passes on the traditions, language, culture, and associated meanings of what it means to be a doctor in our society (Kenny et al., 2003). One of the major transitions from student to full participant within this medical community appears to occur during the internship year as first-year residents assimilate what it truly means to put the needs of the patient above those of the self (E. P. Marlowe, personal communication, June 10, 2015). So much of this knowledge is embedded in tacitly acquired actions and ways of being that the socialization of a physician can be considered a major outcome of a medical education (Goldie, 2012; Kenny et al., 2003).

Developing Confidence as a Teacher

Newly minted doctors, even those who have completed years of training to earn a license to practice, can still be intimidated by the heavy responsibility of teaching the generation who are just behind them in their education as doctors. Dr. Fulco, a hospitalist in internal medicine, describes how he learned to manage his own expectations for the teaching role, and the influence of his former teachers in helping him to shape a philosophy of practice as a teacher:

As a young attending, I would sometimes struggle in my teaching role. I didn't feel like I had the experience or expertise to teach a talented group of residents who were not much younger than I was. But I learned I didn't have to be a content expert and that we could learn content together. It's led me to develop a more informal, collaborative teaching style when I'm teaching on inpatient ward services. I recognize that my learners all bring prior knowledge and I view my role as trying to tease out that knowledge and build on what they already know. Working with learners at differing levels of experience, I often find myself acting as a facilitator, guiding the least experienced to build knowledge by learning from those more experienced. I'm comfortable with power being diffused and truly respect my learner's thoughts. I've been incredibly fortunate to have had a number of amazing teachers who influenced not only my decision to go into academic medicine, but also to play a significant role in my philosophy of teaching and my teaching style.

Learners also provide attending physicians in an academic medical center with the motivation to continue to stay on top of their professional knowledge and skills. Fulco describes the motivation he gains from the teaching role, realizing that he has the potential to influence students and residents, as well as benefit personally from his interactions with them. The reciprocity inherent in developmental relationships first articulated by Kram (1985) has since been confirmed by other scholars as a significant reason for mentoring in organizations (Kram & Ragins, 2007; Lankau & Scandura, 2007). In this example, Fulco explains how he benefits and why he sees this as a unique aspect of his practice as a physician in academic medicine:

While graduating from the combined Internal Medicine/Pediatrics residency, there was a time I thought I would enter community practice. Providing direct patient care is incredibly meaningful and rewarding. *But I found sharing the process with learners made me even more mindful of the importance of patient interactions*... without learners you can get caught up in the chaos and pace of clinical practice ... If I were in private practice, I fear there would be little motivation for me to keep my clinical skills as sharp as possible. I may not remain as up to date or aware of the latest literature in the rapidly changing practice of medicine. Working with students allows me to share my enthusiasm in caring for the hospitalized patient. But probably the main reason I chose to go into academic medicine is that I truly love working with students to share my love of learning and passion for patient care. Learners can provide such great energy in the clinical setting—they really push me to keep learning and literally make me a better clinician.

The mutuality inherent in developmental relationships is one reason for the decision to teach; the desire to give back is another. Erikson's (1959, 1980) early work on developmental stages described the generativity that occurs in midlife for those who find fulfillment in giving back in ways that benefit the younger generation and society. For those who teach in academic medicine, generativity is a strong and rewarding aspect of investing in mentoring and role modeling within the teaching role (Humphrey, 2010).

Developing the Next Generation of Doctors

Dr. Pierce describes the yearning that a physician has to pass on his expertise, and the pride and joy of being able to do so, likening it to the parenting role, a theme Kram (1985) identified in the early research on developmental relationships.

For me, encouraging the development of students is like a father teaching his child to ride a bicycle. There are often insecurities in pedaling without training wheels and skinned knees resulting from a crash on the road. But when the child takes off riding his bike down the street for the first time, there is no greater joy than seeing the expression of pride and accomplishment. *In teaching students or residents, I have a yearning to give what I possess to the learner.* In a recent abdominal surgery, the chief resident was perplexed because the normal anatomy was distorted and a mass was firmly affixed to the left side of the belly. The resident's eyes looked bewildered as she explained her frustration contemplating her next move. "Was she inadequate and undertrained, reaching an insurmountable surgical impossibility?" I wondered. I scrubbed for the surgery and began discussing the anatomy that we could see. She understood the principles and had practiced her surgical skills, but was blocked from further progress. With a few minutes of reassurance, encouragement, and guidance, she resumed operating. She was initially tentative then gained greater confidence as she dissected the tumor from the pelvic wall. After the mass was excised and the surgery complete, I saw again the smile and countenance of a child who had ridden her bike for the first time. *"I knew I could do that. Thanks for the help!"*

Traditionally, mentoring relationships, particularly dyadic ones involving a more senior mentor and a junior learner, contain aspects of the parent–child dynamic described in Dr. Pierce's surgical encounter. Kram (1985) found that relationships were developmental when they were mutually beneficial, not a one-way giving or receiving. This mutuality has been further refined in the Stone Center's work in developing the relational-cultural theory of mentoring (Fletcher & Ragins, 2007). In Pierce's example, both individuals found fulfillment in their roles as teacher and learner: the trainee expressed pride and a sense of accomplishment upon successfully completing a difficult surgery, and the mentor expressed his joy at her being able to do so. Kram's (1985) research indicated that mentor and mentee would often liken their relationship to a significant familial one from earlier years in which "psychological mechanisms, shaped by earlier life experiences, give a particular importance, character, and potency to a developmental relationship" (p. 69). In this way, the generativity associated with developing the skills and knowledge of a young doctor resembles the care of the parent for the child, wanting her to develop into a fully competent surgeon. Similarly, Dr. Fulco, a hospitalist in internal medicine, expresses the desire to mentor the next generation of doctors as rewarding because it contributes to the development of future health care providers:

> The mentoring relationships that develop in academic medicine are so rewarding. Seeing students and residents grow over time—from medical school through residency and sometimes [becoming] faculty is an incredibly gratifying feeling. Like many teachers, my hope is that in some way I may be making the world a better place by teaching the next generation of health care providers.

Learning From Negative Role Models in the Hidden Curriculum

Occasionally, the influence of role models is not positive. Negative role models have been identified as nonetheless an important aspect of learning how not to act, and how not to behave in the literature on mentoring and role modeling (Gibson, 1995; Wear et al., 2009). Within medical education, this aspect of "passing on" undesirable and unprofessional behaviors is considered to be part of the hidden curriculum, an unintended consequence of observation of poor role models within the medical education environment. Some scholars claim that the hidden curriculum, that which is not explicitly taught but is learned through informal and incidental learning encounters, overshadows much of what the formal curriculum attempts to impart, particularly when it comes to learning about professional ways of engaging with patients, families, and colleagues in the health professions. As Kenny et al. (2003) note, "role modeling remains one crucial area where standards are elusive and where repeated negative learning experiences may adversely impact the development of professionalism in medical students and residents" (p. 1203).

At least two of the physician coauthors vividly recall memorable encounters with educators who provided lessons of what not to do or how not to engage with a patient. Dr. Matherly notes that observation of role models does not end with the conclusion of a formal educational experience, but is something that continues throughout one's professional career as a method for extracting valuable lessons about how to be a more effective teacher:

> As I have moved forward in my training, I find myself looking critically at different teachers' techniques. I have watched world leaders in a subject completely fail at getting a point across because they spend too much time showing off the depths of their vast knowledge without tailoring the teaching to their audience. The end result of this is that the learner feels overwhelmed and dumb or simply in awe of the speaker without gaining any tangible knowledge. I have watched enthusiastic lecturers present their material in such a scattered manner that the audience is lost. I have learned from these experiences and used them to make myself a stronger teacher.

In an incident he still vividly remembers, Dr. Garber describes what he learned about being attuned to the needs of the learner from the powerful example of a teacher who did not seem to care. This example of negative role modeling is a memory that has stayed with Garber and he uses it to inform his own actions about how a teacher should behave. With this negative example of role modeling and personal recollection of its effects, Garber not only strives to identify with the learners' needs, but he also makes a special effort to "walk in their shoes." As a young attending physician who is relatively new to academic medicine, he uses this episode to inform a developing philosophy of practice for teaching that includes being a different kind of role model for his learners.

> While I can highlight many excellent teachers and mentors, I can also remember the teachers who were unable to connect with me as a learner and were poor teaching models. My science lab instructor made an impact on me for all the wrong reasons. While chemistry was not the most thrilling of topics to teach, he did not seem to care about us as learners. He would often explain complex topics too quickly, flashing slides faster than anyone could read or take notes, and he would not entertain questions during the lecture or at the end of class. As learners, we tried to adapt to his teaching style, a seemingly impossible task that led many of us to bring voice recorders to class in order to listen to the lecture again later at our own pace. It was extremely challenging and frustrating. I felt discouraged and as though I was set up to fail, not succeed. *I will never forget this experience, which is the antithesis of what I try to do in creating a teaching style and learning environment.* While I may be a relatively new teacher, I feel as though I have a fresh perspective on what works best in

these clinical settings and what pitfalls, difficult topics, and issues my fellow medical students and residents will struggle with during their training. I feel as though I can put myself in my learners' shoes, whether it is their first week of medical school or their last few days of residency.

The ability to empathize with learners is significant within the psychosocial functions of a developmental relationship. Guillemin and Gillam (2015) describe the emotionally laden environment of clinical care as taking a special toll on healthcare providers, as well as their patients. Learning to deal with the emotional content of clinical practice is an important aspect of developing a professional identity that involves influencing trainees, and being influenced by them, as well.

Influencing and Being Influenced as a Learner

This desire to influence doctors-in-training by becoming a physician-educator did not emerge as a fully fleshed out idea for many chapter co-authors when they first began their medical careers. It was, instead, part of their own trajectory of growth as a medical professional that emerged through the influence of teachers as role models and mentors. The reasons for this early lack of identification with the teaching role were diverse: not envisioning themselves as the "expert" educator, or not wanting to relinquish the personal contact with patients by sharing the role of physician with trainees. Dr. Hemrajani, an internist, describes her initial reluctance to imagine a career as a medical educator and the influence of a role model who taught her what it truly meant to care for patients:

> On entering medical school, my major focus was to become a physician to care directly for patients each and every day; I did not envision teaching students or residents as a part of my future endeavors. At the time, I would have thought of that learner as a distancing measure between my patients and me. The medical school I attended was a brand new school . . . It was in this setting that my eyes were opened to the value of a good teacher because of the way my teachers inspired and molded me into the physician I wanted to be. They didn't just teach me history or physical exam skills; they taught me about the art of medicine. One of my Family Medicine preceptors taught me what it meant to care for patients like friends. Almost anyone can teach a simple fact that a learner will remember right after being told it, but only some teachers can create a valuable connection between what they are trying to teach and the learner's experience to create a lasting effect.

Occasionally, it is the role modeling of physician parents who influence the desire to teach in academic medicine. "Legacy" physicians are those who enter their training as the sons and daughters of physicians. Within the medical profession, following in the footsteps of mom or dad is not uncommon. Medically-trained parents can have enormous influence on career decisions of their children; they can also be inspiring teachers as well as larger-than-life role models and mentors. Dr. Lee recalls the memory of his father as a teacher and the influence he had on him:

> My father was often known for using the phrase, "I don't know, what you think?" He would use this phrase with surgical residents and students. Of course, he would already know the answer, but would use this to develop thought and reasoning skills within his learners. He would also use this with me and my sister, and we would groan and ask him to just tell us the answer. He was well known for constantly asking questions of the residents and would tell us that this was his Socratic method. To this day, his former trainees tell me how much my father's teaching influenced them and how much they appreciated his method of teaching. I think my parents' appreciation for academics and teaching stuck with me as I was considering my career, as well.

When faced with a parent who was well-known for his pioneering work as a transplant surgeon, the experiences others had under the influence of his father as a teacher contributed to Dr. Lee's sense of his father as a role model:

> One of the comments I hear about my father as a teacher that sticks with me is how he taught. When I was a [medical] student, the surgeons were famous for being hard-nosed, and, at times, downright mean and intimidating. They would "pimp" [an aggressive form of incessant questioning] you endlessly, and would even challenge each other ruthlessly in their Death and Complications conference. One of the comments that I have often heard about my father, which has greatly influenced me, is that he was never rude or condescending toward students or residents. He was famous for keeping his cool and calmly and quietly asking questions and encouraging his learners to reason through answers. Once they had answered, he would praise what was correct and quietly encourage his learners to try again if they were incorrect. One of his former students told me that my father had a quiet confidence that commanded the respect of his students and peers. He did not need to rant or rave or use gimmicks to teach. I hope to one day achieve that same sort of quiet confidence that allows me to engage my learners and also instill in them the same quiet confidence about what they have learned.

The relationship with a father can also be a little daunting for the physician-educator who aspires to become like him. Dr. Lee expresses both awe and appreciation for the many role models in his life, including the influence of his physician parents. Significantly, what he extracts from these relationships is the desire to not ever let his learners down, but to be responsible to them as learners.

I am often intimidated by the thought that I need to measure up to the expectations of my learners. I sometimes wonder if my teachers over the years had that same sense of intimidation or intense feeling of responsibility. I have developed an increasingly strong feeling of not wanting to let my students down. I want them to have a meaningful experience that helps them transform themselves. When I look back at my most valued teachers, including my parents, I think that they had these feelings and a strong sense of responsibility towards their learners.

APPRECIATING MENTORS AND ROLE MODELS: THE SUM OF MY LEARNING

These illustrations of mentoring and role modeling are descriptions from the lived experiences of physician-educators, all of whom have chosen to pursue their medical careers in a teaching hospital. They were asked to write a paper as part of a professional development course about the experiences that contributed to career decisions to teach in academic medicine. For many of them, what emerged was a description of the major, and life-changing, influence of role models and mentors on their own career choices, as well as their own desires to pass on what they had received during their medical education.

While the function of role modeling is well-documented in the medical education literature (Cruess et al., 2015; Cruess, Cruess, & Steinert, 2008; Kenny et al., 2003; Maudsley, 2001; Passi et al., 2013; Wright et al., 1998), role modeling, as a particular psychosocial element within developmental relationships, is an underrepresented and under-researched concept within the extensive body of research and practice on mentoring across disciplines and areas of practice (Lankau & Scandura, 2007). For physicians, however, role modeling appears to be an essential experience that enables them to become doctors. It involves extracting skills, knowledge, attitudes, values, and ethical beliefs through the extensive apprenticeship of clinical training. More importantly, it results in the formation of a professional identity that is transmitted from generation to generation about what it means to be a physician in our society (Goldie, 2012; Wald, 2015). For those who are exemplars and represent the noble qualities associated with this profession, this identity embraces selfless care for patients and the mantra to do no harm. Dr. Brock describes the cumulative effect of a lifetime of influential role models and mentors, reflecting on their significance for her development as a person, as well as a teacher and a surgeon.

What if Margaret Brock hadn't instilled in me in early life the value of teaching? What if Wilma Bowie hadn't made mathematical problem solving engaging and fun? What if Gwen McCall hadn't made the words of Shakespeare and

Dickens come alive for us by having us read and perform them, and discover their meaning? What if Tom Nassar (intimidating though he was) hadn't made us discover how atoms and molecules work and how they become the substance of all things? What if Steve Cohen hadn't shown me how to stop hemorrhage in a pelvis, and then made sure that I could do it independently? What if my resident hadn't put a laparoscopic instrument through a transverse colon, causing an injury that made crystal clear the moral imperative for our department that we ensure the skills mastery of our trainees prior to operating room experience? We are the sum of our experiences, and I am in no small measure the sum of what I learned from the great teachers in my life. I teach because it is so gratifying to have a similar place in the lives of my students . . . because it is a necessary part of carrying on the legacy of my profession.

AUTHORS' NOTE

This chapter originally appeared as The Influence of Mentors and Role Models on Teaching and Learning in Academic Medicine in *Mentoring in Formal and Informal Contexts* (2016), edited by Kathy Peno, Elaine M. Silva Mangiante, and Rita A. Kenahan, published by Information Age Publishing.

REFERENCES

Bandura, A. (1986). *Social foundations of thought and action: A social cognitive theory.* Englewood Cliffs, NJ: Prentice Hall.

Bell, A. P. (1970). Role modelship and interaction in adolescence and young adulthood. *Developmental Psychology, 2*(1), 123–128.

Cruess, R. L., Cruess, S. R., Boudreau, D., Snell, L., & Steinert, Y. (2015). A schematic representation of the professional identity formation and socialization of medical students and residents: A guide for medical educators. *Academic Medicine, 90*(6), 718–724. https://doi.org/10.1097/ACM.0000000000000700

Cruess, S. R., Cruess, R. L., & Steinert, Y. (2008). Role modelling—Making the most of a powerful teaching strategy. *British Medical Journal, 336,* 718–721. https://doi.org/10.1136/bmj.39503.757847.BE

Erikson, E. H. (1959/1980). *Identity and the life cycle.* New York, NY: Norton.

Fletcher, J. K. (1996). A relational approach to the protean worker. In D. T. Hall & Associates (Eds.), *The career is dead—long live the career: A relational approach to careers* (pp. 105–131). San Francisco, CA: Jossey-Bass.

Fletcher, J. K., & Ragins, B. R. (2007). Stone Center Relational Cultural Theory: A window on relational mentoring. In B. R. Ragins & K. E. Kram (Eds.), *The handbook of mentoring at work: Theory, research, and practice* (pp. 373–399). Thousand Oaks, CA: SAGE.

Gibson, D. E. (1995). *Individual idols, organizational ideals: Role models in organizations.* Available from ProQuest Dissertations & Theses Global. (Order No. 9601397)

Gibson, D. E., & Cordova, D. L. (1999). Women's and men's role models: The importance of exemplars. In A. J. Murrell, F. J. Crosby, & R. J. Ely (Eds.), *Mentoring dilemmas: Developmental relationships within multicultural organizations* (pp. 121–141). Mahwah, NJ: Erlbaum.

Goldie, J. (2012). The formation of professional identity in medical students: Considerations for educators. *Medical Teacher, 34*(9), e641–e648. https://doi.org/10.3 109/0142159X.2012.687476

Guillemin, M., & Gillam, L. (2015). Emotions, narratives, and ethical mindfulness. *Academic Medicine, 90*(6), 726–731.

Hafferty, F. W. (1998). Beyond curriculum reform: Confronting medicine's hidden curriculum. *Academic Medicine, 73*(4), 403–407.

Hafferty, F. W., & Franks, R. (1994). The hidden curriculum, ethics teaching, and the structure of medical education. *Academic Medicine, 69*(11), 861–871.

Heflin, M. T., Pinheiro, S., Kaminetzky, C. P., & McNeill D. (2009). 'So you want to be a clinician-educator...': Designing a clinician-educator curriculum for internal medicine residents. *Medical Teacher, 31*(6), e233–e240.

Holden, M. D., Buck, E., Luk, J., Ambriz, F., Boisaubin, E. V., Clark, M. A.,...Dalrymple, J. L. (2015, June). Professional identity formation: Creating a longitudinal framework through TIME (Transformation in Medical Education). *Academic Medicine, 90*(6), 761–767.

Humphrey, H. J. (2010). Fundamentals of mentoring and professional development. In H. J. Humphrey (Ed.), *Mentoring in academic medicine* (pp. 35–50). Chicago, IL: American College of Physicians.

Jochemsen-van der Leeuw, H. G. A., van Dijk, N., van Etten-Jamaludin, F. S., & Wieringa-de Waard, M. (2013). The attributes of the clinical trainer as role model: A systemic review of the literature. *Academic Medicine, 88*(1), 26–34.

Kelman, H. C. (1961). Processes of opinion change. *Public Opinion Quarterly, 25,* 57–78.

Kenny, N. P., Mann, K. V., & MacLeod, H. (2003). Role modeling in physicians' professional formation: Reconsidering an essential but untapped educational strategy. *Academic Medicine, 78*(12), 1203–1210.

Kenny, N. P., Mann, K. V., Wrixon, W., MacLeod, H., & Coles, C. (2002, August). *See one, do one, teach one: Role models and the CanMEDS Competencies.* Paper presented at the Association for Medical Education in Europe (AIMEE) Conference, Lisbon, Portugal.

Kohlberg, L. (1963). Moral development and identification. In H. W. Stevenson (Ed.), *Child psychology: The sixty-second yearbook of the national society for the study of education* (Part I; pp. 277–332). Chicago, IL: University of Chicago Press.

Kram, K. E. (1985). *Mentoring at work: Developmental relationships in organizational life* (2nd ed). Landam, MD: University Press of America.

Kram, K. E., & Hall, D. T. (1996). Mentoring in the context of diversity and turbulence. In E. E. Kossek & S. A. Lobel (Eds.), *Managing diversity: Human resource strategies for transforming the workplace* (pp. 108–136). Cambridge, MA: Blackwell Business.

Kram, K. E., & Ragins, B. R. (2007). The landscape of mentoring in the 21st century. In B. R. Ragins & K. E. Kram (Eds.), *The handbook of mentoring at work: Theory, research, and practice* (pp. 659–692). Thousand Oaks, CA: SAGE.

Lankau, M. J., & Scandura, T. A. (2007). Mentoring as a forum for personal learning in organizations. In B. R. Ragins & K. E. Kram (Eds.), *The handbook of mentoring at work: Theory, research, and practice* (pp. 95–122). Thousand Oaks, CA: SAGE.

Lave, J., & Wenger. E. (1991). *Situated learning: Legitimate peripheral participation.* Cambridge, England: Cambridge University Press.

Maudsley, R. F. (2001). Role models and the learning environment: Essential elements in effective medical education. *Academic Medicine, 76*(5), 432–434.

McCauley, C. D., & Douglas, C. A. (1998). Developmental relationships. In D. D. McCauley, R. S. Moxley, & E. Van Velsor, E. (Eds.), *Handbook of leadership development* (pp. 160–193). Greensboro, NC: The Center for Creative Leadership.

Mirhaghi, A., Moonaghi, K., Sharafi, S., & Zeydi, A. (2015). Role modeling: A precious heritage in medical education. *Scientific Journal of the Faculty of Medicine in Nis, 32*(1), 31–42. https://doi.org/10.1515/afmnai-2015-0003

Passi, V., Johnson, S., Peile, E., Wright, S., Hafferty, F., & Johnson, N. (2013). Doctor role modelling in medical education: BEME Guide No. 27. *Medical Teacher, 35*(9), e1422–e1436.

Schor, S. M. (1997). Separate and unequal: The nature of women's and men's career-building relationships. *Business Horizons, 40*(5), 51–58.

Wald, H. S. (2015). Professional identity (trans)formation in medical education: Reflection, relationship, resilience. *Academic Medicine, 90*(6), 701–706. https://doi.org/10.1097/ACM.0000000000000731

Walen, T., & Walsh, W. (2011). Going beyond duty hours: A focus on patient safety. In *The 2011 ACGME duty hour standards: Enhancing quality of care, supervision, and resident professional development* (pp. 69–74). Chicago, IL: Accreditation Council for Graduate Medical Education.

Wear, D., Aultman, J. M., Zarconi, J., & Varley, J. D. (2009). Derogatory and cynical humour directed towards patients: Views of residents and attending doctors. *Medical Education, 43*(1), 34–41. https://doi.org/10.1111/j.1365-2923.2008.03171.x

Whitman, N. A., & Schwenk, T. L. (1987). *The physician as teacher.* Salt Lake City, UT: Whitman Associates.

Wright, S., Wong, A., & Newell, C. (1997). The impact of role models on medical students. *Journal of General Internal Medicine, 12*(1), 53–56.

Wright, S. M., Kern, D. E., Kolodner, K., Howard, D. M., & Brancati, F. L. (1998). Attributes of excellent attending-physician role models. *The New England Journal of Medicine, 339*(27), 1986–1993.

CHAPTER 7

VOLUNTEERISM WITH VULNERABLE POPULATIONS

A Catalyst for Professional Identity Formation

Christopher Keith Brown, Jr.
Virginia Commonwealth University School of Medicine

ABSTRACT

Professional identity formation is a socialization process in which medical students begin to see themselves as physicians. Volunteerism can play a critical role in how students identify as physicians through positive experiences within the hidden curriculum. In particular, volunteerism with vulnerable populations after a service learning experience can serve as a catalyst to professional identity formation that is largely transformative in nature. A student volunteer may even begin to incorporate these newfound ideals of service to those most vulnerable in society into future career plans. This chapter will discuss my personal experience in volunteering with members of the home-

Transformative Learning in Healthcare and Helping Professions Education, pages 129–151

less population and the critical educational experiences that have led me to embrace service to the underserved.

Homelessness. Poverty. High school dropout. Drug dealer. These words alone carry with them a weight that can evoke a wide range of emotions. The judgments they imply can vary from a sense of charity to pity or even fear. Some people, whether through experience or prejudice, may even use "homeless" as the single identifier of a person and forget that homelessness is something that a person experiences which may or may not be permanent. Those who view homelessness in this way may never come into contact with anyone living in public housing; certainly, they may be among the many who never once step foot in a public housing unit themselves. Their only exposure to vulnerable populations may be limited to a news story of a theft, murder, or drug deal that ended in violence. For others, homelessness can be a first-hand experience, a constant threat, or even a day-to-day reality of life. The housing unit directly next door to where drug use and other illegal activities occur may be the only semblance of safety and security for a young child growing up in a single parent home.

I would describe my exposure to individuals from medically underserved populations, those experiencing homelessness and living in poverty, as very limited until moving to Richmond, Virginia 3 years before I began medical school. My volunteer experience at a free clinic that serves Richmond's medically underserved population has nurtured what I now consider a calling to address health inequities and disparities faced by this population. Having never been homeless, my only notion of what homelessness meant was much more of an internal battle of etiquette while walking past a person sitting on the street rather than a true interaction at all. "Do I have cash? Is giving cash even appropriate? Am I in the wrong if this person uses the money for alcohol or drugs? Should I just go to get food from a store for the homeless person instead?" It was not until I volunteered at the local free clinic prior to medical school that I had my initial meaningful interaction with those experiencing homelessness or others whose choices included not going to the doctor's office when needed because they would miss out on wages to provide for a family.

In this role of patient advocate, I had the opportunity to hear the stories and challenges faced by those who came to the clinic. During the time I was there, the clinic was nearing capacity and a financial screening process was in place so that only eight new individuals were able to become patients each week. As part of the screening process, potential patients had to complete a packet of background information that included providing their last six pay stubs. With an overwhelming number of people applying, many were turned away multiple times. I saw the personal toll this can take when, often, they were taking precious time off from work to apply to qualify. Without work there was no pay, and with no pay, these low-income families put themselves in further financial risk. It was challenging to watch and participate in this process because the need for medical care within the underserved population is so immense, and yet we, as a clinic, were so limited in our capacity to respond.

One man in particular who was experiencing homelessness was in the process of organizing his information to apply to be a patient at the free clinic. When I met with him, he shared his story of being homeless, including the difficulties of managing medications while living on the streets, and the frustrations he felt trying to coordinate his application and subsequent care. This man's venting session marked the beginning of my developmental journey as a future physician whose plans now include caring for the underserved. It is a journey I am still on, although, now, much more intentionally. This man unknowingly challenged me to grasp the magnitude of factors that influence one's health. I began to discover the interconnectedness of a person's health and the overall health of a community. After hearing his story, I began to question how medical care is delivered, the shortcomings of medicine, and my future role as a physician.

While attending graduate school in Norfolk, Virginia, and then medical school at Virginia Commonwealth University (VCU) School of Medicine in Richmond, I sought out opportunities to volunteer with the homeless community as a student coordinator for two different local shelter programs. With these experiences, I have talked with people who are homeless about their accessibility to, and their perceptions of, healthcare. The connection I developed with the homeless community influenced my decision to join the International, Inner City, Rural Preceptorship (I2CRP) program at VCU. This program supplements the traditional medical education curriculum by focusing on topics surrounding medically underserved populations and the delivery of healthcare. Through this program, I have learned about health inequities and the multifaceted, exacerbating factors that contribute to poor health outcomes, particularly those that occur for people who live in the East End of Richmond. All cities have sub-communities with high concentrations of poverty that are often characterized by a drastically different life expectancy for their residents when compared to neighborhoods only a few miles away. Like many cities, this is the situation in Richmond, Virginia where the concentrated poverty of the East End paints a remarkably different picture of life than in other communities within the greater Richmond area.

I have learned many things since volunteering at the clinic, but, most importantly, I learned that homeless people are really just people experiencing homelessness. Unemployed people living in poverty are faced with many factors that contribute to their situation and are in need of further support to succeed. Unfortunately, homelessness is a major risk factor for many disease states. This chapter will focus on how volunteerism with individuals who are medically underserved can serve as a catalyst for the formation of professional identity for a physician during training. In it, I will share characteristics of vulnerable populations and, in particular, characteristics of people who live in the East End of Richmond, a community in close proximity to my school. I will address my own evolving sense of professional identity and the transformative learning that I have experienced in working with members of these medically underserved communities.

A BRIEF LITERATURE
REVIEW ON VULNERABLE POPULATIONS

As defined by Aday (2001), vulnerable populations are people who are at risk of poor psychological, physical, or social health. The demographics that fit Aday's definition of vulnerability include people with mental illness or chronic disease, people with a history of substance abuse or suicidality, and people who have experienced homelessness or have refugee status. Ultimately, Aday's definition of vulnerable populations also describes people facing economic hardship and individuals who are also uninsured. Bethell, Fiorillo, Knickman, and Lansky (2002) describe the heightened contribution of social factors faced by vulnerable populations and the lack of opportunities for education. Sadly, more recent research indicates that little has changed in the composition of those considered most vulnerable in our society (Henry, Watt, Rosenthal, Shivji, & Abt Associates, 2017; Montgomery, Szymkowiak, Marcus, Howard, & Culhane, 2016; Shi & Stevens, 2010). Members of vulnerable populations also face challenges obtaining and securing long-term medical follow-up care. Scholars have found that within the homeless population, the effects of multiple social and economic factors result in significantly poorer health outcomes than those in the general population (Barrow, Herman, Córdova, & Struening, 1999; Henry et al., 2017; Montgomery et al., 2016; Shi & Stevens, 2010).

Homelessness

On a typical night in the United States, more than 553,000 people are without shelter due to short-term or long-term homelessness (Henry et al., 2017). Although homelessness is more often a temporary condition rather than a chronic long-term state, the mortality rate faced by urban homeless individuals has been found to be approximately 10 times that of the general population (Roncarati et al., 2018). A status of homelessness compounds the effects of substance abuse, mental illness, and other health conditions to result in a disproportionate mortality rate and burden of disease when compared to that of the general population (Barrow et al., 1999; Morrison, 2009; Feodor Nilsson, Laursen, Hjorthøj, & Nordentoft, 2018). A study conducted by the United States Conference of Mayors (2007) reported that approximately 37% of people who are homeless have substance use disorders. Whether substance abuse was a consequence of or a contributing factor to homelessness, there is still an emerging health issue that results.

Maslow's Hierarchy of Needs and the Homeless Population

Maslow's (1970) seminal theory of human development is based on motivations. The theory suggests that basic needs, such as food, water, shelter, and security must be secured prior to addressing the higher needs that humans have, such as self-esteem, love, and a sense of belonging. Considering Maslow's theory, individuals facing homelessness are more likely to be focused on securing food, water, and shelter than achieving higher order needs like self-esteem. People experiencing homelessness are faced with many potential barriers to receiving healthcare that contribute to the health disparities they face. Food insecurity is a significant barrier for many and something that has been found to delay the regular use of healthcare resources while leading to increases in acute care utilization and hospitalization (Baggett et al., 2011; Kushel, Gupta, Gee, & Haas, 2006). Mental health conditions, lack of transportation, language and literacy barriers, absence of consistent contact information, and an inability to provide required documentation are all barriers to successful Medicaid enrollment that are commonly experienced by people who are homeless (DiPietro, Knopf, Artiga, & Arguello, 2012).

Keeping Maslow's (1970) hierarchy of needs in mind, there are inherent basic human needs that are undercut by being homeless in today's society. For example, lack of rest from concerns about personal security while living on the streets is a common concern. These realities of homelessness directly undermine basic needs of safety and psychological well-being. The progression from basic needs to self-fulfillment may never be fully realized due to the barriers associated with homelessness.

Health of Vulnerable Populations

Aday (2001) reports that vulnerable populations have compound healthcare needs that require extensive resources because their health issues are often serious or life-threatening. This is illustrated by the positive association between income and life expectancy (Braveman & Egerter, 2008). People lacking health insurance have been found to be less likely to engage in any medical care, they have lower rates of follow-up care, and they also fill fewer prescriptions (Hadley, 2007). Minority groups self-report lower health status and lower rates of health insurance participation, as well as higher cost barriers to access healthcare (Zimmerman et al., 2016). Shi and Stevens's (2010) study found a significant relationship between uninsured status and the delay or absence of engaging healthcare, which, while not surprising, does not bode well for those who are considered most vulnerable in our society.

Unfortunately, the issue of health disparities faced by many of America's vulnerable populations is not isolated to one or two causes, but, instead, is the result of multiple factors that compound the problem. These include uninsured status in addition to poor educational attainment, low-income households, and unsafe living environments, which all play a role in poor health outcomes (Jiang, Ekono, & Skinner, 2016; Shi & Stevens, 2010; Zimmerman et al., 2016). Heron and colleagues (2009) found that when adults do not obtain a high school diploma, they have an age-adjusted death rate that is more than two and a half times higher than that of individuals who have college educations. Disparities in education are also connected to risky health behaviors that people engage in prior to death. The Centers for Disease Control (2004) reports that the less formal education a person has, the more likely that person is to smoke cigarettes, an unhealthy behavior that contributes to many disease states. While lack of education is associated with engaging in riskier behaviors, Zimmerman and her colleagues (2016) found that obtaining additional education services as a path to higher income can influence health status and overall access to care.

Low-income families, defined as those living at 200% of the federal poverty level, and families living at the poverty level have an increased exposure to factors that increase the risk of poor health outcomes (American Psychological Association, 2018; Jiang et al., 2016). Poverty experienced during childhood negatively influences a child's cognitive and behavioral development (Duncan, Brooks-Gunn, & Klebanov, 1994). Urban environments with high concentrations of poverty increase the challenge of healthcare delivery because many viable options for living a healthy life are not possible. In an urban landscape, a food desert is defined as a community where at least 500 people or 33% of the population live more than a mile from a grocery store (American Nutrition Association, 2011). The effect of food deserts on health is compounded by poverty which increases access issues to grocery stores outside of the community. In addition, diets that are low in fresh produce have been linked to diabetes, obesity, hypertension, and heart disease (United States Department of Agriculture, 2016). When considering the interconnectedness of these factors, it is easy to appreciate the complexities that underlie health disparities among America's vulnerable populations. Consider a person who lives in an unsafe environment who is isolated within a food desert and without regular transportation. The chance that person will feel comfortable pursuing outdoor exercise or having access to healthy foods is greatly diminished as a consequence of his or her lived environment, ultimately resulting in poor health outcomes, the potential for chronic disease, and diminished quality of life.

In addition, exposure to violence has been documented as a cause of psychological distress for caregivers as well as a significant factor in the internalizing and externalizing behaviors of distress in children (Kaslow et al., 2003). Adverse childhood experiences including abuse, neglect, exposure to mental illness, a caregiver's addiction or imprisonment among caregivers, as well as growing up in a single-parent household have been linked to persistent chronic diseases that onset in adulthood (Felitti et al., 1998). According to Felitti and colleagues, these chronic diseases include substance abuse, depression, and suicidality, in addition to heart disease, cancer, and chronic lung and liver disease. The Institute of Medicine (2013) has linked limited access to healthcare, poor health behaviors, and the socioeconomic aspects of poverty, income inequality, and low social mobility to lower life expectancies. Someone who never graduated from high school, is in poverty, and resides in an urban environment that has elevated levels of crime and inaccessibility to healthy food options faces a disproportionate number of health risk factors. This constellation of risk factors is part of the lived experience of members of vulnerable populations including the homeless population and many who live in the East End of the City of Richmond (Zimmerman et al., 2016).

A Contrasting View of the East End of Richmond

Richmond, Virginia is a city rich with history and economic opportunity for most of its residents. Richmond is the capital of Virginia, and is home to the corporate headquarters of 10 Fortune 500 companies as well as one of the 12, regional Federal Reserve Banks in the United States. The city boasts a high-rise downtown skyline of financial institutions, legal firms, and investment firms, with numerous parks and restaurants in the vicinity. Two well-respected universities and several large community colleges claim Richmond as home, and the greater metropolitan area abounds with historical sites, museums, and a wide variety of cultural and sports events (All About Richmond, n.d.).

Richmond's modern history has mirrored the unique and volatile history of the United States South. The Civil War, Jim Crow, and Civil Rights era set the stage for much of the racial, socioeconomic, and geographic landscape within Richmond City today. Current data show that the greater Richmond metropolitan area is home to 1.27 million people with an average household income of approximately $63,000 and a poverty rate of 11.9% (Data USA, 2018). Within the much smaller boundaries of Richmond City, however, pockets of poverty, including those seen in the East End of Richmond, have historical roots that contribute to the strikingly different median household income of approximately $41,000, with a poverty rate of 25.4% (Data USA, 2018).

Richmond, Virginia is home to the VCU Health System, which not only serves the greater Richmond area, but is also considered a safety net hospital and the only Level I trauma center serving central Virginia. A safety net hospital is defined as one that provides a significant amount of care to members of vulnerable populations, people with Medicaid or who are uninsured (Institute of Medicine, 2000). Virginia Commonwealth University, a school of more than 31,000 students, is integrated throughout the city with its academic and health sciences campuses and has invested in Richmond with undergraduate, graduate, and professional program facilities that have contributed to much of the revitalization of the city's downtown area. VCU's dedication to community engagement has earned the university the Carnegie Foundation's Community Engagement classification, a designation shared by only 27 other public universities with medical centers (Porter, 2018). This university has fostered my passion for addressing health inequities in my future career in medicine.

A report by the VCU Center on Society and Health (Zimmerman et al., 2016) examined the implications of health from social factors faced by the residents of Richmond City in comparison to surrounding county neighborhoods. The report details findings consistent with risk factors faced by not only the homeless population as a whole, but also residents of the East End of Richmond. Strikingly, the report cites a 20-year difference in life expectancy for residents of Richmond City when compared to the surrounding metropolitan area. This life expectancy differential results from many factors relating to poverty, crime, lack of educational attainment, and poor economic opportunity for the city's residents. According to Zimmerman and her colleagues, more than a third of Richmond City's African American adult residents have not completed high school, while 58.7% do not have education beyond high school. These scholars also state that the City of Richmond has the highest violent crime rate reported among large Virginia cities and a higher crime rate when compared to comparable cities in the United States, as well as a nonviolent crime rate that is twice the nonviolent crime rate in the state of Virginia. It is in this milieu of social and economic factors that extreme disparities in health and well-being exist for many of the City's residents.

PROFESSIONAL IDENTITY FORMATION
FOR PHYSICIANS IN TRAINING

Professional identity formation, also known as professional identity development in medical education, is a dynamic socialization process that transforms a lay person into a competent, humanistic physician with a unique identity and set of core values (Goldie, 2012; Holden et al., 2015; Wald, 2015; Wald et al., 2015). This process is fostered by reflection on moral subject matter, both privately and through structured experiences within the medical education curriculum (Phillips, Fawn, & Hayes, 2002). In an effort to create a "normative definition" of professionalism in medicine, Swick (2000) developed a list of behaviors that encompass professionalism, behaviors that reinforce the importance of having a moral code and commitment to the profession. Among them are the ideals of maintaining high ethical standards, being accountable in interactions with patients, and having core values of honesty, integrity, compassion, altruism, respect, and trustworthiness.

Although multiple definitions of professionalism exist, each with slightly refined value sets, Inui (2003) emphasizes the importance of educators who commit to role modeling that occurs during daily events to create a positive impact on the student. Inui believed that the professional identity formation that occurs through experiences within medical education is deeply rooted in the culture of medicine in which emphasis on patient interests over self-interest becomes an ingrained way of thinking and acting. However, Holden and his colleagues (2012) found that sometimes the formal curriculum on professionalism is not matched by lived experiences in which students apply principles of professionalism in the clinical setting. Hafferty (1998) described this as the "hidden curriculum" of medical education in which less professional behaviors are observed and tacitly absorbed by students, undermining the ideals of an altruistic professional identity. Both the workplace and the social environments in which a student learns can strongly influence a medical student's development of professional behaviors (van der Zwet et al., 2011), a process that continues beyond formal education.

Applying to medical school often marks the beginning of this socialization by establishing contact with physicians through shadowing experiences; these provide the medical school applicant with a broader picture of what a career in medicine will be like. Volunteer experiences offer insight into specific issues that are present within the community and can help shape the future physician's interests and aspirations. The applicant, through this premedical school socialization process, begins to gain a deeper understanding of the expectations for physicians in society.

Acceptance into medical school then marks the beginning of a transformative process in which students become physicians through social interactions with other students, faculty, physicians, and patients, all of whom contribute to shape professional identity outside of the formal curriculum (van Mook et al., 2009). Social interactions can be most important through role modeling since these relationships have the potential to form student attitudes within the profession (Lublin, 1992). Through relationships and hands-on training, learners repeat behaviors that they witness; these have a powerful influence on their future as physicians. Role modeling relationships form a large part of the hidden curriculum and hold potential to be both positive and negative learning experiences (Hafferty, 1998; Wilkinson et al., 2006). Goldie (2012) found that professional identity formation is influenced more by these aspects of the informal curriculum than the formal curriculum.

Throughout the medical school experience, students can feel a loss of humanity as they gain professional skills (Rabow, Evans, & Remen, 2013), leading Hojat et al. (2009) to assert that "the devil is in the third year" in the decline of medical student empathy (p. 1182). Rabow and colleagues' (2013) study of third-year trainee written reflections indicated that 50% of them focused on power-hierarchy issues within medical training and 30% focused on the dehumanization of the patient. These negative experiences can be detrimental to student learners' professional identity formation because of the power of their influence within the hidden curriculum. Students participating in Rabow et al.'s study reported that in an effort to be seen as professional, they felt that they had to separate themselves from their creativity and spirituality. The researchers interpreted this as the repression of key features of student identities that help to explain depression and negative outlooks that can develop during training. Burnout, a symptom of emotional exhaustion and depersonalization, and signs of depression have been identified in over half of U.S. medical students at a substantially higher rate than their peers who are not in medical training (Dyrbye, Thomas, & Shanafelt, 2006; IsHak et al., 2013; West, Shanafelt, & Kolars, 2011).

Although there are alarming rates of depression and burnout in the medical student population, only a third of students are likely to pursue care for their symptoms, according to Dyrbye and colleagues (2015). This lack of self-care is ultimately linked to higher rates of depression, less desire to work with medically-underserved populations, and decreased empathy and unprofessional behavior that could lead to increased malpractice and medical errors (Dyrbye et al., 2010; Dyrbye et al., 2014; Shanafelt, Bradley, Wipf, & Back, 2002; Thomas et al., 2007). Alternatively, positive experiences and role modeling have shown potential to mitigate the burnout that may stem from negative experiences within the hidden curriculum (Baker & Sen, 2016). Irby, Cooke, & O'Brien (2010) advocate for a restructuring of medical education to support professional identity formation through a more positive environment, providing support for Goldie's (2012) assertion that volunteerism connects learners with the humanistic aspects of medicine to promote empathy and self-identification with the profession.

Medical students are often exposed to patients with whom they lack experience, particularly members of vulnerable populations, including those experiencing homelessness. In learning to provide proper care for patients, the opportunity exists to understand the significant role of social determinants of health that are much more pronounced within vulnerable populations. If a medical student can critically reflect on his or her status in relation to the people who are among the medically underserved, and shift previously held beliefs and assumptions, transformative learning may be possible (Mezirow, 1991, 2012).

The Role of Transformative Learning in Professional Identity Formation

Transformative learning can be defined as a process that leads us to question our previously held views about ourselves and the world in which we live (Cranton, 2016; Mezirow, 1991, 2012). According to Mezirow (1991), who first proposed this theory of learning in 1978, only in adulthood are we able to revise the tacitly acquired beliefs, values, and assumptions that were assimilated uncritically from caregivers, authority figures, and formative experiences during childhood. Thus, he held that learning was a formative experience for children, but potentially transformative in adulthood through critical reflection and critical self-reflection as adults become aware of the limitations of their previously-held perspectives.

Cranton (2016), as well as Mezirow (1991), describe the nature of a disorienting experience as the point at which preconceived notions are challenged by experience or newly gained awareness of a situation. Cranton (2016) expresses the need for self-reflection and self-determination as critical to transformative learning so that we might become free of distorted views about ourselves and our world (p. 11). Through critical examination of our own experiences, a learner has the opportunity to develop professionally. The process of reflecting can come in many forms, usually involves dialogue with others, and can be fostered through authentic relationships and greater awareness of context within learning (Taylor, 2009). Premise reflection requires that learners question why they hold a particular perspective, while transformation occurs when the revised perspective changes the approach to future interactions (Cranton, 2016).

Service Learning as a Pathway
to Professional Identity Formation

In an investigation of the potential for transformative learning among students engaged in service learning experiences, Hullender and colleagues (2015) found that changes in the lens through which one sees the world require time, space, and appropriate support as scaffolding. By examining students' reflective writing, these authors found that without the purposeful reflection and examination of one's own role in a situation, transformative learning may not come to full fruition. Kiely (2005), who also examined student reflections in service learning experiences but in an international context, proposed a five-stage model in which internal events within the learner's mind can result in a transformative process to create the necessary time, space, and support needed.

First, the learner must engage in what Kiely (2005) terms "contextual border crossing" (p. 9). He describes contextual border crossing as the opportunity for diverse perspectives to occur; it is the actual volunteerism experience itself in which the learner puts himself or herself in a new role and connects with a new population. What the learner makes of this experience is often determined by personal, historical, and programmatic aspects of the experience, as well as the student's own position in society as determined by race, class, gender, nationality, and other structural elements. Dissonance occurs when "much of what students see, feel, touch, hear, and participate in is new and incongruent with their frame of reference or world-view" (p. 10).

While all levels of dissonance can result in some level of reexamination, Kiely (2005) asserts that high-intensity dissonance such as witnessing extreme forms of poverty, hunger, scarcity, and disease can have a larger impact on the learner and require the time and space afterwards to process, as confirmed by Hullender et al. (2015). This high intensity dissonance cannot be reconciled through reflection or participation in service work alone, according to Kiely (2005), but remains with the learner long after returning home to influence relationships, lifestyle, and consumption habits, as well as worldview. Personalization occurs when learners connect the poverty they see within their volunteerism with the experience and motivations of real people. The chance to meet the people and hear their stories resonates with the volunteer much more than a reflexive classroom-based experience. This emotional response and personalization becomes a bridge to the population and provides the necessary context to understand the challenges they face. The learner, through critical reflection, is then able to reflect and reevaluate underlying social issues that lead to what he or she experienced. If transformation occurs, the learner ultimately develops an understanding of causes, possible solutions, and current issues affecting the service learning community.

The last crucial component of Kiely's (2005) model is when a moral obligation and attachment develops between the learner and the population with whom he or she volunteered, an attachment that calls the learner to action. Meaningful service then becomes a theme that allows students to identify volunteer experiences as transformative (Hullender et al., 2015). If a learner can develop a deeper understanding of social issues faced by a community, he or she is more likely to address social or medical disparities faced by a particular population in future work. Transformative learning, similar to professional identity formation, is dynamic and requires connection to others and relationship formation (Kiely, 2005; Taylor, 2009). Hullender et al. (2015) found that positive relationships between community partners and students can enhance the overall learning experience by encouraging the questioning of previously held assumptions in an effort to generate solutions to underlying needs. The professional development of a student becomes an opportunity to understand social issues from a first-hand perspective and critically reexamine oneself to address issues faced by that population.

The Impact of Volunteerism on My Professional Identity Formation

Following my volunteer experience at a free clinic, I pursued further volunteer experiences that connected me to the homeless in Richmond. I had achieved a level of understanding of the struggles and comorbidities within the homeless population from my learning experiences in medical school in the I2CRP program. I wanted to further understand my role as a future physician who will be treating vulnerable individuals, families, and groups. At first, while volunteering in shelter programs and clinics, I was unsure of how to act appropriately so that they perceived me as someone who saw them as individuals and not as symbols of homelessness. It was not until after one of my peers was faced with the question of "Are you too good to eat with us?" during the dinner hour that I felt I had a better understanding of my role. I now saw myself as a peer to the shelter residents and, although not homeless, someone who felt a sense of belonging and community with them after sharing a meal together. We had the opportunity to discuss the services the student-run clinic had brought to the shelter that night, engage them in conversations about their health, and also learn of factors that have influenced them in their life situations.

Hearing the Stories of the Homeless

Many of the stories shared by the shelter residents revolved around the concern for safety associated with displacement and lack of security in obtaining resources for daily living; these are some of a human's basic needs. From conversations with residents, the decision to leave a residence and become homeless was often due to concerns for personal safety in which there was more perceived safety in the streets than in staying within their homes. If a person had not become homeless because of a worse situation at home, it was often because that person could no longer afford to pay rent.

Without developing a personal connection with the residents, I would have never heard these stories nor had a context with which I could understand the risk factors faced by this vulnerable population and the subsequent health issues they faced. I now feel like I have a better understanding of the elevated prevalence of substance use disorders and mental health illnesses within the homeless population. More importantly, I can now see how there is a critical opportunity for medical providers to use the sense of community present by engaging with members of the homeless population to connect with them more effectively. I see this as an opportunity to mitigate some of the disproportionate burden of health risks that individuals who are homeless face. The stories of the shelter residents, their lack of choices, and, often, their feelings of being trapped by their circumstances helped shed light on the challenges of healthcare delivery within this population that I can now better appreciate during my career. Most importantly, I learned that these challenges were frustrating to the person who was homeless in that they could not engage the healthcare system in the way in which they wanted.

Many residents shared that they were between jobs; the vast majority of jobs they reported were seasonal. I met a painter who was able to support himself during the warmer months with food and housing; however, in the winter months, he would lose all sources of income. Another was a truck driver who only had work when his company had a need for additional drivers. The uncertainty of long-term employment status led him to go without money and, therefore, to forego food and shelter, as well. I saw examples of Maslow's (1970) hierarchy of needs at play in conversations with these residents. They described their time with regular income as anyone else would, with goals and future plans. When they described their current status, however, they discussed ways in which their lives were put on hold until they could earn money to provide for themselves again.

Many residents discussed how important and comforting it was to get a hotel room for a night. The shelter residents became animated whenever discussing this and I could see the excitement in their eyes. They described how there is nothing in the world like getting a hot shower and a comfortable bed in a hotel room that was completely to themselves. From my experience when residents stay in shelters, they generally sleep in a large, open, collective room. There is no privacy, no opportunity to let one's guard down and truly feel fully secure. I saw the hotel room as evidence that their basic needs were successfully addressed in an escape from any associated trauma from living in an unsafe environment.

The challenge for healthcare providers occurs when a person who is homeless has a chronic medical condition, such as hypertension, and must be compliant with medications. There is a high probability that a homeless person will become noncompliant with medications due to homeless status. If this person has just enough money to get a hotel room on a particularly challenging evening due to any number of factors, but also needs to save that money to purchase needed medication, he or she must decide between satisfying a basic need to feel secure with the need to remain compliant on medications. This situation can lead to noncompliance, especially if the person experiences no symptoms from not taking medication for hypertension, "the silent killer." Reconciling the desire to satisfy basic human needs against medical management with preventive care is often lost among members of the homeless community. Medical issues within the homeless population also extend to the meals that shelters provide. If someone has hypertension, hyperlipidemia, or coronary artery disease and is known to be noncompliant with medications, but the shelter is serving fried chicken and mashed potatoes that night, the shelter resident has little choice. The person may be doing more physical harm to the body that is then compounded by the potential for nonadherence to medications and the difficulty obtaining follow-up care at a physician's office.

One person's story of homelessness highlighted the trauma that can occur from staying in a shelter. He had just moved from a different state in search of a new job opportunity. During the day, he worked for a company, and at night, he went to the local shelter until he had enough money to rent his own apartment. He was paid in cash, and without a bank account, he always had a substantial amount of cash in his possession. He felt very unsafe at the shelter. Other residents would get into fights, and personal items were stolen regularly, all of which contributed to an environment that precipitated a state of chronic stress. Fortunately, his employer helped him navigate his housing situation, and he has since been renting an apartment with his family. His story illustrates some of the associated chronic stress trauma that those who are homeless face. Another resident's story illustrates how easily and unfortunately people can become homeless.

She had become divorced and experienced depression. Over the course of her marriage, she did not work and lived as a homemaker. She described her life since the divorce as being hit by waves that included being evicted, having her family dog die, and becoming homeless without any applicable job experience or computer skills. Her story, although tragic, showed the resilience that can come from facing severe adversity. At the time I met her, she was taking computer courses at the public library to learn how to apply for jobs. Her story influenced me the most because of how abruptly her life changed to lead her to homelessness. I also discovered that her story is not uncommon as many people living in poverty face the danger of becoming homeless.

Appreciating the Challenges of Living in the East End

The Peter Paul Development Center (PPDC) is an invaluable resource that focuses on childhood development in an effort to empower the East End of Richmond community. The Center makes a large impact by addressing many of the social issues that plague surrounding neighborhoods. As an educational exercise, the I2CRP program toured the East End of Richmond and participated in a discussion and reflection with the executive director of the PPDC. One of the most striking facts after experiencing the lived environment for people of the East End was the realization that individuals living here were expected, on average, to live 20 years less than people living in the greater metropolitan area. As the executive director of the PPDC put it, that makes a 45-year-old living in the East End a senior citizen. This tour provided me with the story that really adds life to any one of those striking statistics that describe the East End of Richmond.

Situated in a food desert, this area of little economic opportunity is home to a high concentration of the City's community housing developments in Richmond's East End. The children from these neighborhoods are raised with few examples of positive role models, fewer expectations of future success, and a heavy shadow that a home address will follow them wherever they go. The neighborhoods have gangs that are not isolated to the streets. There is one elementary, one middle school, and one high school to serve the entire area. When these children attend school, all the social factors at play daily in their lives and within their communities also attend school. The middle school has had five different principals in the last 7 years, so there is even a lack of a consistency from adult leaders at school. The preschool in the area has been closed, which puts children from the area at a disadvantage when they attend kindergarten without ever having been in a structured classroom before then.

This is a community that appears plagued by stagnation and a sense of inherent predestiny. Curb appeal is absent from the community, and unwelcoming steel bars greet you over windows and doors in the neighborhood. Several years ago, there was a large shootout over a drug deal that ended badly and a subsequent fire within the building. Today, several years later, that same building still has boards where windows once were. Driving through the area, I felt the trauma that community members face: It is in the buildings and on the streets. We heard stories of how numb the community is to the trauma they are facing when children run to see who is shooting rather than hide because they are scared. Subtle reminders of the city's history of segregation are built into the community. Physically separating the East End from the downtown area are the Richmond City Jail, a major interstate highway traveling north and south through Virginia, and another larger hill upon which Richmond is built. I could feel the weight of the community and could appreciate the danger that the residents face, but, most importantly, I now experienced those 20 years of life expectancy very differently. I saw those years in the context of the environment and the risk factors the people face every day. I have never seen poverty like I did while in the East End, and it will forever change the way I plan to practice medicine.

Envisioning My Career As a Physician

Thoughts were racing through my mind that afternoon we spent in the East End of Richmond. Where do I as a future physician fit into this picture? What can I do that addresses the root cause of these issues while practicing medicine? During our reflection, the executive director of the PPDC challenged each of us to "unapologetically show up" throughout our careers for members of vulnerable populations facing health disparities and inequities. He spoke of accountability and service and investment so that the community can build upon itself. His words coupled with my newfound understanding of the multi-faceted challenges that the East End faces helped me to envision my role in addressing these issues over the course of my career. The issues faced by the East End of Richmond are not necessarily unique. Themes similar to these can be seen in many socially and economically deprived communities in America, communities facing disproportionate burdens of health and significantly lower life expectancies.

I see a career in medicine in which a physician can challenge communities, serve in strong community partnerships, and invest in the community to address many of the risk factors that lead to poor health outcomes. I see an advocacy role for physicians in all of the conversations that take place about the community to alter the presence of drugs and alcohol, violence, inadequate public planning that results in food desserts, and issues within education. I see physicians as playing a large role in encouraging sound childhood development and education. I do not see these things as isolated from health or from each other. An additional challenge exists within medical education in which only 20 students from a class of approximately 200 had an opportunity to witness firsthand a community ravaged by factors that result in such a low life expectancy. Shockingly, it is a community that is only one and a half miles away from the VCU School of Medicine.

CONCLUSION

Reflecting on my volunteer experiences in a free clinic with the homeless population and participating in an extracurricular academic program that emphasized addressing the medical needs of vulnerable populations, I now recognize that my learning has been transformative, in keeping with Mezirow's (1991) theory. A transformative process has occurred that will influence the way in which I practice medicine in the future. Communicating with members of the homeless population and witnessing the community conditions of the East End of Richmond have given me a unique context to critically reflect on the many shortcomings of the healthcare delivery system when I consider my future role as a physician. Without volunteerism, I would not have gained a deeper understanding of the internal conflicts that vulnerable populations face when trying to secure basic needs. Ultimately, without connecting with members of the homeless community and learning of the disparities faced by these residents of Richmond, I do not think my perspective on practicing medicine would have undergone this transformative change.

There have been several positive role models within my medical education, instructors who focused on humanism in medicine and the importance of the affective domains of medical education. They have influenced me deeply during these experiences. I also acknowledge the restorative power that volunteerism can have to mitigate some of my own feelings of burnout throughout my academic journey thus far. The importance of critical reflection and conversations with fellow students and faculty members on my experiences cannot be overstated in the shift in my worldview. Without reflection on my tour of the East End of Richmond, I would not have heard the voices of community leaders describing their own experiences and their vision of the future to have physicians who work to address health disparities in their community. This process has led me to see changes within my own developing professional identity in which I now see myself as a future physician who will be treating members of vulnerable populations. It is by recognizing the influence of these previous experiences that I look to the future and an opportunity to address health disparities faced by vulnerable members within my community.

AUTHOR NOTE

This chapter would not have been possible without the direct support of Dr. Terry Carter. Her dedication and commitment to the education of current and future physicians has greatly influenced me while on my educational journey. I have benefited considerably from her direct guidance and example of how medical education can enrich the student experience to support a lifetime of learning. I am also thankful for the many educators who have invested in my career by encouraging me to consider the role of medicine in addressing health disparities. Their impact will continue to shape generations of physicians and health professionals who are better equipped to handle the needs of our most vulnerable populations.

REFERENCES

Aday, L. A. (2001, February). *At risk in America: The health and health care needs of vulnerable populations in the United States* (2nd ed.). San Francisco, CA: Jossey-Bass.

All About Richmond. (n.d.). Richmond, VA: Virginia Commonwealth University. Retrieved from https://www.vcu.edu/life-at-vcu/all-about-richmond/

American Nutrition Association. (2011, October 12). USDA defines food deserts. *Nutrition Digest, 38*(2). Retrieved from http://americannutritionassociation.org/newsletter/usda-defines-food-deserts

American Psychological Association. (2018). Work, stress, & health & socioeconomic status. Retrieved from http://www.apa.org/pi/ses/resources/publications/work-stress-health.aspx

Baggett, T. P., Singer, D. E., Rao, S. R., O'Connell, J. J., Bharel, M., & Rigotti, N. A. (2011). Food insufficiency and health services utilization in a national sample of homeless adults. *Journal of General Internal Medicine, 26*(6), 627–634. https://doi.org/10.1007/s11606-011-1638-4

Baker, K., & Sen, S. (2016, June). Healing medicine's future: Prioritizing physician trainee mental health. *American Medical Association Journal of Ethics, 18*(6), 604–613. https://doi.org/10.1001/journalofethics.2016.18.6.medu1-1606

Barrow, S. M., Herman, D. B., Córdova, P., & Struening, E. L. (1999). Mortality among homeless shelter residents in New York City. *American Journal of Public Health, 89*(4), 529–534.

Bethell, C., Fiorillo, J., Knickman, J., & Lansky, D. (2002, January 1). *A portrait of the chronically ill in America, 2001.* Princeton, NJ: Robert Wood Johnson Foundation. Retrieved from https://www.issuelab.org/resource/a-portrait-of-the-chronically-ill-in-america-2001.html

Braveman, P., & Egerter, S. (2008). *Overcoming obstacles to health: Report from the Robert Wood Johnson Foundation on the Commission to Build a Healthier America.* Princeton, NJ: Robert Wood Johnson Foundation. Retrieved from http://www.commissiononhealth.org/PDF/ObstaclesToHealth-Report.pdf

Centers for Disease Control and Prevention (CDC). (2004, May 28). Cigarette smoking among adults—United States—2002. *MMWR Morbidity and Mortally Weekly Report, 53*(20), 427–431.

Cranton, P. (2016). *Understanding and promoting transformative learning* (3rd ed). Sterling, VA: Stylus.

Data USA. (n.d.). *Richmond, VA metro area & Richmond City, VA comparison.* Retrieved from https://datausa.io/profile/geo/richmond-va-metro-area/?compare=richmond-city-va

DiPietro, B., Knopf, S., Artiga, S., & Arguello, R. (2012, September). *Medicaid coverage and care for the homeless population: Key lessons to consider for the 2014 Medicaid expansion*. Kaiser Commission on Medicaid and the Uninsured. Menlo Park, CA: The Henry J. Kaiser Foundation. Retrieved from https://www.kff.org/health-reform/report/medicaid-coverage-and-care-for-the-homeless/

Duncan, G. J., Brooks-Gunn, J., & Klebanov, K. P. (1994, April). Economic deprivation and early childhood development. *Child Development, 65*(2), 296–318.

Dyrbye, L. N., Eacker, A., Durning, S. J., Brazeau, C., Moutier, C., Massie, F. S.,...Shanafelt, T. D. (2015). The impact of stigma and personal experiences on the help-seeking behaviors of medical students with burnout. *Academic Medicine, 90*(7), 961–969.

Dyrbye, L. N., Massie, F. S., Eacker, A., Harper, W., Power, D., Durning, S. J.,...Shanafelt, T. D. (2010). Relationship between burnout and professional conduct and attitudes among US medical students. *Journal of the American Medical Association, 304*(11), 1173–1180. https://doi.org/10.1001/jama.2010.1318

Dyrbye, L. N., Thomas, M. R., & Shanafelt, T. D. (2006, April). Systematic review of depression, anxiety, and other indicators of psychological distress among U.S. and Canadian medical students. *Academic Medicine, 81*(4), 354–373.

Dyrbye, L. N., West, C. P., Satele, D., Boone, S., Tan, L., Sloan, J., & Shanafelt, T. D. (2014, March). Burnout among U.S. medical students, residents, and early career physicians relative to the general U.S. population. *Academic Medicine, 89*(3), 443–451. https://doi.org/10.1097/ACM.0000000000000134

Felitti, V. J., Anda, R. F., Nordenberg, D., Williamson, D. F., Spitze, A. M., Edwards, V.,...Marks, J. S. (1998). Relationship of childhood abuse and household dysfunction to many of the leading causes of death in adults. The Adverse Childhood Experiences (ACE) Study. *American Journal of Preventative Medicine, 14*(4), 245–258.

Feodor Nilsson, S., Laursen, T. M., Hjorthøj, C., & Nordentoft, M. (2018). Homelessness as a predictor of mortality: An 11-year register-based cohort study. *Social Psychiatry and Psychiatric Epidemiology, 53*(1), 63–75. https://doi.org/10.1007/s00127-017-1456-z

Goldie, J. (2012). The formation of professional identity in medical students: Considerations for educators. *Medical Teacher, 34*(9), e641–648. https://doi.org/10.3109/0142159X.2012.687476

Hadley, J. (2007, March). Insurance coverage, medical care use, and short-term health changes following an unintentional injury or the onset of a chronic condition. *Journal of the American Medical Association, 297*(10), 1073–1084. https://doi.org/10.1001/jama.297.10.1073

Hafferty, F. W. (1998, April). Beyond curriculum reform: Confronting medicine's hidden curriculum. *Academic Medicine, 73*(4), 403–407.

Henry, M., Watt, R., Rosenthal, L., Shivji, A., & Abt Associates. (2017, December). *The 2017 annual homeless assessment report (AHAR) to Congress: Part I: Point-in-time estimates of homelessness*. Washington, DC: The U.S. Department of Housing and Urban Development Office of Community Planning and Development.

Heron, M., Hoyert, D. L., Murphy, S. L., Xu, J., Kochanek, K. D., Tejada-Vera, B. (2009, April 17). Deaths: Final data for 2006. *National Vital Statistics Report, 57*(14), 1–134.

Holden, M., Buck, E., Clark, M., Szauter, K., & Trumble, J. (2012). Professional identity formation in medical education: the convergence of multiple domains. *Healthcare Ethics Committee Forum, 24*(4), 245–255. https://doi.org/10.1007/s10730-012-9197-6

Holden, M. D., Buck, E., Luk, J., Ambriz, F., Boisaubin, E. V., Clark, M. A.,...Dalrymple, J. L. (2015). Professional identity formation: Creating a longitudinal framework through TIME (Transformation in Medical Education). *Academic Medicine, 90*(6), 761–767.

Hojat, M., Vergare, M. J., Maxwell, K., Brainard, G., Herrine, S. K., Isenberg, G. A.,...Gonella, J. S. (2009). The devil is in the third year: A longitudinal study of erosion of empathy in medical school. *Academic Medicine, 84*(9), 1182–1191. https://doi.org/10.1097/ACM.0b013e3181b17e55

Hullender, R., Hinck, S., Wood-Nartker, J., Burton, T., & Bowlby, S. (2015). Evidences of transformative learning in service-learning reflections. *Journal of the Scholarship of Teaching and Learning, 15*(4), 58–82. Retrieved from https://files.eric.ed.gov/fulltext/EJ1074817.pdf

Institute of Medicine. (2000). *America's healthcare safety net: Intact but endangered.* Washington, DC: National Academy Press.

Institute of Medicine. (2013). *U.S. health in international perspective: Shorter lives, poorer health.* Washington, DC: National Academy Press. Retrieved from http://www.nap.edu/13497

Inui, T. S. (2003). *A flag in the wind: Educating for professionalism in medicine.* Washington, DC: Association of American Medical Colleges. Retrieved from https://members.aamc.org/eweb/upload/A%20Flag%20in%20the%20Wind%20Report.pdf

Irby, D. M., Cooke, M., & O'Brien, B. C. (2010). Calls for reform of medical education by the Carnegie Foundation for the Advancement of Teaching: 1910 and 2010. *Academic Medicine, 85*(2), 220–227. https://doi.org/10.1097/ACM.0b013e3181c88449

IsHak, W., Nikravesh, R., Lederer, S., Perry, R., Ogunyemi, D., & Bernstein, C. (2013). Burnout in medical students: A systematic review. *The Clinical Teacher, 10*(4), 242–245. https://doi.org/10.1111/tct.12014

Jiang, Y., Ekono, M., & Skinner, C. (2016). *Basic facts about low-income children: Children under 18 years, 2014.* New York, NY: National Center for Children in Poverty. Mailman School of Public Health, Columbia University. Retrieved from http://www.nccp.org/publications/pub_1145.html

Kaslow, N. J., Heron, S., Roberts, D. K., Thompson, M., Guessous, O., & Jones, C. (2003). Family and community factors that predict internalizing and externalizing symptoms in low-income, African-American children. *Annals of the New York Academy of Sciences, 1008*(1), 55–68. https://doi.org/10.1196/annals.1301.007

Kiely, R. (2005). A transformative learning model for service-learning: A longitudinal case study. *Michigan Journal of Community Service Learning, 12*(1), 5–22. Retrieved from http://hdl.handle.net/2027/spo.3239521.0012.101

Kushel, M. B., Gupta, R., Gee, L., & Haas, J. S. (2006). Housing instability and food insecurity as barriers to health care among low-income Americans. *Journal of General Internal Medicine, 21*(1), 71–77. https://doi.org/10.1111/j.1525-1497.2005.00278.x

Lublin, J. R. (1992). Role modelling: A case study in general practice. *Medical Education, 26*(2), 116–122. https://doi.org/10.1111/j.1365-2923.1992.tb00136.x

Maslow, A. H. (1970). *Motivation and personality* (2nd ed.). New York, NY: Harper & Row.

Mezirow, J. (1991). *Transformative dimensions of adult learning.* San Francisco, CA: Jossey-Bass.

Mezirow, J. (2012). Learning to think like an adult: Core concepts of transformation theory. In E. W. Taylor, P. Cranton, & Associates (Eds.), *The handbook of transformative learning: Theory, research, and practice* (pp. 73–95). San Francisco, CA: Jossey-Bass.

Montgomery, A. E., Szymkowiak, D., Marcus, J., Howard, P., & Culhane, D. P. (2016). Homelessness, unsheltered status, and risk factors for mortality: Findings from the 100,000 homes campaign. *Public Health Report, 131*(6), 765–772. https://doi.org/10.1177/0033354916667501

Morrison, D. S. (2009). Homelessness as an independent risk factor for mortality: Results from a retrospective cohort study. *International Journal of Epidemiology, 38*(3), 877–883. https://doi.org/10.1093/ije/dyp160

Phillips, D., Fawns, R., & Hayes, B. (2002). From personal reflection to social positioning: The development of a transformational model of professional education in midwifery. *Nursing Inquiry, 9*(4), 239–249. https://doi.org/10.1046/j.1440-1800.2002.00145.x

Porter, M. (2018). VCU receives Carnegie Community Engagement Classification. Retrieved from https://community.vcu.edu/news-and-events/education/vcu-receives-carnegie-foundation-2015-community-engagement-classification.html

Rabow, M. W., Evans, C. N., & Remen, R. N. (2013). Professional formation and deformation: Repression of personal values and qualities in medical education. *Family Medicine, 45*(1), 13–18.

Roncarati, J. S., Baggett, T. P., O'Connell, J. J., Hwang, S. W., Cook, E. F., Krieger, N., & Sorensen, G. (2018). Mortality among unsheltered homeless in Boston, Massachusetts, 2000–2009. *Journal of the American Medical Association, Internal Medicine, 178*(9), 1242–1248. https://doi.org/10.1001/jamainternmed.2018.2924

Shanafelt, T. D., Bradley, K. A., Wipf, J. E., & Back, A. L. (2002). Burnout and self-reported patient care in an Internal Medicine residency program. *Annals of Internal Medicine, 136*(5), 358–367.

Shi, L., & Stevens, G. D. (2010). *Vulnerable populations in the United States* (2nd ed.). San Francisco, CA: Jossey-Bass.

Swick, H. M. (2000). Toward a normative definition of medical professionalism. *Academic Medicine, 75*(6), 612–616.

Taylor, E. W. (2009). Fostering transformative learning. In J. Mezirow, E. W. Taylor, & Associates (Eds.), *Transformative learning in practice: Insights from community, workplace, and higher education* (pp. 3–17). San Francisco, CA: Jossey-Bass.

Thomas, M. R., Dyrbye, L. N., Huntington, J. L., Lawson, K. L., Novotny, P. J., Sloan, J. A., & Shanafelt. (2007). How do distress and well-being relate to medical student empathy? A multicenter study. *Journal of General Internal Medicine,* *22*(2), 177–183. https://doi.org/10.1007/s11606-006-0039-6

United States Conference of Mayors. (2007). *A status report on hunger and homelessness in America's cities: A 23 city survey.* Retrieved from http://www.ncdsv.org/images/USCM_Hunger-homelessness-Survey-in-America%27s-Cities_12%20 2007.pdf

United States Department of Agriculture. (2016). *Why is it important to eat vegetables?* Retrieved from https://www.choosemyplate.gov/vegetables-nutrients-health

van der Zwet, J., Zwietering, P. J., Teunissen, P. W., van der Vleuten, C. P., & Scherpbier, A. J. (2011, August). Workplace learning from a socio-cultural perspective: Creating developmental space during the general practice clerkship. *Advances in Health Science Education, 16*(3), 359-379. doi:10.1007/s10459-010-9268-x.

van Mook, W. N., van Luijk, S. J., de Grave, W., O'Sullivan, H., Wass, V., Schuwirth, L. W., & van der Vleuten, C. P. (2009). Teaching and learning professional behavior in practice. *European Journal of Internal Medicine, 20*(5), e105–e111. https://doi.org/10.1016/j.ejim.2009.01.003

Wald, H. S. (2015). Professional identity (trans)formation in medical education: Reflection, relationship, resilience. *Academic Medicine, 90*(6), 701–706. https://doi.org/10.1097/ACM.0000000000000731

Wald, H. S., Anthony, D., Hutchinson, T. A., Liben, S., Smilovitch, M., & Donato, A. A. (2015). Professional identity formation in medical education for humanistic, resilient physicians: Pedagogic strategies for bridging theory to practice. *Academic Medicine, 90*(6), 753–760.

West, C. P., Shanafelt, T. D., & Kolars, J. C. (2011). Quality of life, burnout, educational debt, and medical knowledge among Internal Medicine residents. *Journal of the American Medical Association, 306*(9), 952–960. https://doi.org/10.1001/jama.2011.1247

Wilkinson, T. J., Gill, D. J., Fitzjohn J., Palmer, C. L., & Mulder, R. T. (2006). The impact on students of adverse experiences during medical school. *Medical Teacher, 28*(2), 129–135. https://doi.org/10.1080/01421590600607195

Zimmerman, E., Haley, A., Walker, A., Woolf, S., Nguyen, K., Shue, W., . . . Chapman, D. (2016, Spring). *Health Equity in Richmond, Virginia.* Richmond, VA: Virginia Commonwealth University Center on Society and Health. Retrieved from https://societyhealth.vcu.edu/media/society-health/pdf/RVAHealthEquity FINAL.pdf

CHAPTER 8

CASE STUDY OF A SCIENCE TEACHER'S PROFESSIONAL IDENTITY DEVELOPMENT ACROSS A CAREER

Elaine Mangiante
Salve Regina University

ABSTRACT

This chapter describes findings from a case study of a sixth-grade science teacher's perceptions of her professional identity development over the course of her career. Ms. Garvey (pseudonym) began as a novice teacher with no experience or training in science education; however, during her career she took responsibility for her transformative learning and became an expert teacher and district leader in science and sustainability education. This narrative outlines Ms. Garvey's characteristics and activities at each stage from novice to expert. In addition, the results pinpoint key factors that influenced her professional identity development and that transformed her view of herself and her teaching from a didactic, textbook-guided instructor to an empowered educator who created student-centered, real-world, inquiry-based learning opportunities aligned with the current reform-based vision for science education.

Transformative Learning in Healthcare and Helping Professions Education, pages 153–174

A person's perception of identity as a professional in a given field can affect both self-efficacy and the willingness to implement reforms or innovations in practice settings (Beijaard, Verloop, & Vermunt, 2000). In the field of education, with the expectation that teachers adopt reforms to improve students' learning outcomes (Goodson & Numan, 2002; Moore Johnson, 2004), teachers' perception of their professional identity can impact their ability to cope with and implement instructional approaches that may differ from their own educational experiences. For example, elementary teachers, in particular, face challenges in adopting science education reforms. The framework developed by the National Research Council (NRC) for the current science education standards, Next Generation Science Standards (NGSS), emphasizes that teachers provide learner-centered opportunities for students to acquire understanding of scientific ideas through inquiry-based learning (NRC, 2012). Such a strategy involves posing questions and conducting investigations, as well as constructing and critiquing explanations about scientific phenomena in the real world (NGSS Lead States, 2013; NRC, 1996; NRC, 2012). However, research studies have documented that for elementary teachers, low self-efficacy in teaching science (Smith & Southerland, 2007; Smolleck & Yoder, 2008), limited science content knowledge (Davis, 2003; Newton & Newton, 2001), and lack of exposure to inquiry-based learning methods during their own schooling (Wallace & Louden, 1992) can impact identity as a science teacher and motivation in teaching reform-based science.

The purpose of this study was to examine the perceptions of professional identity development by an adult learner over the course of a career. In this case, the professional learner was an exemplary sixth-grade science teacher. Ms. Garvey (pseudonym) began as a novice elementary teacher with no experience or training in science education. However, during her career she became an expert teacher and district leader in science and sustainability education. This narrative presents features of her professional identity development over time in transforming her view of herself and her teaching from a didactic, textbook-guided instructor to an empowered educator who created student-centered, real-world, inquiry-based learning opportunities aligned with the vision for science education (NRC, 2012). The following questions guided this study: How did one exemplary sixth grade teacher of science describe her professional identity development across different phases of her science teaching career? What factors influenced the teacher's professional identity development as a science teacher?

BACKGROUND AND LITERATURE REVIEW

The concept of teacher professional identity encompasses one's image of self (Knowles, 1992) within the roles the teacher feels obliged to play

(Volkmann & Anderson, 1998) and the dynamic process of self-evaluation to continually form and reform this self-identity over time (Cooper & Olson, 1996). From the field of medical education, Ewan (1988) defined professional identity as a "self-image which permits feelings of personal adequacy and satisfaction in the performance of the expected role" (p. 85). The expected role for an effective teacher involves a range of domains including technical knowledge of content, practical or communicative knowledge of facilitation and collaborative learning, and emancipatory knowledge of critical questioning and strategies to promote students' examination of alternative views (Cranton, 2016). These teacher competencies are consistent with the recommended teacher roles advocated in the national science standards that emphasize providing students with constructivist learning opportunities to generate explanations and evidence-based arguments (NRC, 2012). As suggested by Cranton (2016), transformative learning may be necessary for teachers to perceive themselves as adequate and satisfied with their identity in the science teaching role (p. 81).

A science teacher's identity develops through affinity for the role and a set of specific educational practices as well as through discourse with others about one's beliefs and actions for teaching (Gee, 2000; Varelas, House, & Wenzel, 2005). From research in elementary teachers' identity development in teaching science, Settlage, Southerland, Smith, and Ceglie (2009) reported that novice teachers tend to have an affinity for science lessons designed to entertain students as well as engage in classroom discourse that privileges teacher delivery of activities over student learning. Settlage et al. have posited that novice teachers are often over-confident in their abilities, which can blind them to self-doubt. Yet, Wheatley (2002) argues that self-doubt can serve as a force that fosters teachers' reflection, evaluation, and revision of teaching practices and promote identity development with legitimate confidence in reform-based teaching.

In addition, Day et al. (2006) claim that teachers' professional identities develop through interactions in the professional realm from external expectations of teachers (i.e., educational policies or workplace requirements), the situated dimension (i.e., the localized context of the school or student characteristics), and the personal dimension (i.e., a teacher's values and life outside of school). Their research revealed that teacher identity development depended not only on the range of learning opportunities provided by school leaders, but also on teachers' awareness and ability to manage their needs and concerns in these dimensions.

CONCEPTUAL FRAMEWORKS

Two conceptual frameworks guided this study to address each of the research questions. For the first framework, Berliner (2004) applies the Dreyfus and Dreyfus (1986) five stage adult skill acquisition model (novice, advanced beginner, competent, proficient, and expert) to the field of education by describing teachers' professional development at different career stages. This model provided a guide to identify Ms. Garvey's reported stages of development across her career. Berliner noted that novice teachers in their first year tend to follow learned procedures inflexibly without considering the context, such as the needs of individual students. Second or third year teachers at the advanced beginner stage can recognize similarities across student situations and identify when to ignore procedures or rules; however, they may still struggle with determining the relative importance or outcomes of instructional strategies. According to Berliner, many third, fourth, and fifth year teachers attain the level of becoming competent in their ability to make instructional decisions based on student characteristics. However, some teachers plateau at this stage by adhering to a personal, inflexible perspective for instructional choices. After 5 years or more, a smaller number of teachers reach the proficient level with the ability to replace learned procedures with situational intuition; yet, their decisions still require analysis of the situation and deliberation. From thousands of hours of reflective teaching experience, more in-depth knowledge, and an awareness of different ways to help individual students learn, Berliner asserts that a few teachers attain the expert stage; their teaching and interactions are intuitive and fluid without requiring conscious decision-making.

The second framework details possible factors that could have influenced Ms. Garvey's professional identity development throughout the stages of her career. From a review of literature on teacher professional identity, Beijaard, Meijer, and Verloop (2004) identified four essential features for teachers' professional identity development:

1. An *ongoing process* of reflection, interpretation, and reinterpretation of experiences. The teacher's interpretation from this process involves not only the perception of his or her identity in the moment, but also an anticipated identity of who the teacher wants to become (Conway, 2001).
2. An involvement of both the *person and context*. Teachers' own attitudes intersect with expected professional behaviors in a school culture, yet teachers may develop their own teaching perspective within that context (Feiman-Nemser & Floden, 1986).
3. An influence of the teachers' *sub-identities* from different contexts and relationships. A teacher's sub-identities harmonize to varying

extents; change in expectations or work environment can pose potential conflicts (Connelly & Clandinin, 1999).

4. The element of a teacher's *agency* in the activity of learning. Teachers' professional identity development depends on their efforts in constructing an understanding of the teacher role, both individually and collaboratively (Coldron & Smith, 1999).

These features for teachers' professional identity development provide a framework to examine possible factors that influenced Ms. Garvey's transformation as a teacher of science across her career. Through the ongoing habit of mind of reflecting on personal attitudes, sub-identities, and agency in addition to relational and work contexts (Beijaard et al., 2004), the teacher may experience the transformative process of increasing self-awareness, critically evaluating assumptions about teaching and learning, generating alternatives, and developing an informed teaching practice (Cranton, 2016).

METHODOLOGY

Case study methodology (Merriam, 1998) was used to gain an in-depth view of one teacher's perception of her professional identity development in science teaching as she progressed through her career. Case studies allow for an "intensive, holistic description and analysis of a single unit" of study such as the phenomenon experienced by an individual (Merriam, 1998, p. 12). This methodology permits the researcher to discover an individual's meaning made from the experience.

Participant

Ms. Garvey, a retired sixth grade teacher of science, had worked in the same suburban school district in a northeastern state for 31 years and taught science for 25 of those years. She majored in special education and elementary teacher education in her preservice training. Early in her career, Ms. Garvey taught third grade for 2 years and self-contained special education in Grades Kindergarten, 1, 3, and 4 for 3 years before taking a sixth grade general education position. One year later, she agreed to be the sixth grade science teacher for her team since no other teacher felt comfortable teaching science. With limited science content knowledge or awareness of science education pedagogy, Ms. Garvey embarked on a career in science education. Over time, she developed in-depth units involving her students in real world experimentation with aquaculture, hydroponics, and sustainable farming while collaborating with community members, farmers, and university researchers. As a result, she became the district teacher leader for K–8 science education. Ms. Garvey was chosen purposefully for this study as an information-rich, extreme case participant (Patton, 2002) to explore her perceptions of factors that supported her professional identity development as an exemplary science teacher who provided rigorous, authentic learning experiences for her students.

Data Sources and Analysis

The data sources included four, hour-and-a-half interviews during her first year of retirement using Belli's (1998) event history calendar approach to assist Ms. Garvey in reconstructing her autobiography and description of her professional identity development. The trustworthiness of retrospective reporting depends on a participant's ability to accurately report past events (Belli, 1998) since there can be memory limitations (Jobe, Tourangeau, & Smith, 1993; Schwarz, 2007). However, Belli cited evidence of participants' increase in response quality from the use of an event history calendar to assist respondents in reconstructing their autobiographies more accurately. An event history calendar provides a structure for respondents to "consider various events that constitute their personal pasts as contained within broader thematic streams of events" (p. 394). Ms. Garvey and I created an event history calendar together by first identifying key events chronologically in her personal life to remind her of events in her teaching. Through face-to face interviewing using the timeline as a visual cue, I encouraged Ms. Garvey's retrieval of her perceptions associated with personal events and professional experiences. This process allowed Ms. Garvey to self-correct reports as she plotted her teaching practice and her professional identity development over time.

Data collection and analysis for this study was an iterative process that required seeking clarification of developing patterns during succeeding interviews (Merriam, 1998). From a repeated and systematic examination of the data and the event history calendar, data were coded to identify Ms. Garvey's perception of (a) her teaching practice from novice to expert (Berliner, 2004) and (b) her professional identity development across her career. Using constant comparison analysis (Glaser & Strauss, 1967), categories were examined for patterns of factors that influenced Ms. Garvey's professional identity development. By providing detailed description of the results from this study of one adult learner, readers can determine the applicability of the claims to their own contexts.

RESULTS

The results are presented in two sections. The first section outlines Ms. Garvey's characteristics and activities at each stage from novice to expert (Berliner, 2004; Dreyfus & Dreyfus, 1986) in conjunction with a description of her perception of her professional identity. The second section describes factors impacting her professional identity development across her career that emerged from Ms. Garvey's reports.

Transitions in Career

The data indicated that Ms. Garvey made shifts in her professional practice throughout her teaching career. Table 8.1 depicts a compressed version of the event history calendar developed with Ms. Garvey showing time periods across her career with respective stages of development, teaching practices, and perceptions of her professional identity. From Ms. Garvey's description of her developing skills in science teaching, the data showed a progression from teacher-directed instruction to an increasingly student-centered learning practice.

When comparing the approaches that guided Ms. Garvey's teaching with the characteristics of the Dreyfus and Dreyfus (1986) stages for adult skill acquisition, a correlation emerged suggesting not only that her professional identity changed over time, but also the professional development she sought shifted to align with her perception of what was needed at the time for her own growth as a teacher. For example, during Ms. Garvey's first year of teaching science, she viewed herself as a novice. She explained:

> I had never taught science. So when I stepped up to the plate, it was a science book with read the chapter, answer the questions...I did that for the first year and I wasn't thrilled with it...I learned quickly that that certainly wasn't the way to be teaching science. I was bored. I knew there was a connection if I had passion, they would feel passion, but I didn't have passion that first year.

From Ms. Garvey's displeasure with her professional identity of teaching inflexibly from a textbook, she described herself as "restless" and sought out a 2-week summer workshop to learn ways to engage her students in science learning activities. She explained that as a child she "really disliked school and didn't like sitting in a chair, but this workshop never lost my attention and I wanted my kids to have this experience." Ms. Garvey had learned strategies from this workshop that were "child-oriented, but at a higher level of thinking, much higher than the book" and students would be able to "experiment and talk about what they were discovering." She explained, "I took the initiative on my own...because I needed to grow"

TABLE 8.1 Compressed Version of Ms. Garvey's Event History Calendar

Year(s) Teaching Science	Stage of Adult Skill Acquisition	Teaching Practices	Evidence of Her Teaching and Her Perception of Her Professional Identity
1	Novice—inflexible following of procedures	Didactic teacher-directed instruction	Taught from science textbook "Never taught science," "bored," "restless," "I needed to grow."
2–3	Advanced Beginner—beginning awareness of students' needs	Addition of brief hands-on activities for student engagement	Attended a science activities workshop—incorporated in oceanography unit "I took initiative on my own." "I embraced change."
4–7	Competent—responsible for own teaching perspective	Incorporation of singular real-world experiences into science unit	Included half-day research cruise and shore-side investigations with oceanography unit "I was willing to grow and learn about oceanography."
8–13	Proficient—intuitive, yet deliberate decision-making	In-class investigations connected with ecological issues and analysis of global data	District leader of K–8 science Brought water quality investigations into the classroom Sought out global warming data "I did it on my own." "I wanted more data, I wanted a higher level."
14–25	Expert—fluid, flexible decision-making from experience and intuition	Use of continuous in-class real-world research by students	Offered students sustainability experiments: a. Salmon and oyster restoration, b. Endangered Dominique chickens, c. Aquaculture, and d. Hydroponics (NASA grant). "By the end of my career, I was beyond expert."

and subsequently "walked out of there a completely different teacher." As a result, in her second and third years of teaching science (advanced beginner stage), Ms. Garvey explained, "I embraced change . . . I started to design my own lessons to help students learn, and that was the beginning of me branching out." She included short activities into her oceanography unit to promote students' questioning, observations, expression of ideas, and curiosity about scientific phenomena.

As Ms. Garvey assumed more responsibility in refining her oceanography unit in her fourth year of science teaching (competent stage), she adopted the perspective that the students needed to experience authentic techniques used for ocean research by participating in a half-day research cruise on the bay or by conducting shoreside investigations. To prepare students for these field trips, Ms. Garvey sought out content information and science lesson ideas from an organization focused on ocean health and from practitioners such as fishermen to learn "what was going on with the ocean"; she was "willing to grow and learn about oceanography." A pattern emerged in Ms. Garvey's professional identity—she saw herself as an initiator who would educate herself by contacting and learning from individuals in the field rather than relying on typical professional development opportunities provided by a district. She felt that "someone could not be a good teacher if they did not know and like their subject matter."

During Ms. Garvey's eighth year when she was chosen as district leader for Grades K–8 science, two events led her to take on a more self-directed and influential role. First, since funds were eliminated for half-day field trips, she assumed the responsibility of bringing ocean water quality experiments into the classroom as a part of the students' learning experiences. Next, commercial science kits became available for K–6 teachers, and the district called upon her expertise to evaluate the kits to "get the elementary teachers more involved in science." She recommended their adoption since the kits provided guidance for novice elementary teachers or teachers who feared teaching science. However, given the level to which Ms. Garvey had developed her science teaching, she personally wanted more in-depth content, investigations, and real-world applications to enhance the kit lessons. As a teacher in the proficient stage, she identified what she needed and deliberately sought out a workshop that provided her with current data on global conditions, energy use, and sea-level rise. She explained,

> I did it on my own . . . I loved that workshop because it gave me environmental [sic] accurate information. It gave me hard data that was taking me hours to find. It was great because it was global and I could present a graph to kids and have them analyse it.

During this stage, Ms. Garvey viewed her professional identity as a change-agent promoting students' environmental literacy. Her science instruction reflected her expectation that students should be involved in investigations to explore current issues facing ecosystems as well as analyze real-world data about environmental conditions in different countries.

Finally, in her last 11 years of teaching as an expert, from years of experience refining her science units, Ms. Garvey assumed a more robust approach that immersed students in continuous real-world research through collaboration with scientists, universities, state initiatives, and community members. At this point in her career, she described her professional identity as "above expert." Her science teaching had become a fluid process of adopting authentic learning opportunities including research with salmon and oyster restoration, endangered Dominique chickens, aquaculture, and hydroponics. She explained, "My whole curriculum revolved around things that I was absolutely passionate about—not just because they meant something to me, but because I believed in sustainability of the world and children are going to sustain the world." She had attained a sense of satisfaction from accomplishing her vision of creating a learning laboratory in which students engaged in inquiry of authentic questions related to sustainability for the community and their own lives.

Key Themes From Ms. Garvey's Professional Identity Development

Six themes emerged from Ms. Garvey's description of her career that provide insight into factors impacting her professional identity development and transformation as a science teacher. The sections that follow describe each of the themes: encouragement and support from fellow teachers and administration, self-evaluation of professional needs, self-efficacy and trust in own instincts, self-motivation to seek more in-depth content knowledge, personal investment from incorporating passions and experience with teaching, and self-determined meaningful mission.

Encouragement and Support
From Fellow Teachers and Administration

A major factor contributing to Ms. Garvey's identity development was the support she received from fellow teachers and her administration. Ms. Garvey described an example early in her career:

> I was very fortunate my very first year there when I was a long-term sub in a resource room. The woman that I took her place looked at me and she said, "You can do this. Do what you do best." She had total faith in me...In the very first time meeting with her, she entrusted that I, as an individual, was capable of understanding and knowing what to do best.

This level of trust and support also pervaded her interactions with teachers throughout her career. She described the collegial spirit of the teaching team:

> We always shared. If I was having a hard time with a child, I would think nothing of saying, "Where am I going wrong? What worked? What do you know

that I don't know?" It was so productive. The communication was incredible . . . It was all about doing what worked best for the child.

Ms. Garvey felt that the spirit of the collaboration among educators in the school reinforced her own personal philosophy about teaching that "it was all about the kids."

In addition, Ms. Garvey felt the administration respected her professional judgments for science teaching. She noted, "I was always supported by the administration for science and that was empowering. They knew that everything I asked for was getting used and was for the kids." Ms. Garvey explained that her principal "gave me freedom." She was able to design science units to meet the goals of the district curriculum, "but I wasn't told what it had to be." Evidence of district support for her work was their willingness to secure a $200,000 NASA grant for hydroponics and aquaculture projects in the last 3 years of her teaching. The tangible and intangible support from Ms. Garvey's district provided her with autonomy to explore her passions and confidence to develop in-depth science units aligned with the national standards for students to engage in real-world experimentation.

However, Ms. Garvey also explained that later in her career, with the onset of standardized testing, the administration eliminated the previous practice of seeking teacher input regarding professional development and made decisions focused on raising district scores. She noted that the topics often did not relate to science, and she noted her reaction to these decisions:

> So, I would sit there and personally I was insulted because I thought my time was more important than to be sitting there doing something that I couldn't take back to the classroom and use. So, I found that offensive.

Ms. Garvey felt conflicted with the district approach to teachers' professional development since she had come to value her own judgment and recognition of her needs.

Self-Evaluation of Professional Needs

Throughout her career, Ms. Garvey's professional identity in teaching science was strengthened by the initiative she took to evaluate her teaching continuously and to determine the professional development or resources she needed to improve her practice. As early as her first year, Ms. Garvey recognized she needed to learn pedagogical approaches for science teaching and, thus, sought out professional development in science teaching activities for student engagement. Ms. Garvey saw that these activities helped her students "put their heads together to discuss ideas and to listen to each other." Subsequently, with her increased awareness of what was possible for students' science learning, she developed more enriching science units and sought advice from more seasoned teachers as well as information from scientists and fishermen for her oceanography unit. Ms. Garvey's success with seeking out resources on her own to create engaging science lessons shaped her professional view of herself as a self-directed teacher who could evaluate and improve her teaching without relying on professional development from the district.

Self-Efficacy and Trust in Own Instincts

From trial and error, experience, and continual reflection, Ms. Garvey came to trust herself and believe in her ability to help students learn science. She held the professional view of herself that she could tune into the students' needs to guide her instructional decisions. She noted, "I think there's that internal piece in really paying attention and listening and observing kids...I think it also comes with becoming more comfortable within myself and listening to myself." She explained how her background empowered her to connect with students and understand their needs:

> I feel that when I work with kids, there's a magic there. It can be the worse kid. It can be the best kid. It can be the lonely one. I didn't have it easy growing up, and they always say there's good that comes out of bad. Well, I truly believe that and I think so much of my background made me have so much compassion and insight into the children who may have only one parent or who go home and there isn't a meal there. And the children that are really, really smart, but no one is challenging their brains. I just think that there was something magical that connected me to children.

Thus, Ms. Garvey's self-image of her background, compassion, instincts, and reflection shaped her professional identity informing her of how to engage all students in learning.

Self-Motivation to Seek More In-Depth Content Knowledge

Repeatedly throughout her career, Ms. Garvey implemented new learning opportunities for students that required her first to increase her own content knowledge. Her self-motivation and initiative in this regard became an important characteristic of her professional identity. For example, though she had advised the district to adopt commercial science kits to support elementary teachers in teaching science, she noted that the kits involved generic investigations covering science content at a basic level, unrelated to where the students lived. Since Ms. Garvey wanted her students to have more in-depth learning experiences, she knew she needed to gain additional content knowledge for her oceanography unit and, thus, attended a workshop that provided up-to-date data on environmental trends. She noted, "I got really picky about where I was going and what I was doing. I wanted to come away with something that I would really use." For example, she obtained global data about energy use for students to analyze.

It was graphs about carbon levels and which countries were using the most carbon, making the biggest carbon footprint. It was data about ocean levels rising, which areas, countries, and continents were going to have issues first. At that point, because I was doing so much with the Bay, I had all the hands-on pieces, but that gave me hard data that was taking me hours to find and here it was all put in front of me ... They could see that India was making the largest carbon imprint on the world. So, I could always tie science in globally and I think that is really important.

Ms. Garvey understood that to achieve the instructional goals based on the standards, students needed real-world applications for what they were learning. Thus, her personal vision for students' science learning and global understanding drove her to seek more professional development rather than relying on the kit resource.

Personal Investment From Incorporating
Passions and Experience With Teaching

Ms. Garvey's sub-identities from her personal life (i.e., Ms. Garvey volunteered on an organic farm and she was married to a fisherman) were integrated with her professional teaching identity. For example, she brought her personal interests in organic farming, fishing, and sustainable food production into science units. From years 14 to 25, Ms. Garvey's passions fueled her decisions about learning opportunities for students. To provide context for their learning, students investigated the advantages and disadvantages of traditional farming versus organic farming. The authentic issue of food production and the role of microbes in soil became the venue through which students met their learning goals on microorganisms. When a hydroponics facility opened near the local organic farm, Ms. Garvey enlisted support from the hydroponics expert and sought funding from a NASA grant to set up a hydroponics system in her classroom. Students were able to apply their previous learning from an ecosystem's unit to a real farming system by monitoring nutrients, light levels, and pH daily while growing vegetables that they would harvest for their families.

As Ms. Garvey's confidence, knowledge, and resourcefulness increased, she advanced to the expert level by providing students with opportunities to engage in scientific research themselves. For example, she became aware of the state salmon restoration project. The students already were well versed in water quality regimens of testing for oxygen, nitrates, and pH; however, this opportunity allowed students to participate in aquaculture experimentation. Students computed the effect of water temperature on salmon growth and discovered that the colder the water, the slower the growth. Her decision to bring her personal interests into the science curriculum enabled her to envision the local community as a resource to enrich students' learning experiences and make connections for themselves.

Self-Determined Meaningful Mission

According to Ms. Garvey, the driving forces behind her professional identity were her dedication to her students and to sustaining the planet. Ms. Garvey felt responsible to educate students about human and environmental interaction. This mission drove her to seek current data on global conditions to integrate with students' experimentation and concept development so the learning was meaningful. This self-determined mission was reinforced when students would ask, "Did you see on TV about the oil spill in . . . or did you read about China's pollution, or do you know what that's doing to the water?" Ms. Garvey's view of her effectiveness as a teacher was linked to her students' connecting their in-class learning to world events and their own lives.

Likewise, an aspect of her mission was to create a classroom environment in which the students felt safe to share and debate their ideas about the data from their investigations.

> I made it very clear that disagreement was a good thing. I would be walking around and it would be a bantering back and forth of ideas . . . the bottom line is they were working it through, they were discussing it and they were thinking.

Through students' introduction to real-world data and ownership in relevant classroom investigations, Ms. Garvey had created a climate in which the students were committed to their in-class research, willing to debate their proposed explanations, and invested in applying their growing knowledge to world events. These authentic student learning experiences served to bolster Ms. Garvey's professional identity development by giving her a sense of empowerment to achieve her mission. She believed her teaching had an impact on students' view of the world and she hoped this learning would influence their future behaviors and interactions.

DISCUSSION

The results of this study indicated how one elementary teacher described her professional identity development as it progressed from one of limited knowledge to that of an expert practitioner in the field of science education. The development of Ms. Garvey's professional identity across her career was, in large measure, a function of the self-initiative she took to transform her science teaching practice. Though Ms. Garvey was a unique individual who applied her personal interest in environmental sustainability to enrich the learning of her students through real-world investigations, this discussion will address her professional identity development from a broad perspective in order to provide insights for educators of professional learners in other helping disciplines.

Ms. Garvey was a committed adult learner who came to view herself as a capable, competent, and effective teacher of science; it is noteworthy that she maintained her professional efforts up until retirement. This finding is in contrast to research indicating that some educators in the later years of their career become less effective in their teaching and more subject to declining commitment to change efforts (Day, 2008). As noted by researchers in adult development and education, many teachers do not advance beyond the mid-level of competency from adopting and maintaining a rigid personal perspective in teaching (Berliner, 2004; Dreyfus & Dreyfus, 1986).

For Ms. Garvey to develop to the expert stage in science teaching and transform her professional identity from a novice, didactic, textbook instructor to an accomplished science educator, she needed to acquire a range of knowledge domains: technical knowledge in science topics, communicative knowledge of how to engage students actively in collaborative learning, and emancipatory knowledge of how to help students express their thinking and consider alternative ideas through discourse and argumentation with their peers (Cranton, 2016). Yet, the acquisition of these knowledge bases required agency on Ms. Garvey's part (Coldron & Smith, 1999). She was empowered not only through her own internal characteristics of self-reflection, self-efficacy, motivation, personal interests, passions, and self-determined mission, but also through external factors such as administrative and collegial support and respect for her autonomous decision-making (Connelly & Clandinin, 1999; Conway, 2001; Peno & Silva Mangiante, 2014; Short & Rinehart, 1992). These factors promoted her resilience in this transformative learning process (Day & Gu, 2014).

Rogers' learning theory (1983) provides a possible explanation of how Ms. Garvey employed these internal and external factors to transform her professional identity over time. Rogers posited that learners can have significant professional learning gains by evaluating their needs, pursuing meaningful learning opportunities, and incorporating personal interests to deepen their practice. The evidence indicated that Ms. Garvey's professional identity unfolded, in part, from her motivation to reflect on her practice, identify next steps in her development, seek resources to fulfil those needs, and incorporate personal passions from her sub-identities to make learning meaningful. Rogers (1983) noted that self-initiated learning becomes responsible learning through evaluation of one's learning.

> It is when the individual has to take the responsibility for deciding what criteria are important to him, what goals must be achieved, and the extent to which he has achieved those goals, that he truly learns to take responsibility for himself and his directions. (p. 158)

Ms. Garvey's perception of how to transform her science teaching practice involved taking responsibility for seeking out more comprehensive professional development opportunities to increase her content and pedagogical knowledge. Consistent with research indicating the impact of increased science content knowledge on teachers' efficacy and effectiveness in science teaching (Newton & Newton, 2001; Roth et al., 2011), Ms. Garvey knew that she needed to supplement her content knowledge in order to engage students in more complex, interconnected, and meaningful science learning opportunities. Ms. Garvey was aware of the changes to the land and ocean from human activities across the globe and felt it was her responsibility to focus on environmental sustainability. Acquisition of professional subject area knowledge or technical knowledge empowered Ms. Garvey to transform her teaching and strengthen her professional identity as a teacher who promotes environmental responsibility (Beijaard et al., 2000; Cranton, 2016; Klecher & Loadman, 1998).

Ms. Garvey's approach parallels Lange's (2012) call to address issues of social and environmental sustainability in transformative learning, not merely from an emotional response, but by including knowledge in conscious thought. However, Lange cautions that educators cannot assume that activities and content on sustainability will shift students' thinking. Rather, teachers can view their role of promoting discourse as "a mirror against which assumptions are evaluated" with the potential of transforming students' conceptions (p. 205). From Ms. Garvey's own professional development, she came to view her science teacher identity as one that fosters and values students' critical analyses about global issues.

The findings also suggested that Ms. Garvey's role of self-evaluation and personal responsibility (Rogers, 1983) was promoted further when the school supported her efforts in professional growth (Coldron & Smith, 1999; Day & Gu, 2014). From administrators' trust in her decisions and willingness to give her space to collaborate with community specialists to incorporate meaningful applications into the science curriculum, Ms. Garvey felt safe to develop more advanced learning opportunities for her students. This case provides evidence that teachers can be empowered and resilient in their efforts when they perceive that administration respects their judgments and recognizes their accomplishments. Day and Gu (2014) report that when school leaders and collaborative school communities affirm teachers' efforts, teachers develop resilience, commitment to teaching, and the capacity to negotiate stressors in the profession; teachers also provide higher quality learning opportunities for students. Yet, when school structures are not designed for teacher input into decisions that affect their professional capacity building, teachers may become frustrated and feel undervalued. Coldron and Smith (1999) assert:

Any narrowing of "participation" . . . runs the risk of impoverishing dialogue, and turning the vital community of teachers into a blunt tool of policy. Teachers . . . should be empowered to work and debate with fellow practitioners so that they can watch and learn from one another. (pp. 721–722)

Ms. Garvey's case also indicated the internal conflict that educators may feel when the administration closes off teacher input into professional development choices.

Ms. Garvey's professional identity emanated from choices she made for her own adult learning. Through inquiring into her own practice (Conway, 2001), integrating her sub-identities from her personal life, and engaging collaboratively with other professionals within and outside the education community (Connelly & Clandinin, 1999), Ms. Garvey increased her opportunity for professional autonomy and teacher agency (Coldron & Smith, 1999). Such a transformation is not without potential tensions between administration and teachers, particularly given the current emphasis on accountability for student outcomes (Kennedy, 2014). However, the results of this case study of one elementary teacher of science indicated how she was able to develop her professional identity and meet the intent of the science standards for students' deep learning not only from her own self-directed efforts, but also from support and trust by her administration.

CONCLUSION

The evidence from this research indicated that Ms. Garvey took responsibility for her transformative learning to develop her professional identity by increasing her technical knowledge, practical or communicative knowledge, and emancipatory knowledge (Cranton, 2016). For example, by taking the initiative to participate in professional development early in her career, she gained technical knowledge of science content and inquiry-based learning methods. Ms. Garvey developed her practical or communicative knowledge by engaging one-on-one with farmers, fishermen, and others in the community who became her collaborators in learning and her supporters in discovering how to bring real-world investigations into the science classroom. Finally, over the course of her career, Ms. Garvey developed her emancipatory knowledge about teaching by developing skill in questioning students and strategies to promote students' examination of critical global issues. From these efforts, she altered her perspective on what it meant to become a science teacher and gained freedom from traditional didactic pedagogical practices. Ms. Garvey's transformation took place gradually over the course of her 25 years as a science teacher. During this time, her understanding of her role as an expert science teacher was very different from what it was as a novice teacher. Ms. Garvey noted that this realization was freeing for her in that she now felt ownership and agency to develop learning opportunities that provided potentially transformative experiences for her students in keeping with her own experience of transformation.

It is noteworthy that the findings from this study suggest professional identity development of educators may involve more demanding roles for *both* the teachers and the administrators. Ms. Garvey assumed an active role in identifying her needs and seeking out more comprehensive resources to prepare her in developing rigorous science learning opportunities for her students. This study also suggested a critical role for administrators in providing the type of environment necessary for transformative learning to occur and for a resilient professional identity to be formed. The level of openness and trust afforded to Ms. Garvey by administrators was a factor that influenced her willingness to be self-directed in transforming her professional identity.

Though the findings from a single case cannot be generalized to the larger population of educators across a range of helping professions including healthcare, counseling, social work, and education, Ms. Garvey's extreme case may provide some insight into alternative approaches that could be considered for an educator's transformative learning and professional identity development at different stages of a career. The following suggestions emerged from the research of how educators can take responsibility for their professional identity development and how administrators can support the future development of professional learners.

For educators to develop their professional identity with the self-efficacy and competencies of an expert, personal reflection and effort is required (Coldron & Smith, 1999). An educator makes choices of how to develop his or her professional self. However, an educator's "choice is crucially determined by the array of possibilities he or she perceives as available" (p. 715). Those possibilities are envisioned through the different communities in which the educator is a member or could become a member. In the case of Ms. Garvey, she sought out various human resources (Spillane, Diamond, Walker, Halverson, & Jita, 2001; Varelas et al., 2005): (a) an informal collegial learning community with fellow teachers, (b) community content experts, and (c) professional development trainers. Educators seeking to bolster their self-efficacy in a field also could seek out mentors who understand adult learning and stage development (Volkmann & Anderson, 1998) to help them expand their existing vision of education as well as gain confidence in creating personal meaning in their work and for those they educate (Coldron & Smith, 1999).

Administrators can empower educators by giving them the opportunity to identify their own professional needs (Smylie & Evans, 2006) and act to achieve those goals (Rogers, 1983). However, the results suggested that teachers' learning needs may change throughout a career. Rather than providing the typical one-size-fits-all professional development approach (Smith, 2014), administrators could survey educators for the type of content, professional development, and resources they need. Researchers have suggested that by offering tiered sequential professional development opportunities, administrators are able to meet diverse needs of faculty members at different stages in their careers (Coldron & Smith, 1999; Day, 2008). By providing more advanced professional learning opportunities, administrators create a venue from which to identify educational leaders, with similar personal attributes as Ms. Garvey, to serve as human resources to colleagues (Spillane et al., 2001) who could help fellow educators envision a path for their own development and offer a potential community for collaboration. In addition, this approach would allow administrators to call upon educational leaders as resources to offer the next tier of professional development. Finally, administrators could encourage relationship-building with community members and organizations in order for educators to seek out other avenues for learning in their own areas of interest as an alternative form of professional development.

This report of the transformative learning of one exemplary teacher of science who began her career lacking knowledge and confidence in her teaching provides insight for administrators and professionals from a range of educational fields into how her professional identity development is possible. It illuminates how one teacher's choices for adult learning not only strengthened her self-efficacy and influenced the quality of her teaching, but also provided students with meaningful learning experiences that hold the potential to shape their own identities as capable, inquiring citizens.

REFERENCES

Beijaard, D., Meijer, P. C., & Verloop, N. (2004). Reconsidering research on teachers' professional identity. *Teaching and Teacher Education, 20*(2), 107–128.

Beijaard, D., Verloop, N., & Vermunt, J. D. (2000). Teachers' perception of professional identity: An exploratory study from a personal knowledge perspective. *Teaching and Teacher Education, 16*(7), 749–764.

Belli, R. (1998). The structure of autobiographical memory and the event history calendar: Potential improvements in the quality of retrospective reports in surveys. *Memory, 6*(4), 383–406.

Berliner, D. C. (2004). Describing the behavior and documenting the accomplishments of expert teachers. *Bulletin of Science, Technology & Science, 24*(3), 200–212.

Coldron, J., & Smith, R. (1999). Active location in teachers' construction of their professional identities. *Journal of Curriculum Studies, 31*(6), 711–726.

Connelly, F. M., & Clandinin, D. J. (1999). *Shaping a professional identity: Stories of education practice.* London, England: Althouse Press.

Conway, P. (2001). Anticipatory reflection while learning to teach: From a temporally truncated to a temporally distributed model of reflection in teacher education. *Teaching and Teacher Education, 17*(1), 89–106.

Cooper, K., & Olson, M. R. (1996). The multiple 'I's' of teacher identity. In M. Kompf, W. R. Bond, D. Dworet, & R. T. Boak (Eds.), *Changing research and practice: Teachers' professionalism, identities and knowledge* (pp. 78–89). London, England: The Falmer Press.

Cranton, P. (2016). *Understanding and promoting transformative learning: A guide to theory and practice* (3rd ed.). Sterling, VA: Stylus.

Davis, K. S. (2003). "Change is hard": What science teachers are telling us about reform and teacher learning of innovative practices. *Science Education, 87*(1), 3–20.

Day, C. (2008). Committed for life? Variations in teachers' work, lives, and effectiveness. *Journal of Educational Change, 9*(3), 243–260.

Day, C., & Gu, Q. (2014). *Resilient teachers, resilient schools.* Oxford, England: Routledge.

Day, C., Stobart, G., Sammons, P., Kington, A., Gu, Q., Smees, R., & Mujtaba, T. (2006). *Variation in teachers' work, lives and effectiveness.* London, England: Department of Education and Skills.

Dreyfus, H. L., & Dreyfus, S. E. (1986). *Mind over machine: The power of human intuition and expertise in the era of the computer.* New York, NY: Free Press.

Ewan, C. (1988). Becoming a doctor. In K. Cox and C. Ewan (Eds.), *The medical teacher* (pp. 83–87). Edinburgh, Scotland: Churchill Livingstone.

Feiman-Nemser, S., & Floden, R. E. (1986). The cultures of teaching. In M. C. Wittrock (Ed.), *Handbook of research on teaching* (pp. 505–526). New York, NY: Macmillan.

Gee, J. P. (2000). Identity as an analytic lens for research in education. *Review of Research in Education, 25*(1), 99–125.

Glaser, B., & Strauss, A. L. (1967). *The discovery of grounded theory: Strategies for qualitative research.* Chicago, IL: Aldine.

Goodson, I. F., & Numan, U. (2002). Teachers' life worlds, agency and policy contexts. *Teachers and Teaching: Theory and Practice, 8*(3), 269–277.

Jobe, J. B., Tourangeau, R., & Smith, A. F. (1993). Contributions of survey research to the understanding of memory. *Applied Cognitive Psychology, 7*(7), 567–584.

Kennedy, A. (2014). Models of continuing professional development: A framework for analysis. *Professional Development in Education, 40*(3), 336–351.

Klecher, B. M., & Loadman, W. E. (1998). Another look at the dimensionality of the School Participant Empowerment Scale. *Educational and Psychological Measurement, 58*(6), 944–954.

Knowles, G. J. (1992). Models for understanding pre-service and beginning teachers' biographies: Illustrations from case studies. In I. F. Goodson (Ed.), *Studying teachers' lives* (pp. 99–152). London, England: Routledge.

Lange, E. A. (2012). Transforming transformative learning through sustainability and the new science. In E. W. Taylor, P. Cranton, & Associates (Eds.), *The handbook of transformative learning: Theory, research, and practice* (pp. 195–211). San Francisco, CA: Jossey-Bass.

Merriam, S. B. (1998). *Qualitative research and case study applications in education.* San Francisco, CA: Jossey-Bass.

Moore Johnson, S. (2004). *Finders keepers: Helping new teachers survive and thrive in our schools.* San Francisco, CA: Jossey-Bass.

National Research Council. (1996). *National science education standards*. Washington, DC: National Academic Press.

National Research Council. (2012). *A framework for K–12 science education: Practices, crosscutting concepts, and core ideas*. Washington, DC: National Academies Press.

Newton, D. P., & Newton, L. D. (2001). Subject content knowledge and teacher talk in the primary science classroom. *European Journal of Teacher Education, 24*(3), 369–378.

NGSS Lead States. (2013). *Next generation science standards: For states by states*. Washington, DC: Achieve Inc.

Patton, M. Q. (2002). *Qualitative research & evaluation methods* (3rd ed.). Thousand Oaks, CA: SAGE.

Peno, K., & Silva Mangiante, E. (2014). Rear view mirror: A retrospective by retired teachers on learning to teach from novice to expert. In C. J. Boden & K. P. King (Eds.), *Developing and sustaining adult learners* (pp. 335–356). Charlotte, NC: Information Age.

Rogers, C. R. (1983). *Freedom to learn for the 80's*. Columbus, OH: Merrill.

Roth, K. J., Garnier, H. E., Chen, C., Lemmens, M., Schwille, K., & Wickler, N. I. Z. (2011). Videotaped lesson analysis: Effective science PD for teacher and student learning. *Journal of research in science teaching, 48*(2), 117–148.

Schwarz, N. (2007). Retrospective and concurrent self-reports: The rationale for real-time data capture. In A. A. Stone, S. S. Shiffman, A. Atienza, & L. Nebeling (Eds.), *The science of real-time data capture: Self-reports in health research* (pp. 11–26). New York, NY: Oxford University Press.

Settlage, J., Southerland, S. A., Smith, L. K., & Ceglie, R. (2009). Constructing a doubt-free teaching self: Self-efficacy, teacher identity, and science instruction within diverse settings. *Journal of Research in Science Teaching, 46*(1), 102–125.

Short, P. M., & Rinehart, J. S. (1992). School participant empowerment scale: Assessment of level of empowerment in the school environment. *Educational and Psychological Measurement, 52*(4), 951–961.

Smith, G. (2014). An innovative model of professional development to enhance the teaching and learning of primary science in Irish schools. *Professional Development in Education, 40*(3), 467–487.

Smith, L. K., & Southerland, S. A. (2007). Reforming practice or modifying reforms? Elementary teachers' response to the tools of reform. *Journal of Research in Science Teaching, 44*(3), 396–423.

Smolleck, L. A., & Yoder, E. P. (2008). Further development and validation of the Teaching Science as Inquiry (TSI) instrument. *School Science and Mathematics, 108*(7), 291–297.

Smylie, M. A., & Evans, A. E. (2006). Social capital and the problem of implementation. In M. I. Honig (Ed.), *New directions in education policy implementation: Confronting complexity* (pp. 187–208). Albany, NY: The State University of New York Press.

Spillane, J. P., Diamond, J. B., Walker, L. J., Halverson, R., & Jita, L. (2001). Urban school leadership for elementary science instruction: Identifying and activating resources in an undervalued school subject. *Journal of Research in Science Teaching, 38*(8), 918–940.

Varelas, M., House, R., & Wenzel, S. (2005). Beginning teachers immersed into science: Scientist and science teacher identities. *Science Education, 89*(3), 492–516.

Volkmann, M. J., & Anderson, M. A. (1998). Creating professional identity: Dilemmas and metaphors of a first-year chemistry teacher. *Science Education, 82*(3), 293–310.

Wallace, J., & Louden, W. (1992). Science teaching and teachers' knowledge: Prospects for reform of elementary classrooms. *Science Education, 76*(5), 507–521.

Wheatley, K. F. (2002). The potential benefits of teacher efficacy doubts for educational reform. *Teaching and Teacher Education, 18*(1), 5–22.

CHAPTER 9

USING TRANSFORMATIONAL LEARNING AS A FRAMEWORK FOR MEDICAL STUDENT REMEDIATION EXPERIENCES AND PROFESSIONAL IDENTITY FORMATION

Pamela O'Callaghan
University of South Florida

Kelly E. McCarthy
University of South Florida

Deborah J. DeWaay
University of South Florida

ABSTRACT

The transformation from a novice student to a competent medical professional is a daunting experience. Medical students must demonstrate a considerable

Transformative Learning in Healthcare and Helping Professions Education, pages 175–194
Copyright © 2019 by Information Age Publishing
175

amount of scientific knowledge and develop extensive clinical skills all while establishing their own set of values and commitments to the field of medicine. During this journey, some students develop academic, clinical, or professional deficiencies. Addressing these discrepancies through remediation interventions and other curricular mandates is essential to the development of a student's professional identity and subsequent performance as a physician. While remediation plans are unique to each student, having an established structure to guide the process is helpful to achieve satisfactory results. This chapter utilizes Mezirow's transformational learning theory as a framework for structuring remediation as it provides a holistic approach and encourages attention to critical reflection and dialectical discourse. Each of Mezirow's original 10 phases is explored and stories of struggling students are shared throughout the chapter to illustrate the need for, and use of, transformational learning in remediation. By utilizing remediation as a transformational experience, students are better equipped to develop the necessary competencies and confidence in their journey to become practicing physicians.

Within this chapter, we present the stories of students who have stumbled during their medical education experience and the simultaneous development of their professional identities through the lens of Mezirow's (1991) transformational learning theory. According to Fuks, Brawer, and Boudreau (2012), "to be a physician requires a transformation of the individual—one does not simply learn to be a physician, one becomes a physician" (p. 124). In simple terms, doctoring cannot be defined by the accumulation of skills, but instead by the interaction between doctor and patient; the process encompasses both the arts and sciences and is driven forward by reflection. In a similar manner, transformative learning is the development of autonomous thinking, based on the interpretation of one's experience guided by reflection (Mezirow, 1996, 1997).

When a student struggles, it creates a divergence between the expectancy to become a skilled clinician and the need to overcome personal challenges (Derderian & Kenkel, 2016). Remediation, however, can serve as a catalyst for students to reflect on what hindered their progress, adjust their frames of reference, and gain heightened potential (Jarvis-Selinger, Pratt, & Regehr, 2012). Therefore, when a medical student faces academic uncertainty, remediation can become a transformative learning experience that bolsters professional identity and academic development.

PROFESSIONAL IDENTITY FORMATION

Medical education is a perpetual process. To practice evidence-based medicine, a clinician must continue to acquire knowledge throughout the years of practice to better incorporate scientific evidence into patient care (Masic,

Miokovic, & Muhamedagic, 2008). Therefore, practicing medicine is a life-long educational endeavor. The formal training in medical education occurs in two separate but related levels that follow successful completion of a baccalaureate degree: undergraduate medical education (UME) and graduate medical education (GME). At the conclusion of UME, students obtain a Doctor of Medicine degree and are referred to as doctors; nonetheless, according to the Federation of State Medical Boards (2018), graduates must complete an additional 1 to 3 years of GME training to receive a medical license and independently practice medicine in the United States. The development of medical knowledge, clinical skills, and professional behavioral standards is critical during medical school because physicians are expected to demonstrate a wide range of abilities and competencies when they begin a GME program for residency training. Therefore, current pedagogical initiatives seek to develop professional identity in medical students to ensure appropriate behavioral responses to the stresses and demands of being a physician (Olive & Abercrombie, 2017).

Professional identity formation has become a cornerstone of medical education and practice (Howe, Smajdor, & Stöckl, 2012). In medical education, professionalism serves as "the foundation of the professional trust and fiduciary relationship between physicians and patients, as well as for the contract between the medical profession and society" (Holden, Buck, Clark, Szauter, & Tumble, 2012, pp. 246–247). Cruess, Cruess, Boudreau, Snell, and Steinert (2014, 2015) postulate that the identity development of a physician is based on a series of characteristics, commitments, and beliefs that are solidified through the completion of practical experiences during education. These events can take place individually, relationally, with close individuals, or collectively, within a larger social group (Luyckx, Schwartz, Goossens, Beyers, & Missotten, 2011). As these experiences build, the student's morals, values, and self-awareness evolve (Branch & Frankel, 2016; Holden et al., 2012).

When students begin their clinical training, professionalism becomes an important element to their professional identity formation (Branch, 2010; Monrouxe, Rees, & Hu, 2011). According to Swick (2000), physicians who have developed a professional identity adhere to moral and ethical standards, put the needs of others first, demonstrate competency in areas of practice, and commit to reflective assessment of practice to direct ongoing scholarship. The process is similar to Mezirow's (1978) phase model of adult learning which involves becoming more reflective, being more open to the perspectives of others, and being less defensive and more accepting of new ideas.

REMEDIATION

The transformation of medical students, many of whom have been trained as "applied scientists" into humanistic physician-healers is a daunting task (Kearsley, 2015). Medical school is an arduous journey for many, with approximately 10% to 15% of students requiring academic remediation in the form of individualized learning plans to achieve competency (Audétat, Lubarsky, Blais, & Charlin, 2013; Guerrasio, Garrity, & Aagaard, 2014; Holland, 2016). Although these students struggle, they still have tremendous potential and can often exceed expectations when previously unperceived weaknesses are addressed (Derderian & Kenkel, 2016). While recognizing students' performance gaps can cause them to self-doubt their abilities, focused interventions can produce global improvements in their performance (Guerrasio et al., 2014). The use of these remediation interventions can serve as a turning point to challenge students in unique ways, especially in relation to their self-image as future physicians.

Cleland et al. (2013), in a systematic review of remediation programs in undergraduate medical education, identified 31 studies that included both a remediation intervention and outcome data. They found conflicting evidence about the effectiveness of remediation, and in studies that included long-term follow-up, improvements were not sustained. Within medical education, it remains unclear how a lack of competence should be addressed before promotion from one academic level to the next (Audétat et al., 2013). The cost of remediation is high, and educational interventions are resource intensive for a small number of learners. Faculty and staff often devote considerable time and effort serving on student promotion committees and discussing student performance at departmental meetings. Finding ways to adapt theory-based methodologies to remediation of medical students is critical because those who exhibit poor clinical judgment, knowledge, or skills may pose a risk of significant harm to the public at large (Durning et al., 2011).

The experiences of struggling medical students are rarely shared among colleagues, administrators, or disseminated to a wider audience. Therefore, we provide descriptive snapshots of the lived experiences of medical students who underwent remediation to illustrate the key learning phases of Mezirow's (1996) theory of transformational learning. While the qualitative examples are not empirical nor intended to be fully representative of all learners, they represent trends and impressions collected over several years while working with students who experienced severe academic difficulty. As there is a call to reform remediation in medical education, the aim of this chapter is to initiate a discussion regarding the potential remediation holds to function as a transformational learning experience for students.

TRANSFORMATIONAL LEARNING
FRAMEWORK FOR REMEDIATION

Mezirow (1997) proposed that transformative learning often follows a stepwise progression, although some scholars have asserted a more recursive or spiraling progress to the change involved (Taylor, 2008). Each of the original phases that Mezirow proposed prepares the learner to become an autonomous thinker, capable of making socially responsible decisions in environments of rapid change (Mezirow, 1997). The outcome of transformative learning can be considered comparable to the goals of medical education: to enable a learner to develop deep levels of cognitive thinking and well-defined affective skills. In medical programs, this is achieved by integrating scientific content with experiential learning opportunities to train students to understand the complex needs of their patients and to determine the best treatment options for care (Oh, Chung, Han, Woo, & Deiter, 2016). This focus is particularly appropriate in apprenticeship learning settings like medicine, "where what is 'learned' is not in the complete control of teacher or learner; it emerges as a consequence of the social interaction, which is shaped by the physical, social and organizational context" (Lingard, 2009, p. 267). Remediation, viewed in terms of transformative learning, provides an opportunity for unsuccessful learners to reformulate the meaning of their experiences (Cranton, 1994) in a specific, intense, and focused environment that embodies compassion for all learners (Ellaway, Chou, & Kalet, 2018). In addition to meaning making, medical education remediation serves as a guide to get students back on course with their journey towards developing the necessary skills and professional identity of a competent physician (Kalet, Chou, & Ellaway, 2017).

Phase 1: A Disorienting Dilemma

Phase 1 of transformative learning occurs when a student experiences a disorienting dilemma. For struggling students, unsatisfactory performance is almost always a jarring event, throwing them off their normal stride in the process. According to Mezirow (1991), these types of learning events are "epochal" and serve as a reference point for a qualitative shift in the student's approach to learning. When the disorienting dilemma involves failure, it exposes the learner's limitations and areas for improvement, causing learners to pause and question their epistemological beliefs (Wittich, Reed, McDonald, Varkey, & Beckman, 2010). However, not all problematic performance brings about a transformation. To facilitate the process, an educator, through the process of remediation, must make students aware of their abilities to improve and assist them as they engage in the transformative learning process (Mezirow, 2009). It is critical for the student to want to improve since this constitutes a starting point to foster transformative learning efforts. It is also important to understand the impact the disorienting dilemma can have on a student's professional identity formation. Jarvis-Selinger et al. (2012) emphasize that, like transformational learning, transitions in professional identity formation are marked by abrupt discontinuities precipitated by a "crisis." Similar to a disorienting dilemma, these events occur when there is a discrepancy between students' understanding of themselves in a professional role and their understanding of the experiences and challenges they are facing.

Although episodes of discontinuity and crises are natural and necessary aspects of the developmental process within professional identity formation, it is essential for educators to help learners manage discontinuities and effectively navigate the transition from one form of identity to another. When medical learners underperform, the crises represent a crucial period of increased vulnerability and heightened potential. Most importantly, professional identity formation must be the focus of attention in parallel with improvement of skills and knowledge during remediation in order to influence the aspiring physician's understanding of what it means to "be" a doctor (Jarvis-Selinger et al., 2012).

The next two steps in the process of transformative learning involve critical reflection. Mezirow (1991) differentiated among three types of reflection on experience: content, process, and premise reflection. Content reflection is thinking about the actual experience itself; process reflection is thinking how to handle the experience; and premise reflection involves reexamining long-held, socially constructed assumptions, beliefs, and values about the experience or problem (Merriam, 2004). Only premise reflection, or critical reflection on assumptions, can lead to transformative learning, according to Mezirow. While critical reflection is a key part of transformational learning, it also serves as a foundation for professional identity formation; it fosters "practical wisdom" for engaging in messy complexities of practice and potentially influences choices of how to act in difficult or morally ambiguous circumstances (Wald, 2015). The transformation process, according to Mezirow, "always involves critical reflection upon the distorted premises sustaining our structure of expectation" (p. 167). Without critical self-reflection, personal and professional identity transformation cannot occur. Therefore, it is important to create opportunities during the remediation process for medical students to critically reflect on the impact of their struggles upon their self-identities before undertaking skill or academic development.

Phase 2: Self-Examination
With Feelings of Guilt or Shame

Phase 2 of the transformative process focuses on critical reflection where the student must self-examine the feelings of shame or guilt that often accompany underperformance. There is an implicit assumption that medical students are predominantly high-functioning and successful; therefore, they are not expected to fail. Patel, Tarrant, Bonas, and Shaw (2015) conducted a qualitative analysis of interviews with medical students who had experienced high-stakes failure and were required to repeat a year of medical school. They identified that the experience of failing a course, clerkship, or licensing exam during medical school can generate significant emotional trauma for the student. In addition, the way in which students comprehend their situation influences the experience of remediation. Critical reflection often generates these emotional responses to poor performance, and at times may reveal feelings of deep inadequacy.

Medical students who lack the ability to see themselves as physicians are characterized by chronic feelings of self-doubt and fear of being discovered as intellectual frauds; this is commonly referred to as "imposter syndrome" (Villwock, Sobin, Koester, & Harris, 2016). Upon starting medical school, students are expected to immerse themselves in the values and behaviors consistent with physicianship. Often, this process requires students to "go through the motions" of being a physician before they can fully embody this role. Struggling students lack a sense of belonging to the professional community of medicine. Despite evidence of being intellectually capable, students suffering from impostor syndrome are unable to internalize a sense of accomplishment, competence, or skill. Most importantly, imposter syndrome can hinder a student's willingness to volunteer answers and information, leading to innate differences in learning style (Villwock et al., 2016). In the vignette below, Sharpless et al. (2015) provide an account of imposter syndrome in which a third-year medical student was asked to reflect on how the role of "pretending" impacts professional life.

We are apprentices, not yet masters. And like the sorcerer's apprentice, it is expected that when we attempt to wear the "magic hat," some havoc will ensue. The educational system acknowledges us as learners who need guidance if we are to fully develop our abilities, and in my experience, this offers some protection against self-doubt. Instead, a different kind of pretending plagues me: pretending that I am finished with the challenges of the apprenticeship process. I am tempted to escape the present moment (with its difficult lessons) and imagine that I have already passed through the fires of medical school and residency, and have emerged on the other side without needing to be burned and shaped by them. If I struggle with pretending, it is not so much with the notion of "fake it 'til I make it," for instructors reassure me that they do not expect perfection. Rather, I struggle with remaining present through this difficult process of PIF [professional identity formation], so I can fully experience what it is like to be ignorant, even as I strive to gain knowledge. (p. 714)

The critical reflection steps in the process of transformative learning embody the key theme of rational discourse. Rationality is about hearing other points of view, examining evidence and reaching consensus to better under the experience of the struggling learner. Entering and progressing through these phases is vital for the student's successful remediation.

Phase 3: A Critical Assessment of Epistemic Assumptions

The focus of Phase 3 is the critical reflection of assumptions, such as one's own beliefs about how to solve problems. Mezirow emphasizes a frame of reference as a way of knowing (Kegan, 2009). Understanding one's philosophical concept of knowledge and the rationality of beliefs is critical to both transformative learning and remediation. In medical education, how students view knowledge will influence their approach to studying and problem solving. Holland (2016), in a critical review of medical students' motivation after failure, proposed that adopting clinically-oriented patterns of knowledge are essential to a student's success. A medical student must move away from a biophysical view of knowledge, focused on the biological and physical factors of a system, towards a more heuristic pattern of understanding which incorporates both theory and practice to learn the skill of clinical reasoning. This is similar to Mezirow's (1991) shift from an instrumental form of learning to communicative learning in which a student begins to understand the psychocultural assumptions related to knowing.

Critical reflection can challenge the established definition of a problem being addressed, and, potentially, reorient a student's problem-solving efforts in a more effective way (Mezirow, 1990). If a student with a biophysical or instrumental belief of knowledge struggles, the student often believes the only way to improve performance is to expand upon the fund of knowledge, as opposed to modifying how knowledge and learning are constructed; such students are more likely to have a maladaptive response to failure (Holland, 2016). Faculty members who are charged with remediation must understand that a student's existing conception of knowledge and learning will shape how that student interprets guidance (Mattick & Knight, 2007). Through critical reflection, the goal is to help students better understand themselves as learners (Mezirow, 1991).

Epistemological transitions are also critical to the development of a professional identity in physicians. Knight and Mattick (2006) propose that a key feature of a physician's professional identity formation occurs when a medical student's epistemological thinking expands beyond the scientific ways of knowing to encompass a humanistic, experiential way of knowing related to each patient's individual experience. This understanding of knowledge is an example of Mezirow's (1991) premise reflection which "makes possible a more inclusive, discriminating, and integrating perspective" (p. 167). Researchers have demonstrated that when medical students begin to value knowledge beyond scientific authority, it improves their clinical reasoning and encourages sincerer attention with patient interactions (Oh et al., 2016). Therefore, remediation should aim to challenge why, what, and how individuals study and view their conception of learning.

Medical students can suspend transformation at this stage, becoming "caught in their own history and reliving it" (Mezirow, 1978, p. 101). Students can become resistant, choosing to focus on instrumental forms of learning because they attribute their weak performance to a lack of knowledge. The practice of medicine often presents as an ill-structured problem; a student must weigh empirical evidence along with subjective evidence, such as a patient's narrative, to generate meaning from the information (Assenheimer, Knox, Nadarajah, & Zimitat, 2016). Some students will focus on increasing their fund of knowledge without changing their existing frames of reference. Although an increase in content knowledge may allow the student to pass an exam, this method impedes the ability to improve clinical reasoning. The following serves as an example for how these behaviors can impede a student's journey to become a physician.

Although Laura Jacobs (a pseudonym) had excelled in college, she found medical school hard going. At the conclusion of her first year as a medical trainee, she had passed all her courses but failed the end-of-year comprehensive exam. The Academic Performance Review Committee voted to have her repeat the first year of training. Laura appealed the decision and was granted an opportunity to move on to the second year of course work. Afraid to acknowledge her own shortcomings, Laura rejected advice to change her learning approach; she subsequently failed the first two courses of year two and was mandated to take a leave of absence and restart year two in the fall. As part of her remediation, Laura was also required to meet with the school's learning specialist. Laura was resistant to take ownership of her academic outcomes. Instead, she blamed the curriculum and other outside influences which she deemed had set her up for failure. Laura had also refused to participate in a study group created as part of her remediation plan.

Although Laura was resistant to change her study approach during the remediation process, eventually she successfully passed all her courses. Next, she began an independent study period to prepare for her first national board examination, commonly referred to as Step 1. Despite reporting a rigorous study schedule, Laura could not pass any practice exams. After extending her study period from two months to four months, she took the exam as required and failed by 15 points. Again, she was required to meet with the learning specialist who recommended a new approach. This new plan incorporated additional resources and required closer monitoring; nonetheless, Laura refused. She insisted that she ran out of time to prepare, but with several additional months for preparation, Laura was confident she could pass. After taking the exam a second time, she failed again. When the learning specialist called to inform her of the results, Laura was shocked. She reported feeling great while taking the exam and felt confident she passed this time, when, in fact, she scored one point lower than her previous attempt. Her inability to pass the exam ultimately resulted in her leaving the program.

This example highlights the importance of critical reflection. Laura was unable to reflect on the issues surrounding her academic difficulties and thus could not develop an effective plan to improve her performance. Merriam (2004) has argued that a certain level of cognitive development is required to be able to engage in the transformative learning process. Mezirow (2000) also commented that not everyone is fully prepared to participate in the process. Therefore, it is imperative that adult educators create "the conditions for and the skills of effective adult reasoning and the disposition for transformative learning—including critical reflection and dialectical discourse" (Mezirow, 2003, p. 62).

Phase 4: Recognition That
the Transformative Process Is a Shared Event

After deep self-reflection, students move to Phase 4 where they must recognize their discontent and realize the process of transformation is not unique to an individual's situation if they are to succeed in remediation efforts. Laura was unable to make this leap in her thinking and her approach to learning, but for those who do, this phase is similar to the concept of common humanity: "Seeing one's experiences as part of the larger human experience rather than seeing them as separating and isolating" (Neff, 2003, p. 89). It is important for students to recognize that others have negotiated similar setbacks successfully. This new awareness validates remediation as a temporary situation, an experience which the student can transcend to become a better, stronger, and more resilient learner. This transformation requires the student to act upon new insights, leading to the next phase. Within medical education remediation, it is important to have an open dialogue with students and remind them that although their struggles have become a part of their education process, they do not define their ability to become successful physicians.

Phase 5: Exploration of Options for New Roles, Relationships, and Actions

Phase 5 represents action as students explore new roles as learners by trying new learning techniques, working within a group of learners, or changing how they acquire new information. Samenow, Worley, Neufeld, Fishel, and Swiggart (2013) provide an example of how to apply transformative learning in a professional development program as a way to correct disruptive physician behavior. The curriculum utilized experiential exercises and role playing to explore and practice new skills and behavior in a safe group process. Program learning objectives for Phase 5 included the discussion of disruptive behavior from the viewpoints of staff, patients, colleagues, and administrators, as well as methods to establish healthy boundaries and the appropriate expression of emotions in the workplace.

Furthermore, Patel et al. (2015) found that during remediation, students need to develop self-awareness to recognize the links between personal growth (and struggles) and their sense of professional competence. Remediation learning plans need to include activities that are designed to boost students' self-efficacy (confidence to achieve specific tasks) for reflective learning alongside development of their professional confidence. The following vignette outlines such a learning plan and subsequent reflection by a former student who had experienced significant setbacks during medical education and had all but lost hope of fulfilling his dream to be a physician.

Abe Johnson (a pseudonym) was an exceptional student. In fact, he was accepted as a high school student to a prestigious seven-year combined BS/MD program. Accelerated combined programs allow students to earn a bachelor's degree in three years and then proceed directly into a four-year medical program. Abe earned his BA degree with highest honor and entered medical school confident his success would continue. Unfortunately, Abe encountered a minor bump in the road at the end of his second year which quickly escalated into multiple failures, lapses in professionalism, and eventually dismissal from the school. The Dean recognized that these events were not a reflection of Abe's ability, but, instead, the result of a series of events, including poorly structured and administered remediation.

Abe was reinstated into the medical school under the condition he follow a rigid learning plan. Abe's learning plan was specifically designed to simultaneously build clinical skill competency and confidence. There was concern that Abe viewed remediation as a never-ending cycle that he could not escape; therefore, his first requirement was to teach physical exam skills to first and second year medical students who had requested extra practice. Abe was astounded that he was allowed to work as a physician educator as he had previously seen himself as an inferior student, often working in isolation. Abe quickly rose to the occasion, expertly preparing for each session; his professionalism and academic performance were exceptional once again. In fact, not only did Abe graduate from medical school, he earned a residency position at a prestigious academic program. The following are edited excerpts from Abe's personal statement for residency, used with permission:

> I am determined, resilient, and humble. After taking a leave of absence (due to remediation), I re-joined my classmates, who were three rotations ahead of me. The [specialty] clerkship was a challenge as my peers performed better than me. . .Although I initially lacked in medical knowledge, I have compensated with hard work, determination, and resilience to build my clinical knowledge, skills, and techniques. The difficulties I experienced. . .taught me that anyone, at any time, can hit a wall. I learned that determination and resilience, mixed with humility, can allow anyone to get back up and carry on toward their dream.

Students who undergo remediation may feel stymied and want to use the same learning techniques and resources they utilized prior to their failure. Therefore, it is important for staff to develop a wide range of support options for students to utilize during the remediation experience and these opportunities should challenge the learner's traditional beliefs of how learning best occurs. As shared in this vignette, the student did not feel equipped, nor did he see the value, in working as a physician educator. However, these experiential learning encounters created a rich environment in which he was driven to improve his content knowledge and gain practical clinical understanding through successful teaching experiences to further develop his professional identity.

Phase 6: Planning a Course of Action

While the former five phases represent the more affective side of remediation, Mezirow's (1991) remaining phases align with the operational side of the remediation process. Formalized remediation is defined by Guerrasio et al. (2014) as additional teaching above and beyond the standard curriculum, individualized to the learner who, without the additional teaching, would not achieve the necessary skills for the profession. In medical education, these interventions serve to fill competency gaps and better prepare students for their future career endeavors. Unfortunately, there is surprisingly little evidence to guide "best practices" for remediation in medical education, and it remains unclear how a lack of competence should be addressed before promotion (Audétat et al., 2013).

When planning a course of action (Phase 6), remediation methods and strategies need to be selected based on the learner's difficulties. Cleland et al. (2013) provided findings that many remedial interventions lack a theoretical foundation; more often than not, interventions amount to providing "more of the same" to the learner's difficulties. In medical education, although academic problems are often mixed, it is clinical reasoning and not knowledge gaps that are involved in most cases. The remediation methods used by teachers are often not perfectly congruent with the nature of these difficulties. Teachers tend to give priority to reading programs and organizational measures instead of correcting specific problems (Audétat, Voirol, Béland, Fernandez, & Sanche, 2015). Consequently, it is imperative for educators to resist the urge to apply a standardized plan; instead, they need to dig deeper to correctly diagnose the unique issues that the student is facing and thus plan an appropriate course of action to address them.

Phases 7 and 8: Implementing a Plan and Trying on New Roles

After an individualized analysis of performance has identified a learner's areas of difficulty, the student begins the learning phase of the remediation plan (Phase 7). It is best to also integrate Phase 8 (simulation of the desired competency) in concert with the acquisition of knowledge and skills. Studies using current medical school assessment frameworks or remediation programs usually explained less than 30% of the variance in the various outcomes used to assess medical student performance (Durning et al., 2011, p. 490). Molloy (2009) cautions that positioning the student as a passive receiver of ineffective teaching strategies may be detrimental to the student's development of a professional identity. Mezirow (1997) suggests that the educator serve as a facilitator or provocateur in order to foster the self-direction and control need for transformative learning. Therefore, it is not surprising that Todres, Tsimtsiou, Sidhu, Stephenson, and Jones (2012) report that students repeating their final year of undergraduate medical education due to inability to meet performance expectations were unable to connect their learning to future practice, despite being at the end of their remediation plan. This exemplifies the crucial role of supportive relationships in fostering transformative learning during the remediation experience (Taylor, 2009). Educators should view the progression of the plan as a fluid process. Check points can be incorporated so that the student and facilitator can reflect on successes and develop alternatives for resources that are ineffective.

Phase 9: Building Competence
and Self-Confidence in New Roles and Relationships

Successful remediation must also build confidence (Phase 9) while addressing competency issues. Mezirow (2000) encourages educators to continuously confirm and support a learner's sense of personal efficacy to take action on reflective insights during the process of transformation. Kalet et al. (2017) proposed that remediation be reframed from punishment and stigma to training that requires the expertise that comes from appreciative coaching to support struggling learners and manage the remediation process. In this vignette from actual experience, the learner describes the effects of an appreciative coaching approach:

> Sam Green (a pseudonym) was an outstanding resident physician. Unfortunately, his residency program was required to terminate him due to unsatisfactory performance on his final board certification exam. After three attempts on Step 3, the hospital would no longer provide oversight for a physician-in-training. This is when Sam was referred to meet with the learning specialist. The residency program spoke highly of Sam's clinical ability, bedside manner, and his desire to work hard and improve. They also offered hope; if Sam could pass the exam in three months, the hospital guaranteed to re-hire him into the program. It was paramount to recognize that Sam had successfully attained many educational milestones to reach this stage of his career in medical education. After analyzing Sam's performance on multiple choice exams and the results of diagnostic neuropsychological testing, it appeared that Sam was not only a slow reader, but also an inefficient reader. He possessed a strong fund of clinical knowledge, but his application of knowledge was clumsy. His previous struggles primed him to apply all possible knowledge to every aspect of a clinical presentation, slowing him down. Furthermore, when he reached a question he could not confidently answer, he would move on to the next question, but continue to think about the previous question. This technique resulted in cognitive overload.

> To address these deficiencies, a learning plan was created to incorporate frequent testing to improve test-taking skills, content review to build retrieval speed, and a mentoring experience to build confidence. Sam also volunteered to help a medical student with a reading disability prepare for an upcoming exam. By methodically reading practice questions with the medical student, Sam developed a standard approach to multiple-choice questions. Building on Sam's strengths increased his self-confidence. By adopting an appreciative approach, Sam was able to identify how he achieved previous exam successes and build his self-efficacy beliefs which led to improved performance on Step 3 and a successful re-entry into his residency training program.

Appreciative coaching is both pragmatic and hopeful, and invites the construction of a powerful, positive future (Carter, 2009). The application of a strengths-based mindset does not ignore "weaknesses" but reframes remediation to focus on a strength that needs developing. In Sam's situation, this was the application of current knowledge in a straightforward manner to improve efficiency. The appreciative approach to building self-confidence shifts the dialogue from deficit terminology and phrases toward the use of affirmative language in order to help the learner develop expectations and identify provocative potential (Cooperrider, Magruder, & Watkins, 2000).

Phase 10: Reintegration of a Revised Perspective Into Life

Phase 10 is the final phase of transformative learning. It occurs when an individual has fully integrated the conditions dictated by the new perspective (Mezirow, 2000). It also represents the conclusion of remediation, when the student is reintegrated into the curriculum equipped with newfound strengths developed from appreciative coaching. These newly developed skills aid students to achieve clinical competency, which is a fundamental objective of medical education and a necessary component of professional identity formation. With increasing competence, learners both feel and are regarded by their peers and instructors as being more secure in their role; thus, they move away from peripheral participation in medicine's community of practice toward full membership (Lave & Wenger, 1991). This perceived competence feeds back into the socialization process, reinforcing an altered sense of self and helps learners to define and stabilize their identity. Alternatively, if an individual does not feel comfortable in the required role or is perceived as lacking important capabilities, professional identity formation may be compromised (Cruess et al., 2015). Hence, after the remediation plan is complete, it is critical for teachers to continue to check-in and support the student as needed until successful reintegration into the program has been achieved.

DISCUSSION

In order to practice medicine successfully, future doctors must meet the necessary curricular benchmarks and competencies while also developing their own professional identity as a physician. Prior research suggests that when medical students fall short in an academic pursuit, especially one directly related to their identity of becoming physicians, they do not give up their goal; instead, they increase their goal-directed efforts to make sure that they are capable of fulfilling the role of a competent doctor

(Brunstein, 2000). Hence, remediation can serve as a transformational event in the professional development of medical students and trainees. Identifying and addressing lapses in skills throughout the curriculum is essential to creating competent and effective physicians. By crafting communications that stress that remediation is normal, and by assigning interventions that are beneficial to identified deficiencies, it may help to enhance a student's self-efficacy and self-compassion as well as aid in the development of the student's professional identity formation.

Medical school is an exigent experience. Students must acquire a vast array of scientific knowledge and clinical skills while also establishing their own set of beliefs and commitments to the field of medicine. During this journey, some students will develop academic, clinical, or professional deficits. Researchers acknowledge there is a need for the development of a comprehensive approach for addressing undergraduate and graduate medical education deficiencies (Audétat et al., 2013; Holland, 2016). Successful completion of remediation and other curricular mandates is critical to the development of a student's professional identity and subsequent performance as a physician (Brunstein & Gollwitzer, 1996; Cruess et al., 2015; Derderian & Kenkel, 2016; Guerrasio et al., 2014). As medical educators, we should try to incorporate the same humanistic approach in remediation situations that we ideally bring to patient care (Ellaway et al., 2018). A non-punitive, reliable, and transparent remediation process supports a culture where all learners can hold themselves and each other to the very highest standards (Kalet et al., 2017).

Applying Mezirow's (1991) theory of transformative learning as the philosophical underpinning for remediation efforts allows a struggling student to gain greater adaptive capacity to capitalize and act on prior knowledge and experience through critical reflection. Viewing remediation from this perspective requires an enlargement of the current paradigm of linear thinking and all too often cynical view of the less-than-competent medical trainee to one that includes a creative and multifaceted approach to "knowing" (Carter, 2009). Although there is a lack of research on transformative learning theory in creating remedial strategies, it is known that instructors enhance a student's learning experience by promoting critical self-reflection and problem solving in simulation scenarios (Evans & Harder, 2013).

Faculty need to be mindful of how students will learn during remediation, and transformative learning theory seems integral as an approach to support students who are not meeting academic or clinical course objectives with developmental opportunities. Furthermore, "transformative learning, facilitated by an appreciative inquiry approach to practice, has the potential to offer those individuals who are struggling with the old assumptions and unproductive behaviors to discover a learning path of possibility, potential and action" (Carter, 2009, p. 211). Following Mezirow's (1991) phases of transformational learning provides a guided path for medical teachers who are seeking solutions to assist students who encounter difficulties during their education. Utilizing this framework can assist the medical community to develop effective remediation plans that create competent and confident physicians.

REFERENCES

Assenheimer, D., Knox, K., Nadarajah, V. D., & Zimitat, C. (2016). Medical students' epistemological beliefs: Implications for curriculum. *Education for Health, 29*(2), 107–112. https://doi.org/10.4103/1357-6283.188748

Audétat, M. C., Lubarsky, S., Blais, J. G., & Charlin, B. (2013). Clinical reasoning: Where do we stand on identifying and remediating difficulties? *Creative Education, 4*(6a), 42–48. https://doi.org/10.4236/ce.2013.46A008

Audétat, M. C., Voirol, C., Béland, N., Fernandez, N., & Sanche, G. (2015). Remediation plans in family medicine residency. *Canadian Family Physician, 61*(9), 425–434.

Branch, W. T. (2010). The road to professionalism: Reflective practice and reflective learning. *Patient Education and Counseling, 80*(3), 327–332. https://doi.org/10.1016/j.pec.2010.04.022

Branch, W. T., & Frankel, R. (2016). Not all stories of professional identity formation are equal: An analysis of formation narratives of highly humanistic physicians. *Patient Education and Counseling, 99*(8), 1394–1399. https://doi.org/10.1016/j.pec.2016.03.018

Brunstein, J. (2000). Motivation and performance following failure: The effortful pursuit of self-defining goals. *Applied Psychology: An International Review, 49*(3), 340–356.

Brunstein, J. C., & Gollwitzer, P. M. (1996). Effects of failure on subsequent performance: The importance of self-defining goals. *Journal of Personality and Social Psychology, 70*(2), 395–407.

Carter, M. T. (2009). *Appreciative inquiry and adult transformative learning as an integrated framework to guide life coaching practice.* Dissertation Abstracts International: Section B; 70/08. No. 3368983. Retrieved from https://pqdtopen.proquest.com/doc/305108676.html?FMT=ABS

Cleland, J., Leggett, H., Sandars, J., Costa, M. J., Patel, R., & Moffat, M. (2013). The remediation challenge: Theoretical and methodological insights from a systematic review. *Medical Education, 47*(3), 242–251. https://doi.org/10.1111/medu.12052

Cooperrider, D., Magruder, J., & Watkins, K. (2000). Appreciative inquiry: A transformative paradigm. *OD Practitioner, 32*(1), 6–12.

Cranton, P. (1994). Self-directed and transformative instructional development. *Journal of Higher Education, 65*(6), 726–744.

Cruess, R. L., Cruess, S. R., Boudreau, J. D., Snell, L., & Steinert, Y. (2014). Reframing medical education to support professional identity formation. *Academic Medicine, 89*(11), 1446–1451. https://doi.org/10.1097/ACM.0000000000000427

Cruess, R. L., Cruess, S. R., Boudreau, J. D., Snell, L., & Steinert, Y. (2015). A schematic representation of the professional identity formation and socialization of medical students and residents: A guide for medical educators. *Academic Medicine, 90*(6), 718–725.

Derderian, C. A., & Kenkel, J. M. (2016). Remediation as a road to competency: Strategies for early identification of the struggling resident and generating the remediation plan. *The Journal of Craniofacial Surgery, 27*(1), 8–12. https://doi.org/10.1097/SCS.0000000000002375

Durning, S., Cleary, T., Sandars, J., Hemmer, P., Kokotailo, P., & Artino, A. (2011). Viewing "strugglers" through a different lens: How a self-regulated learning perspective can help medical educators with assessment and remediation. *Academic Medicine, 86*(4), 488–495. https://doi.org/10.1097/ACM.0b013e31820dc384

Ellaway, R. H., Chou, C. L., & Kalet, A. L. (2018). Situating remediation: Accommodating success and failure in medical education systems. *Academic Medicine, 93*(3), 391–398. https://doi.org/10.1097/ACM.0000000000001855

Evans, C. J., & Harder, N. (2013). A formative approach to student remediation. *Nurse Educator, 38*(4), 147–151. https://doi.org/10.1097/NNE.0b013e318296dd0f

Federation of State Medical Boards. (2018). *State-specific requirements for initial medical licensure.* Retrieved from https://www.fsmb.org/step-3/state-licensure/

Fuks, A., Brawer, J., & Boudreau, J. D. (2012). The foundation of physicianship. *Perspectives in Biology and Medicine, 55*(1), 114–126. https://doi.org/10.1353/pbm.2012.0002

Guerrasio, J., Garrity, M. J., & Aagaard, E. M. (2014). Learner deficits and academic outcomes of medical students, residents, fellows, and attending physicians referred to a remediation program, 2006–2012. *Academic Medicine, 89*(2), 352–358. https://doi.org/10.1097/ACM.0000000000000122

Holden, M., Buck, E., Clark, M., Szauter, K., & Trumble, J. (2012). Professional identity formation in medical education: The convergence of multiple domains. *HEC Forum, 24*(4), 245–255. https://doi.org/10.1007/s10730-012-9197-6

Holland, C. (2016). Critical review: Medical students' motivation after failure. *Advances in Health Science Education, 21*(3), 695–710. https://doi.org/10.1007/s10459-015-9643-8

Howe, A., Smajdor, A., & Stöckl, A. (2012). Towards an understanding of resilience and its relevance to medical training. *Medical Education, 46*(4), 349–356. https://doi.org/10.1111/j.1365-2923.2011.04188.x

Jarvis-Selinger, S., Pratt, D. D., & Regehr, G. (2012). Competency is not enough: Integrating identity formation into the medical education discourse. *Academic Medicine, 87*(9), 1185–1190. https://doi.org/10.1097/ACM.0b013e3182604968

Kalet, A., Chou, C. L., & Ellaway, R. H. (2017). To fail is human: Remediating remediation in medical education. *Perspectives on Medical Education, 6*(6), 418–424. https://doi.org/10.1007/s40037-017-0385-6

Kearsley, J. H. (2015). Transformative learning as the basis for teaching healing. *International Journal of Whole Person Care, 2*(1), 21–37. Retrieved from http://ijwpc.mcgill.ca/article/download/89/30

Kegan, R. (2009). What "form" transforms? A constructive-developmental approach to transformative learning. In K. Illeris (Ed.), *Contemporary theories of learning* (pp. 35–52). New York, NY: Routledge.

Knight, L. V., & Mattick, K. (2006). 'When I first came here, I thought medicine was black and white': Making sense of medical students' ways of knowing. *Social Science & Medicine, 63*(4), 1084–1096.

Lave, J., & Wenger, E. (1991). *Situated learning: Legitimate peripheral participation.* New York, NY: Cambridge University Press.

Lingard, L. (2009). What we see and don't see when we look at 'competence': Notes on a god term. *Advance in Health Science Education, 14*(5), 625–628. https://doi.org/10.1007/s10459-009-9206-y

Luyckx, K., Schwartz, S. J., Goossens, L., Beyers, W., & Missotten, L. (2011). Processes of personal identity formation and evaluation. In S. J. Schwartz, K. Luyckx, & V. L. Vignoles (Eds.), *Handbook of identity theory and research: Structure and processes* (pp. 77–98). New York, NY: Springer.

Masic, I., Miokovic, M., & Muhamedagic, B. (2008). Evidence based medicine—new approaches and challenges. *Acta Informatica Medica, 16*(4), 219–225. https://doi.org/10.5455/aim.2008.16.219-225

Mattick, K., & Knight, L. (2007). High-quality learning: Harder to achieve than we think? *Medical Education, 41*(7), 638–644. https://doi.org/10.1111/j.1365-2923.2007.02783.x

Merriam, S. B. (2004). The role of cognitive development in Mezirow's transformational learning theory. *Adult Education Quarterly, 55*(1), 60–68.

Mezirow, J. (1978). Perspective transformation. *Adult Education Quarterly, 28*(2), 100–110.

Mezirow, J. (1990). How critical reflection triggers transformative learning. In J. Mezirow (Ed.), *Fostering critical reflection in adulthood: A guide to transformative and emancipatory learning* (pp. 1–20). San Francisco, CA: Jossey-Bass.

Mezirow, J. (1991). *Transformative dimensions in adult learning.* San Francisco, CA: Jossey-Bass.

Mezirow, J. (1996). Contemporary paradigms of learning. *Adult Education Quarterly, 46*(3), 158–173.

Mezirow, J. (1997). Transformative learning: Theory to practice. *New Directions for Adult and Continuing Education, 1997*(74), 5–12.

Mezirow, J. (2000). Learning to think like an adult: Core concepts of transformation theory. In J. Mezirow (Ed.), *Learning as transformation: Critical perspectives on a theory in progress* (pp. 3–33). San Francisco, CA: Jossey-Bass.

Mezirow, J. (2003). Transformative learning as discourse. *Journal of Transformative Education, 1*(1), 58–63.

Mezirow, J. (2009). An overview on transformative learning. In K. Illeris (Ed.), *Contemporary theories of learning* (pp. 92–105). New York, NY: Routledge.

Molloy, E. K. (2009). Time to pause: Feedback in clinical education. In C. Delaney & E. K. Molloy (Eds.), *Clinical education in health professions* (pp. 128–146). Sydney, Australia: Elsevier.

Monrouxe, L. V., Rees, C. E., & Hu, W. (2011). Differences in medical students' explicit discourses of professionalism: Acting, representing, becoming. *Medical Education, 45*(6), 585–602. https://doi.org/10.1111/j.1365-2923.2010.03878.x

Neff, K. (2003). Self-compassion: An alternative conceptualization of a healing attitude toward oneself. *Self and Identity, 2*(2), 85–101. https://doi.org/10.1080/15298860309032

Oh, S., Chung, E., Han, E., Woo, Y., & Deiter, K. (2016). The relationship between medical students' epistemological beliefs and achievement on a clinical performance examination. *Korean Journal of Medical Education, 28*(1), 29–34.

Olive, K. E., & Abercrombie, C. L. (2017). Developing a physician's professional identity through medical education. *The American Journal of the Medical Sciences, 353*(2), 101–108.

Patel, R. S., Tarrant, C., Bonas, S., & Shaw, R. L. (2015). Medical students' personal experience of high-stakes failure: Case studies using interpretative phenomenological analysis. *BMC Medical Education, 15*(86), 1–9. https://doi.org/10.1186/s12909-015-0371-9

Samenow, C. P., Worley, L., Neufeld, R., Fishel, T., & Swiggart, W. H. (2013). Transformative learning in a professional development course aimed at addressing disruptive physician behavior: A composite case study. *Academic Medicine, 88*(1), 117–1223.

Sharpless, J., Baldwin, N., Cook, R., Kofman, A., Morley-Fletcher, A., Slotkin, R., & Wald, H. S. (2015). The becoming: Students' reflections on the process of professional identity formation in medical education. *Academic Medicine, 90*(6), 713–717.

Swick, H. M. (2000). Toward a normative definition of medical professionalism. *Academic Medicine, 75*(6), 612–616.

Taylor, E. (2008). Transformative learning theory. *New directions for adult and continuing education, 2008*(119), 5–15. https://doi.org/10.1002/ace.301

Taylor, E. W. (2009). Fostering transformative learning. In J. Mezirow, E. W. Taylor, & Associates (Eds.), *Transformative learning in practice: Insights from community, workplace, and higher education* (pp. 3–17). San Francisco, CA: Jossey-Bass.

Todres, M., Tsimtsiou, Z., Sidhu, K., Stephenson, A., & Jones, R. (2012). Medical students' perceptions of the factors influencing their academic performance: An exploratory interview study with high-achieving and re-sitting medical students. *Medical Teacher, 34*(5), 325–331. https://doi.org/10.3109/0142159X.2012.668626

Villwock, J. A., Sobin, L. B., Koester, L. A., & Harris, T. M. (2016). Impostor syndrome and burnout among American medical students: A pilot study. *International Journal of Medical Education, 7*, 364–369. https://doi.org/10.5116/ijme.5801.eac4

Wald, H. (2015). Professional identity (trans)formation in medical education: Reflection, relationship, resilience. *Academic Medicine, 90*(6), 701–706.

Wittich, C. M., Reed, D. A., McDonald, F. S., Varkey, P., & Beckman, T. J. (2010). Transformative learning: A framework using critical reflection to link the improvement competencies in graduate medical education. *Academic Medicine, 85*(11), 1790–1793. https://doi.org/10.1097/ACM.0b013e3181f54eed

PART III

BUILDING CAPACITY FOR RESILIENCE

CHAPTER 10

OUTDOOR ADVENTURE-BASED GROUP WORK TO PROMOTE COPING AND RESILIENCE AMONG CHILD WELFARE WORKERS

Christine Lynn Norton
Texas State University

Michael J. Schultz
State of Connecticut Department of Children and Families

Amy D. Benton
Texas State University

Cameron Kiosoglous
U.S. Rowing

Carrie J. Boden
Texas State University

Transformative Learning in Healthcare and Helping Professions Education, pages 197–219
Copyright © 2019 by Information Age Publishing
All rights of reproduction in any form reserved.
197

ABSTRACT

This chapter draws attention to high rates of secondary traumatic stress and burnout among child welfare workers nationally. The authors address the need for innovative practices and transformative learning experiences to build coping and resilience among child welfare workers to help them effectively manage the emotional labor of child welfare work. In particular, this chapter focuses on the use of outdoor adventure-based group work as a potential promising practice and presents a case study of an outdoor adventure-based program being implemented by the Wilderness School within the Department of Children and Families in the State of Connecticut. This case example demonstrates how adventure therapy may build team cohesion and reduce the effects of secondary traumatic stress and burnout among child welfare workers.

> *Sara Barth had nightmares about the mounting pile of cases on her desk: children covered in bruises, kids confessing they'd been raped, mothers dead of drug overdoses. She felt like she was drowning, responsible for too many of the state's most helpless children.*
>
> —Galofaro, 2015, para. 1

Engulfed by vicarious trauma, the experience of this case worker exemplifies an all too familiar feeling that child welfare (CW) workers face throughout the United States. Though this is not the only reality experienced by CW workers, it is certainly one of the most problematic, resulting in burnout and staff turnover which, in turn, negatively affects vulnerable children and families (Strolin, McCarthy, & Caringi, 2007). For this reason, this chapter will draw attention to high rates of stress, burnout, and vicarious trauma among CW workers nationally. This problem will be grounded in the larger context of the CW system in America and the challenges faced by CW workers, along with the need for resilient professional identities in this helping profession.

We will address the need for innovative practices and transformative learning experiences to build coping and resilience among CW workers to help them effectively manage the emotional labor of CW work. In particular, this chapter will focus on the use of outdoor adventure-based group work as a potential promising practice and will present a case example of a program being implemented by the Wilderness School within the Department of Children and Families in the State of Connecticut. By providing this case, we hope to inspire a larger dialogue within CW and social services about creative ways to strengthen and sustain the professional identities of those in this helping profession through transformative learning experiences that promote critical self-reflection and constructive change (Brookfield, 1990a, 1990b; Cranton, 1992; Marlowe & Carter, 2016; Taylor, 2008).

THE CHILD WELFARE SYSTEM AND ROLES
OF CHILD WELFARE WORKERS

The purpose, scope, and structure of the CW system in the United States has been the source of rigorous debate and rich collaboration among advocates, courts of law, educators, interdisciplinary professionals, and political leaders for more than a century. The CW system's complex and evolving economic, legal, medical, and psychosocial context has been well-documented and broadly analyzed by practitioners, researchers, and theorists representing a myriad of public institutions and private foundations (Child Welfare League of America, 2013; Popple & Vecchiolla, 2007). This meaningful history and ensuing implications for current policies and practices described in these publications serve as an invaluable backdrop for transformative learning among CW workers. Furthermore, our case example offers tangible support for the ways in which outdoor adventure-based group work can bring about individual resilience and greater team cohesion within and across helping systems.

Social policy in the United States presently defines public CW and child protective services (CPS) as mainly focused on victims of abuse and neglect. Social work is considered to be the profession that is responsible for implementing this policy, even though states and jurisdictions across the nation have varying educational and experiential requirements for entry-level and managerial employment. For the purpose of this chapter, the CW system is considered comprehensively to encompass public and private interdisciplinary professionals from education, healthcare, juvenile courts, law enforcement, and a plethora of community-based agencies. Community-based agencies working with children and families within the context of the CW system generally offer an array of services that emphasize prevention, early intervention, and treatment.

The primary goal of public CPS agencies is to prevent further maltreatment. To achieve this goal, the CPS worker coordinates services with various professionals and community agencies representing three primary groups, including professionals who provide referrals and important information; those who provide authority to take needed actions; and those who provide additional services to help families realize safety, permanency, and well-being (Taylor, Schultz, & Noel, 2007).

CHALLENGES FACED BY CHILD WELFARE WORKERS

Child welfare professionals around the world recognize that abuse and neglect are not isolated phenomena. Families that come to the attention of CPS agencies are most often embedded in multiple systems. These same families have typically experienced intergenerational behavioral health impairments, complicated medical problems, domestic violence, legal issues, poverty, substance abuse, and traumatic reactions to these biological and psychosocial conditions. Moreover, two primary paradoxes often accompany both clients and CW professionals: Clients who need the most help and support are least likely to seek it, since they do not trust the system, and direct care professionals with the least amount of experience and training are those usually called upon to handle the most complicated circumstances at the most challenging of times (during crises, on evenings, nights, weekends, and holidays). Timely and effective collaboration and communication between the multiple professionals who engage with families involved in the CW system are paramount to positive outcomes and are frequent sources of confusion and stress. The roles and responsibilities of public CW professionals are often wrought with conflicted values, competing demands, constant changes, and intensive public scrutiny. Negative reporting by the media leads to public perceptions of CW workers as incompetent, cold, and negligent (Chenot, 2011; Cooper, 2005). Furthermore, there is widespread misunderstanding or lack of awareness about the scope of services provided in the CW system. It is difficult for CW workers to be known only as the people who take children away. An additional impact is reactive policy changes due to high profile cases and public perceptions without input from frontline workers and other stakeholders as to whether the policy change is best for the system (Chenot, 2011; Cooper, 2005).

Nested within an increasingly volatile and uncertain political and socioeconomic context, public CW and related human services organizations are being asked to "do more with less." These same agencies are confronted with the reality of operating within contradictory value systems (Simmons, 2003). The first value entails the importance of advocating for those less fortunate and who are suffering by constructing public systems that intervene and correct the conditions leading to their distress. The second value ensures that these efforts to educate, protect, and support vulnerable persons are conducted without imposing unnecessary legal or social control. The third value assures that those who have suffered pervasive abuse and neglect have opportunities for the same outcomes as those who have had more stable and nurturing lives and relationships. These conflicting value systems and harsh realities can at times create a "damned if you do" (remove a child from a home) and "damned if you don't" (family preservation) situation for CPS agencies, particularly when responding to critical injuries and death (Popple & Vecchiolla, 2007). Thus, the interplay between organizational structure, public value, and interpersonal dynamics requires: (a) astute reflection, (b) reasonable caseloads and workloads for frontline staff, (c) collaboration among responsible leaders, (d) a focus on team-oriented quality and solutions, and (e) a sound supervisory contingent with the capacity to support those in the field in timely ways.

THE TOLL OF EMOTIONAL LABOR

Emotional labor is commonly understood as the affective demands required among helping professionals. According to Caringi, Lawson, and Devlin (2012), "Child welfare workers routinely perform emotional labor in their relationships and interactions with clients" (p. 4). In particular, the emotional labor involved in serving children and families with a multitude of problems within a system defined by conflicting values may result in burnout and secondary traumatic stress. Jayaratne and Chess (1984) found CW to be one of most stressful practice areas within the field of social work. When surveyed along with family service and community mental health workers, CW workers described significantly higher levels of stress as identified through role conflict, role ambiguity, and workload (Jayaratne & Chess, 1984). Along with its impact on workers, stress reduces effective service provision. Work environments with higher levels of perceived stress have been linked to poorer client outcomes (Williams & Glisson, 2013).

Secondary Traumatic Stress and Burnout

Secondary traumatic stress (STS) is defined as a set of reactions to the indirect exposure to trauma experienced by clients (Figley, 2012; National Child Traumatic Stress Network (NCTSN), 2011). Symptoms of STS can include hopelessness, hypervigilance, avoidance, fear, loss of trust, and physical complaints (NCTSN, 2011; Shackleford, 2012). CW workers can experience STS as well as burnout. Burnout comes from prolonged exposure to an unsupportive work environment whereas STS can occur after a single client interaction (Shackleford, 2012). Several studies of behavioral health professionals have indicated significantly higher rates of both burnout and STS for CW workers than other workers (Kim, 2011; Sprang, Craig, & Clark, 2011), including those that report approximately one-third of CW workers suffering from STS (Bride, Jones, & McMaster, 2007; Cornille & Meyers, 1999; Middleton & Potter, 2015). One study of CW workers indicated that 62% had high levels of emotional exhaustion, a key component of burnout (Anderson, 2000; Kim, 2011).

In CW research, work-related stress is often explored through burnout constructs (Ellett, 2009; Mor Barak, Nissly, & Levin, 2001). However, it is important to note that stress and burnout are not synonymous. Burnout is the result of "prolonged and unrelieved stress" (Lait & Wallace, 2002, p. 464). Examination of burnout using the Maslach Burnout Inventory (MBI) is frequently used in studies of turnover among CW workers (Dickinson & Perry, 2002; Drake & Yadama, 1996; Reagh, 1994; Samantrai, 1992). The MBI includes three subscales which measure emotional exhaustion, personal accomplishment, and depersonalization (Dickinson & Perry, 2002; Maslach & Jackson, 1981). The emotional exhaustion subscale reflects the degree to which workers feel they have no more energy for the job. The depersonalization subscale measures the development of cynical attitudes towards and detachment from clients. The personal accomplishment subscale consists of items addressing how workers evaluate themselves and their ability to help clients (Maslach & Jackson, 1981). A study examining the relationship of various job elements to burnout reflected that hours worked and amount of time spent on paperwork predicted burnout, whereas supervisor support and perceptions of success with clients reduced the risk of burnout (Benton, 2010). Researchers suggest that workers may initially report high levels of emotional exhaustion, which, unattended to, leads to increased levels of depersonalization (Kim, 2011; Lizano & Mor Barak, 2015).

Negative Outcomes

The cognitive dissonance caused by STS can impact workers' professional identities. Workers may shut down as they experience a loss of trust of others. Additionally, they may question their role in CW as they lose confidence in their own abilities. Workers who are motivated to enter social work due to a personal history of trauma may be at a higher risk of experiencing STS and its influence on professional identity (McFadden, Campbell, & Taylor, 2015).

Along with harm to the individual worker, each of the constructs discussed here impacts organizational functioning through high levels of turnover and poor service provision. Stress and burnout have been linked to turnover (Barford & Whelton, 2010; O'Donnell & Kirkner, 2009). In one study of CW workers ($n = 1192$), vicarious trauma was a significant predictor on intentions to quit (Middleton & Potter, 2015). Over 50% of participants in this study somewhat agreed with the statement that they would leave their job immediately if offered employment for the same pay but with reduced stress (Middleton & Potter, 2015). Bride and colleagues (2007) also found a correlation between STS and intentions to quit.

Chronic turnover in CW agencies has been linked to longer placements in care and reduced chances of reunification or permanency for children (American Public Human Services Association, 2005; Flower, McDonald, & Sumski, 2005; Hess, Folaron, & Jefferson, 1992). CW workers who experience STS and decide to stay also negatively affect the quality of services provided. Workers may have moved into "survival mode" in their approach to work and the work environment (Dombo & Blome, 2016). The impairments related to STS—hopelessness, loss of trust, and avoidance—reduce a worker's ability to provide competent, consistent services and apply rigorous, thorough decisions.

CURRENT BEST PRACTICES FOR ADDRESSING BURNOUT AND SECONDARY TRAUMATIC STRESS

Sprang et al. (2011) recommend interventions tailored specifically to CW given the significantly higher rates of burnout and STS among CW workers in their study. At this point, many of the strategies utilized to address the problems of STS and burnout among CW workers are preventative, including psychoeducation, preparedness, and planning (Hendricks, 2012). Psychoeducation can help CW workers understand the signs and symptoms of vicarious trauma and burnout, which can lead to early intervention. Preparedness involves being transparent with new hires about the stressors associated with this type of work and teaching coping skills early on to deal with this stress effectively. This includes self-care planning on the part of individual CW workers as well as organizational planning to develop support systems and response strategies. Though all of these prevention strategies are helpful, the reality is that sometimes CW workers still find themselves experiencing secondary trauma and burnout. This is not only true for CW workers but also applies to supervisors who are affected by emotional contagion, in which a person vicariously experiences the emotions of others (Collins-Camargo, 2012; Dill, 2007; Middleton & Potter, 2015).

Specific interventions to address this trauma include strategies used by an individual to build awareness of one's own trauma triggers and the negative impact it creates in a person's life (Hendricks, 2012). CW workers and supervisors may also need help reestablishing balance in their lives by setting boundaries, managing their time more effectively, engaging in self-care, and avoiding negative coping skills (Hendricks, 2012). Engaging in personal therapy also may be a helpful strategy for learning these skills and processing the difficult emotions that accompany secondary trauma and burnout. Research shows that avoiding personal and professional isolation is also important (Bober & Regehr, 2006). This may include opportunities for debriefing, building new relationships, and engaging in spiritual practices. However, to regain balance and connection in their lives, CW workers may also need additional organizational support.

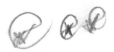

SYSTEMIC, ORGANIZATIONAL APPROACHES
TO PROMOTE TRANSFORMATIVE LEARNING

According to Dombo and Blome (2016), CW agencies are also responsible for addressing burnout and STS. A systemic approach to enacting both prevention and intervention strategies for CW workers has been shown to be the most comprehensive approach. This approach must focus on building resilience—the ability to overcome life's challenges—which is a valuable concept in considering and treating individuals and organizations experiencing trauma and adversity. The State of Connecticut's Office of Organizational Climate and Staff Support offers an example of a resilience and well-being framework for therapeutic and preventive efforts with both clients and staff who have endured severe trauma. This framework avoids simply providing a description of tragic circumstances or a set of techniques to treat or change families and organizations in the aftermath of tragedy and heartache. Instead, it uses a strengths-based approach that enables interdisciplinary CW staff and community partners to draw out the abilities and potential in each other. This framework also encourages an active process of learning and growth on personal and professional dimensions. As families, helping organizations, and professional staff all increase their capacity to rebound from immediate crises and weather persistent stress, they also gain vital resources to deal more effectively with future challenges. Thus, in building organizational resilience among professionals, every learning moment is also a preventive measure.

One of the most effective ways of building organizational resilience is through effective supervision. Supervisor support can ameliorate the role ambiguity that workers often feel that then leads to emotional exhaustion (Lizano & Mor Barak, 2015). Supervisors also provide space for emotional release, debriefing, and reflection (Kadushin & Harkness, 2014). Critical reflection groups have also been used to help manage the emotional labor of CW work (Smith et al., 2016). These "involve small peer groups working together to assist one another to reflect on concrete examples of practice that are identified by practitioners to be significant" (Smith et al., 2016, p. 4). These outlets are invaluable for CW workers, who often feel isolated and disconnected, and they help create a positive organizational culture that can help them manage the strain of emotional labor. To do so, organizations need to attend to workers' affective states and look for ways to help workers express and regulate affect in the context of the workplace.

The Role of Transformative Learning

Though the best practices listed above have been shown to be effective strategies for addressing burnout and secondary trauma among CW workers,

Transformative
Learning

professional stress and staff turnover continue to plague the CW system (Lizano & Mor Barak, 2012). We assert that a new framework of transformative learning is needed to engage CW workers in experiences that build resilient professional identities and enhance coping skills. Transformative learning is the process of revising the meaning of experiences (Mezirow, 1978) through critical reflection and self-reflection on "disorienting dilemmas" (Mezirow, 1991, 2012) and critical incidents (Brookfield, 1990b). Building on Habermas' (1973) and Freire's (1970) constructs of communicative and emancipatory learning, Mezirow (1991, 2012) developed transformative learning theory to conceptualize how changes occur in the assumptions, belief systems, values, and mindsets of an adult. Instances of transformative learning may move an adult towards a more inclusive, discriminating, self-reflective, and integrative frame of reference (Merriam & Brockett, 2007; Mezirow, 1978). Transformative learning changes people (Clark, 1993) in ways that they and others can identify. The transformative process, however, is not complete until the person has chosen to act on the new meanings or understandings (Mezirow, 1991, 2012).

For CW workers, transformative learning is a crucial building block for the creation and maintenance of a resilient professional identity because it can help them acquire the skill and habit of critical reflection. Schön's (1987) seminal work on becoming a reflective practitioner has influenced social work education with the development of a number of programs to prepare CW professionals. In one bachelor's of social work program in Australia, social work students learn how to practice critical self-reflection in their final year of professional preparation. Similarly, in a social work preparation program in the United Kingdom, critical reflection assists students with reframing knowledge and assumptions to prepare them to work with oppressed groups (McCusker, 2013). In the United States, an arts-based approach to critical reflection assists students with deconstructing main-stream media representations that serve to perpetuate stereotypes and hegemonic structures (Desyllas & Sinclair, 2014). In addition to these programs, efforts that aim to foster transformative learning among child care workers can teach the skills and habits of critical reflection by modeling critical thinking skills that will enable CW workers to reflect on their own frames of reference and consider those of their clients, as well. These reflections could provide revised meaning schemes for dominant discourses, taken-for-granted assumptions, causal attributions, and other sensemaking around issues of power and identity. They also could impel professionals to facilitate personal and social transformation and to promote the movement for social justice.

Transformative learning is a result of reflective practice and is central to the development of an authentic professional identity (Cranton & King, 2003). Professional identity is strengthened as these behaviors become more intuitive and deliberate. Through deliberate practice, behaviors soon match values, and values match identity (Branch & Frankel, 2016). Professional identity includes the knowledge, skills, and abilities one needs to be a member of a community of practice as well as the values and behaviors associated with the profession (Cruess, Cruess, Boudreau, Snell, & Steinert, 2015; Levinson, Darrow, & Klein, 1986; Kegan, 1982). The capacity for transformative learning, cultivated as a skill and habit during professional preparation, can become part of one's professional identity, which in turn can improve resilience and coping strategies for those in healthcare and the helping professions, as illustrated in this book. This is particularly important for CW workers, who are especially susceptible to compassion fatigue, burnout, and STS (Kim, 2011; Sprang et al., 2011).

Resiliency and Coping Skills Needed Among Child Welfare Professionals

The specific considerations, skills, and resilience strategies needed by CPS workers and supervisors as they navigate complex social systems have been noted by practitioners and researchers in a number of related fields, including behavioral health, CW, education, juvenile justice, pediatrics, medical science, substance abuse, and trauma. The primary principles and practices of brief, family-centered, solution-oriented, and structural family therapy approaches have predominated the research (Berg & Kelly, 2000; Caringi, Lawson, & Devlin, 2012; De Jong & Berg, 1998; Minuchin, 1974; Minuchin, Colapinto, & Minuchin, 1998). A summary of basic skills recommended for CPS workers has emerged from this eclectic, strengths-based theoretical framework that includes the following:

1. An ability to forge positive professional alliances with families, colleagues, supervisors, and other key players in the helping system.
2. The capacity to tolerate and effectively manage intensive family and organizational stress.
3. An ability and willingness to resolve interpersonal conflicts in constructive ways.
4. An acute awareness and understanding of family organization and patterns of interaction.
5. An ability to effectively intervene in these patterns of interaction through collaborative planning, teamwork, and on-going revision of solution-oriented activities.
6. An ability to accurately assess the influence of the larger system on the family's functioning.
7. An ability to effectively coordinate professional activities with the family and helping system.

8. A willingness to utilize supervision and constructive feedback to become more aware of one's strengths and limitations while developing a professional style.
9. A keen awareness of the impact of age, culture, development, ethnicity, gender, race, sexuality, and traumatic experience on personal and professional encounters.
10. An ability to create documentation that adequately reflects and communicates the quality of interactions with clients and colleagues in a timely fashion.
11. The ability to effectively manage the emotional labor associated with CW work.

OUTDOOR ADVENTURE-BASED GROUP WORK AS A LEARNING STRATEGY

Participation in professional development training and retreats has been used to recruit and retain CW workers (Fox, Miller, & Barbee, 2003; Landsman, 2007); however, little research exists in the area of applying outdoor adventure to the training of helping professionals. One study of recent nursing graduates found that they gained confidence, competence, and leadership skills by participating in outdoor adventure activities (Greer-Day, Medland, Watson, & Bojak 2015); however, no research has been done in this area with CW workers.

In general, therapeutic outdoor adventure experiences have targeted youth and young adult clients, with research showing enhanced intrapersonal and interpersonal growth and healthy psychosocial functioning (Norton et al, 2014). Also known as adventure-based group work (ABGW), this type of intervention involves the physical engagement of participants and the intentional use of cooperative games, problem solving initiatives, challenges, and adventure activities, often in an outdoor setting (Newes & Bandoroff, 2004). Adventure-based group work has been used to promote social skills (Tucker, 2009), enhance self-concept and perception of competence in major life skills, and foster group cohesion (Norton & Tucker, 2010). All of these things are essential for providing CW workers transformative learning opportunities to reflect on their personal and professional challenges. Several features of adventure-based group work stand out for their relevance to CW workers.

The first is the connection between ABGW and experiential learning (Norton et al., 2014). Kolb's (1984) experiential learning cycle incorporates action, reflection, and integration as key elements of the learning process, has broad application in adventure-based group work, and can aid in the critical reflection required for transformative learning. According to Norton et al. (2014), the application of experiential learning in therapeutic settings "provides direct, hands-on adventure experiences that engage clients [in this case, CW professionals] as active participants in the therapeutic process, elicit[s] motivation. . .and provide[s] opportunities for reflection and transfer of learning" (p. 47). In addition, Alvarez and Stauffer (2001) believe that the use of experiential learning in outdoor adventure-based activities can facilitate change and build community. The learning from these adventure experiences can become a catalyst for processing and creating new behaviors and transferring skills learned through the ABGW experience for use in the work environment and in daily life (Newes & Bandoroff, 2004). These new behaviors may help foster greater coping and resilience as CW workers make the metaphoric connection between the ABGW experience and their professional lives.

The second key feature of ABGW that may help CW workers establish resilient professional identities is an emphasis on inclusion and diversity. Research has shown that ABGW may be an effective approach for building culturally-responsive communities of support (Zlotnik, DePanfilis, Daining, & McDermott Lane, 2005). Specifically, Norton and Tucker (2010) found that adventure-based group work has the ability to bring diverse people together and address diversity issues in a way that empowers participants. Though CW worker demographics often reflect those within their states, national data show that CW workers are most often female and white, except in urban areas (Barth, Lloyd, Christ, Chapman, & Dickinson, 2008). However, regardless of diversity within the CW workforce, issues of race, class, and other markers of diversity often arise in these settings in which CW workers interact with clients and community members.

Finally, ABGW is gaining new ground in the realm of trauma recovery. Through a trauma-informed approach to outdoor adventure, participants can be "kinesthetically engaged on cognitive, affective, and behavioral levels" (Gass, Gillis, & Russell, 2012, p. 1) to examine the impact of trauma symptoms in a safe setting. Norton, Tucker, Farnham, Borroel, and Pelletier (2017) found that participation in a trauma-informed adventure therapy program for youth and families affected by abuse led to a decrease in trauma symptoms and an increase in family functioning. Though this study focused on clients' trauma recovery, ABGW may also be a vehicle for decreasing secondary traumatic stress among CW workers. To explore this hypothesis and connect theory to practice, this chapter offers a case example of a trauma-informed support program for CW workers in the State of Connecticut that demonstrates the power of transformational learning through outdoor adventure.

THE CASE OF THE WILDERNESS SCHOOL

The Connecticut State Department of Children and Families (DCF) established the Office of Organizational Climate and Staff Support in January of 2016. The Department's commitment to family-centered and trauma-informed care recognizes that the physiological and psychosocial effects of exposure to trauma and violence extend beyond those directly affected. Preventing and limiting the harmful effects of primary and secondary stress requires an organizational climate of active and astute leadership, fairness and equity, interpersonal safety, indisputable trust, and a vibrant team approach. Though a range of trauma-informed interventions are offered, this chapter will focus on adventure-based group work offered at the Wilderness School.

The Experience

The Connecticut DCF Wilderness School has maintained a high level of established adolescent and community programming that has spanned 42 years and is expanding its capacity to serve DCF leadership and staff teams across the state. During the past year, the Office and Wilderness School have facilitated several team-building and transformative leadership experiences for more than 1,600 interdisciplinary staff within the context of outdoor education and group work. The Wilderness School established a three-part process with DCF staff to maximize learning and reinforce progress in the everyday employment settings of participants. The process includes: (a) an orientation meeting with leadership and the designated staff cohort in their local area to develop rapport and clarify goals, logistics, questions, and expectations; (b) a customized Wilderness School experience based on the initial orientation and goal-setting process; and (c) follow-up sessions in the local area to solidify changes, transfer-of-learning, and ongoing team support. These sequences of engagement and intervention have yielded positive connections within and across programs, enhanced morale, and increased productivity.

The Crisis Intervention

During the late Fall and early Winter of 2015, one field office—housing approximately 120 interdisciplinary staff—experienced several high-profile fatalities of infants and children that were involved with the Department's services at the time of their deaths. These critical incidents took place within a few weeks of one another. The field office is nested within a diverse urban environment and historically responds to frequent allegations of abuse and neglect as well as intergenerational domestic violence, mental health impairments, poverty, and substance abuse problems, among others. In addition to the intensive media attention that surrounded two particular cases involving the death of a child, child advocates and political leaders were quick to cast blame on the Department's handling of the cases by calling for independent investigations "to clarify the facts." Each case concurrently involved an internal investigation resulting in significant changes in leadership. Office morale hit an all-time low and staff felt overwhelmed and under-supported, while the routine barrage of new cases kept coming.

For many that work in the CW system, these are not unusual scenarios. Field office leadership reached out to the department office for guidance and support, recognizing that the multiple stresses and rapid changes in leadership were compromising relationships among interdisciplinary team members. Following a sequence of meetings with the local leadership and social work supervisors, it was determined that the office as a whole would benefit from adventure-based group work experiences at the Wilderness School. Three specific cohorts (approximately 30 participants in each one) were established to cover the majority of full-time staff in the office, with the understanding that these subgroups would be brought together in their field office once each team participated in Wilderness School activities.

Before arriving at the Wilderness School, each group received an orientation in their field office. In addition to providing information and a context for collaboration, the orientation served to reduce anxiety and apprehension for many of the staff who were less than comfortable in a rural and rustic place. Because the Wilderness School rests in a beautiful and natural part of the state, the grounds are well-suited for a range of mindfulness exercises, large and small group discussions, and socialization. These activities reinforce the notion that the best tool a professional can use is the self. The hallmark of healthy organizational functioning is creating space for all staff to make use of "their sense of self" in the helping context.

The Wilderness School is located in the northwest corner of the State of Connecticut and rests on approximately 12 acres. The Wilderness School has adapted the models of Outward Bound Schools as a foundation for work with students and their families. The principles and practices of social group work and family therapy enrich therapeutic programming. The Wilderness School is licensed by the State of Connecticut's Office of Child Development. Even though the School's focus with CW professionals is qualitatively different than its work with youth and families, the core components of outdoor experiential learning remain intact.

Five full-time and year-round interdisciplinary staff with education and training in outdoor experiential education, clinical social work, counseling, marriage and family therapy, and clinical psychology serve as administrators and supervisors. Four of the full-time staff are certified in Wilderness

First Responder (WFR), Cardiopulmonary Resuscitation (CPR), and Water Safety through the American Red Cross. Twenty-eight seasonal staff with knowledge and interest in outdoor education and experiential learning are integral to programming during the spring, summer, and fall. Program staff have previous experience in Outward Bound, National Outdoor Leadership, and affiliated Wilderness Education Associations. The majority of seasonal staff are enrolled in undergraduate and graduate level training in education, ecological studies, human services, and social work. Each seasonal staff member receives individual and group supervision with one of the full-time staff.

All full-time and seasonal staff receive comprehensive education and training in the spring prior to their involvement with students, their families, and DCF staff. Content areas align with program options and include: (a) broad overview of the DCF; (b) overview of the Wilderness School philosophy, relational approaches, and policies and procedures; (c) group theory and practice; (d) family-centered and trauma-effective principles and practices; (e) cultural humility and diversity; (f) student supervision; (g) course area knowledge; (h) backpacking; (i) rock-climbing; (j) canoeing and water safety; (k) ropes course elements; (l) team-building games and facilitation; (m) briefing and debriefing techniques; (n) logistical systems; (o) course planning and preparation; (p) vehicle and trailer driving; (q) medication administration; (r) enrollment practices and procedures; (s) field-based food systems; and (t) staff expectations for community living and wellness.

The main campus houses a large community room with full kitchen facilities that is used year-round. Twelve additional cabin-style buildings are used for administrative offices, lodging, and housing for equipment. The grounds are well-maintained in a wooded area with walking trails and a fresh-water pond. The program course area follows the Appalachian Trail corridor of the Taconic and Berkshire mountain ranges of Connecticut and Massachusetts. Programming for DCF staff takes place on the main campus and in most of Connecticut's State Parks that are in close proximity to field offices for hiking, canoeing, rock-climbing, and team-building activities.

The initial orientation established a springboard of safety and trust with a 90-minute introductory ritual. This facilitated group conversation included two basic questions for participants: (a) "What do you hope to gain by being here today?"; and (b) "What do you hope the team will learn today that you can carry back to your office?" Typically, the facilitator expanded upon each response to clarify points of view and engage staff in a dialogue. Then, the respondent is asked to select the next person whose opinion they would like to hear or asks for a volunteer to respond to the same questions. The process encourages explicit views, spontaneity, and playfulness as the discussion flows freely, binding the team together along the way. In each of the three participating staff groups, a meaningful level of group cohesion developed quickly during this phase of the experience, setting the tone for the day.

The Wilderness School's interventions with the field offices deliberately leave space between activities for leisure time and bonding. The "challenge by choice" value system empowers individuals and groups to actively decide what they would like from the group and what they are willing to contribute to the group during the team-building day. The focus on the individual's present experience with her team often brings forth a concurrent sense of autonomy and belonging, deepening affiliations, and providing levels of emotional safety and trust.

Following the introductions and 20 minutes of leisure time, each of the three groups engaged in large group activities designed to be fun, promote connection, and require movement. These activities involved recognition of physical limitations and each member's relative level of comfort with structured engagement with colleagues. After each activity, participants briefly reflected on their experiences, and facilitators tied these reflections to the goals and objectives identified in the orientation and introductory exercises.

Lunch and mealtimes are meaningful rituals at the Wilderness School. Each of the three groups brought food to share that is representative of their family-of-origin or current family context. Organizing the lunch and food selection prior to their arrival at the Wilderness School mirrors the many ways in which the team interacts and nurtures one another. Deeply insightful connections between the personal identity and professional identity abounded during this phase of the intervention. It was common to hear staff express that they had acquired "a deeper understanding and appreciation of their colleagues" as the meal evolved. By and large, the Wilderness School leaves space for approximately 75 minutes for lunch, conversation, and leisure with groups of this size, approximately 30 people.

The afternoon moved very quickly with physical activity, involving games to promote cooperation and movement ("Mail Call," "Alaskan Baseball," and "People to People"). Mail Call and People to People connect pairs of team members via guiding questions. Pairs hold brief conversations guided by focused topics such as one's favorite vacation location, restaurant, film, music, wellness activity, and so forth. Wilderness School staff develop questions based on the team's goals and level of cohesion, including those that can be more provocative in nature. Pairs rotate every 5 minutes to ensure that the team members are having one-to-one contact with several others. Alaskan baseball is a team-oriented game that divides the whole group into two parts. This is a very active game that involves competition, running, throwing objects, and working together by moving objects among team members (over a shoulder, between legs and so forth).

An important aspect of the afternoon is the "solo experience." The solo experience is a mindfulness activity encompassing 45 minutes of individual time at a lake with options to meditate, journal, draw, or focus on sights, sounds, thoughts, and emotions. Individual time stimulates reflection and relaxation, and it affords staff an opportunity to bridge the experience of the day with the stresses and strains of professional lives and relationships. This is a time of creativity, and several staff were able to reframe the complexities of their work into possibilities for hope and greater collaboration. These activities were followed by a facilitated circle to close the day. Although each group is unique, feedback about the day has been consistent. Staff shared moving experiences of mutual learning, reciprocal support, and admiration for their colleagues. In the highly respectful and insightful connections that developed, staff members found the motivation to share their lives with each other as professionals and human beings. During the debriefing session, staff were able and willing to challenge their previous assumptions, expand their thinking, and recognize the common beliefs and values they share as a team.

Each team and most members talked about the experiences of hope and possibility they would carry forth and described the day at the Wilderness School as "rejuvenating mind, body, and spirit." Feedback from leadership and colleagues in their field offices indicated that each group returned with tangible increases in healthy energy and unity. Evaluations and feedback at the 4-week follow-up indicated that the respective teams believed they were providing more compassionate care to clients and collaborating with one another more effectively as a team as a result of the experience. Many participants indicated that they were more mindful of self-care (diet, exercise, and work-life balance) and felt better connected to their colleagues.

DISCUSSION AND CONCLUSION

This case example explores how adventure-based group work can provide a transformative learning experience for CW workers that fosters resilience, coping, and cohesion among workers, even in the face of crisis. Child welfare workers who participated in ABGW felt a sense of personal and community renewal. They had the opportunity to build connections and increase rapport among one another as a group. As individuals, transformative learning occurred as they were able to build resilience and coping strategies to cope with the STS they often face in their roles as CW workers. In many ways, the program offered at the Wilderness School created a safe space in which workers could find respite from the emotional labor of the CW system. The experience also provided space for critical reflection by connecting personal and professional values, leading to the development of a more resilient professional identity.

The case example provided shows that adventure-based group work experience must be reinforced and linked to the day-to-day interactions in the CW system to sustain healthy changes and team cohesion. This is no easy task. The moment-to-moment grind and complexity of CW work is pervasive and relentless. Accordingly, in our case example, several subsequent sessions in the field office were held in large and small groups to solidify changes post-program and to build resilience and keep momentum going. This type of follow-up is critical for the results of individual transformative learning to become integrated into the overall organizational culture.

We believe that these types of programs can be replicated in other CW systems, especially because many of the stressors CW workers experience are the same all around the nation. Ironically, the dramatic events associated with the death of several children in a short period of time and the resulting negative backlash that the CW system faced were a catalyst for transformative learning to occur, and this could be true in other CW systems. However, it is important for other professionals who wish to replicate this type of intervention to note that these sessions included a wide-range of forums, such as: (a) focused sessions with leadership and social work supervisors about the interplay of organizational structure, public values, and interpersonal dynamics; (b) seminars for staff with regard to their "use of self" as an instrument for personal and professional efficacy and growth; (c) seminars on self-care and wellness, with an emphasis on mindfulness with strategies for utilizing nature as a healing force; (d) facilitated conversations about emotional labor, global stress, and race relations; and (e) cross-team collaboration to enhance relationships, communication, and office culture.

Likewise, replicability requires broad organizational support for this type of intervention. A trauma-informed organizational culture that prioritizes wellness is more likely to provide the time and resources needed for CW staff to engage in this type of community-building experience. Clearly, future research is needed to empirically validate the role that ABGW has in decreasing burnout and secondary traumatic stress; however, the Wilderness School appears to be a viable step in a series of ongoing development efforts to build resilient professional identities and coping skills among CW workers.

AUTHOR NOTE

The authors of this chapter would like to acknowledge the efforts of those who support and facilitate the work of the Connecticut DCF Wilderness School: Commissioner Joette Katz, Deputy Commissioner Michael Williams, Regional Administrator Vannessa Dorantes, Area Director Kelly McVey, former Program Director Eugene Marchand, and three Field Supervisors in alphabetical order: Bonnie Sterpka, Kim Thorne-Kaunelis, and Aaron Wiebe.

REFERENCES

Alvarez, A. G., & Stauffer, G. A. (2001). Musings on adventure therapy. *Journal of Experiential Education, 24*(2), 85–91. https://doi.org/10.1177/105382590102400205

American Public Human Services Association. (2005). *Report from the 2004 Child Welfare Workforce Survey: State agency findings.* Washington, DC: Author.

Anderson, D. G. (2000). Coping strategies and burnout among veteran child protection workers. *Child Abuse & Neglect, 24*(6), 839–848.

Barford, S.W., & Whelton, W. J. (2010). Understanding burnout in child and youth care workers. *Child & Youth Care Forum, 39*(4), 271–287.

Barth, R. P., Lloyd, E. C., Christ, S. L., Chapman, M. V., & Dickinson, N. S. (2008). Child welfare worker characteristics and job satisfaction: A national study. *Social Work, 53*(3), 199–209.

Benton, A. D. (2010). *Why do they stay? Building a conceptual model to understand worker retention and turnover in public child welfare.* Dissertation Abstracts International: Section A, 72/06. No. 3448983. Retrieved from https://pqdtopen.proquest.com/doc/861731085.html?FMT=ABS

Berg, I. K., & Kelly, S. (2000). *Building solutions in child protective services.* New York, NY: Norton.

Bober, T., & Regehr, C. (2006). Strategies for reducing secondary or vicarious trauma: Do they work? *Brief Treatment and Crisis Intervention, 6*(1), 1–9.

Branch, W., & Frankel, R. (2016). Not all stories of professional identity formation are equal: An analysis of formation narratives of highly humanistic physicians. *Patient Education & Counseling, 99*(8), 1394–1399. https://doi.org/10.1016/j.pec.2016.03.018

Bride, B., Jones, J., & MacMaster, S. (2007). Correlates of secondary traumatic stress in child protective services workers. *Journal of Evidence-Based Social Work, 4*(3/4), 69–80.

Brookfield, S. (1990a). *The skillful teacher: On technique, trust, and responsiveness in the classroom.* San Francisco, CA: Jossey-Bass.

Brookfield, S. (1990b). Using critical incidents to explore learner's assumptions. In J. Mezirow & Associates (Eds.), *Fostering critical reflection in adulthood: A guide to transformative and emancipatory learning* (pp. 177–193). San Francisco, CA: Jossey-Bass.

Caringi, J. C., Lawson, H. A., & Devlin, M. (2012). Planning for emotional labor and secondary traumatic stress in child welfare organizations. *Journal of Family Strengths, 12*(1), 11–25.

Chenot, D. (2011). The vicious cycle: Recurrent interactions among the media, politicians, the public, and child welfare services organizations. *Journal of Public Child Welfare, 5*(2/3), 167–184.

Child Welfare League of America. (2013). *CWLA executive summary: National blueprint for excellence in child welfare.* Retrieved from http://www.cwla.org/wp-content/uploads/2013/12/BlueprintExecutiveSummary1.pdf

Clark, M. C. (1993). Transformational learning. *New Directions for Adult and Continuing Education, 1993*(57), 47–56. San Francisco, CA: Jossey-Bass.

Collins-Camargo, C. (2012). Secondary traumatic stress and supervisors: The forgotten victims. In T. LaLiberte & T. Crudo (Eds.), *CW360: Secondary trauma and the child welfare workforce* (Spring, pp. 8–9). Retrieved from http://centerforchildwelfare.fmhi.usf.edu/kb/TraumaInformedCare/CW360-2ndary-Trauma_2012.pdf

Cooper, L. D. (2005). Implications of media scrutiny for a child protection agency. *Journal of Sociology and Social Welfare, 32*(3), 107–121.

Cornille, T. A., & Meyers, T. W. (1999). Secondary traumatic stress among child protective service workers: Prevalence, severity and predictive factors. *Traumatology, 5*(1), 15–31.

Cranton, P. (1992). *Working with adult learners.* Middletown, OH: Wall & Emerson.

Cranton, P., & King, K. P. (2003). Transformative learning as a professional development goal. *New Directions for Adult and Continuing Education, 2003*(98), 31–38.

Cruess, R. L., Cruess, S. R., Boudreau, J. D., Snell, L., & Steinert, Y. (2015). A schematic representation of the professional identity formation and socialization of medical students and residents: A guide for medical educators. *Academic Medicine, 90*(6), 718–725.

De Jong, P., & Berg, I. K. (1998). *Interviewing for solutions.* Pacific Grove, CA: Brooks-Cole.

Desyllas, M. C., & Sinclair, A. (2014). Zine-making as a pedagogical tool for transformative learning in social work education. *Social Work Education, 30*(3), 296–316.

Dickinson, N., & Perry, R. (2002). Factors influencing the retention of specially educated public child welfare workers. *Journal of Health and Social Policy, 15*(3/4), 89–103.

Dill, K. (2007). Impact of stressors on front-line child welfare supervisors. *The Clinical Supervisor, 26*(1/2), 177–193.

Dombo, E., & Blome, W. (2016). Vicarious trauma in child welfare workers: A study of organizational responses. *Journal of Public Child Welfare, 10*(5), 505–523.

Drake, B., & Yadama, G. (1996). A structural equation model of burnout and job exit among child protective services workers. *Social Work Research, 20*(3), 179–187.

Ellett, A. (2009). Intentions to remain employed in child welfare: The role of human caring, self-efficacy beliefs, and professional organizational culture. *Children and Youth Services Review, 31*(1), 78–88.

Figley. (2012). Helping that hurts: Child welfare secondary traumatic stress reactions. In T. LaLiberte & T. Crudo (Eds.), *CW360: Secondary trauma and the child welfare workforce* (Spring, pp. 4–5). Retrieved from http://centerforchildwelfare.fmhi.usf.edu/kb/TraumaInformedCare/CW360-2ndaryTrauma_2012.pdf

Flower, C., McDonald, J., & Sumski, M. (2005). *Review of turnover in Milwaukee County private agency child welfare ongoing case management staff.* Retrieved from http://fsm.builtbymighty.com/uploads/misc/Flower_Permanency_Study_in_Milwaukee_05.pdf

Fox, S. R., Miller, V. P., & Barbee, A. P. (2003). Finding and keeping child welfare workers: Effective use of training and professional development. *Journal of Human Behavior in the Social Environment, 7*(1/2), 67–81.

Freire, P. (1970). *Pedagogy of the oppressed.* New York, NY: Herder & Herder.

Galofaro, C. (2015, February 6). Social worker turnover leads to high caseloads. *The Courier Journal*. Retrieved from http://www.courier-journal.com/story/news/local/2015/02/06/social-worker-turnover-leads-high-caseloads/22983561/

Gass, M. A., Gillis, L., & Russell, K. C. (2012). *Adventure therapy: Theory, research, and practice*. New York, NY: Routledge.

Greer-Day, S., Medland, J., Watson, L., & Bojak, S. (2015). Outdoor adventure program builds confidence and competence to help new graduate RNs become "every day" leaders at the point of care. *Journal for Nurses in Professional Development, 31*(1), 40–46.

Habermas, J. (1973). *Knowledge and human interests*. London, England: Heineman.

Hendricks, A. (2012). Secondary traumatic stress in child welfare: Multi-level prevention and intervention strategies. In T. LaLiberte & T. Crudo (Eds.), *CW360: Secondary trauma and the child welfare workforce* (Spring, pp. 12–13). Retrieved from http://centerforchildwelfare.fmhi.usf.edu/kb/TraumaInformedCare/CW360-2ndaryTrauma_2012.pdf

Hess, P. M., Folaron, G., & Jefferson, A. B. (1992). Effectiveness of family reunification services: An innovative evaluative model. *Social Work, 37*(4), 304–311.

Jayaratne, S., & Chess, W. (1984). Job satisfaction, burnout, and turnover: A national study. *Social Work, 29*(5), 448–553.

Kadushin, A., & Harkness, D. (2014). *Supervision in social work*. New York, NY: Columbia University Press.

Kegan, R. (1982). *The evolving self: Problem and process in human development*. Cambridge, MA: Harvard University Press.

Kim, H. (2011). Job conditions, unmet expectations, and burnout in public child welfare workers: How different from other social workers? *Children and Youth Services Review, 33*(2), 358–367.

Kolb, D. (1984). *Experiential learning: Experience as the source of learning and development*. Englewood Cliffs, NJ: Prentice Hall.

Lait, J., & Wallace, J. (2002). Stress at work: A study of organizational-professional conflict and unmet expectations. *Industrial Relations, 57*(3), 463–487.

Landsman, M. (2007). Supporting child welfare supervisors to improve worker retention. *Child Welfare, 86*(2), 105–124.

Levinson, D. J., Darrow, C. N., & Klein, E. B. (1986). *The seasons of a man's life*. New York, NY: Ballantine Books.

Lizano E. L., & Mor Barak, M. E. (2012). Workplace demands and resources as antecedents of job burnout among public child welfare workers: A longitudinal study. *Children and Youth Services Review, 34*(9), 1769–1976.

Lizano, E. L., & Mor Barak, M. (2015). Job burnout and affective wellbeing: A longitudinal study of burnout and job satisfaction among public child welfare workers. *Children and Youth Services Review, 55*, 18–28.

Marlowe, E., & Carter, T. (2016). The role of transformative learning in fostering identity development among learners in professional education programs of study. *Adult Education Research Conference*. Retrieved from http://newprairiepress.org/aerc/2016/roundtables/11

Maslach, C., & Jackson, S. (1981). The measurement of experienced burnout. *Journal of Occupational Behavior, 2*(2), 99–113.

McCusker, P. (2013). Harnessing the potential of constructive developmental pedagogy to achieve transformative learning in social work education. *Journal of Transformative Education, 11*(1), 3–25.

McFadden, P., Campbell, A., & Taylor, B. (2015). Resilience and burnout in child protection social work: Individual and organizational themes from a systematic literature review. *British Journal of Social Work, 45*(5), 1546–1563.

Merriam, S. B., & Brockett, R. G. (2007). *The profession and practice of adult education: An introduction.* San Francisco, CA: Jossey-Bass.

Mezirow, J. (1978). Perspective transformation. *Adult Education Quarterly, 28*(2), 100–110.

Mezirow, J. (1991). *Transformative dimensions of adult learning.* San Francisco, CA: Wiley.

Mezirow, J. (2012). Learning to think like an adult: Core concepts of transformation theory. In E. Taylor, P. Cranton, & Associates (Eds.), *The handbook of transformative learning* (pp. 73–95). San Francisco, CA: Jossey-Bass.

Middleton, J., & Potter, C. (2015). Relationship between vicarious traumatization and turnover among child welfare professionals. *Journal of Public Child Welfare, 9*(2), 195–216.

Minuchin, S. (1974). *Families and family therapy.* Cambridge, MA: Harvard University Press.

Minuchin, P., Colapinto, J., & Minuchin, S. (1998). *Working with families of the poor.* New York, NY: Guilford Press.

Mor Barak, M., Nissly, J., & Levin, A. (2001). Antecedents to retention and turnover among child welfare, social work, and other human service employees: What can we learn from past research? A review and meta-analysis. *Social Service Review, 75*(4), 625–661.

National Child Traumatic Stress Network. (2011). *Secondary traumatic stress: A fact sheet for child-serving professionals.* Los Angeles, CA: National Center for Child Traumatic Stress.

Newes, S., & Bandoroff, S. (2004). What is adventure therapy? In S. Newes & S. Bandoroff (Eds.), *Coming of age: The evolving field of adventure therapy* (pp. 1–30). Boulder, CO: The Association for Experiential Education.

Norton, C. L., & Tucker, A. (2010). New heights: Adventure based group work in social work education and practice. *Groupwork, 20*(2), 24–44.

Norton, C. L., Tucker, A., Russell, K. C., Bettmann, J. E., Gass, M. A., Gillis, H. L., & Behrens, E. (2014). Adventure therapy with youth. *Journal of Experiential Education, 37*(1), 46–59.

Norton, C. L., Tucker, A. R., Farnham, M., Borroel, F., & Pelletier, A. (2017). Family enrichment adventure therapy: A mixed methods study examining the impact of trauma-informed adventure therapy on children and families affected by abuse. *Journal of Child and Adolescent Trauma, 12*(1), 85–95. https://doi.org/10.1007/s40653-017-0133-4

O'Donnell, J., & Kirkner, S. (2009). A longitudinal study of factors influencing the retention of Title IV-E master's of social work graduates in public child welfare. *Journal of Public Child Welfare, 3*(1), 64–86.

Popple, P., & Vecchiolla, F. (Eds.). (2007). *Child welfare social work: An introduction.* Boston, MA: Allyn & Bacon.

Reagh, R. (1994). Public child welfare professionals: Those who stay. *Journal of Sociology & Social Welfare, 21*(3), 69–78.

Samantrai, K. (1992). Factors in the decision to leave: Retaining social workers with MSWs in public child welfare. *Social Work, 37*(5), 454–458.

Schön, D. A. (1987). *Educating the reflective practitioner: Toward a new design for teaching and learning in the professions.* San Francisco, CA: Jossey-Bass.

Shackleford, K. (2012). Occupational hazards of work in child welfare: Direct trauma, secondary trauma and burnout. In T. LaLiberte & T. Crudo (Eds.), *CW360: Secondary trauma and the child welfare workforce* (Spring, pp. 6–7). Retrieved from http://centerforchildwelfare.fmhi.usf.edu/kb/Trauma InformedCare/CW360-2ndaryTrauma_2012.pdf

Simmons, B. (2003). *Child welfare ethics and values.* Berkeley, CA: California Social Work Education Center. Retrieved from http://bayareaacademy.org/wp-content/uploads/2016/10/Trainer_Ethics_Values.pdf

Smith, M., Cree, V. E., MacRae, R., Sharp, D., Wallace, E., & O'Halloran, S. (2016). Social suffering: Changing organisational culture in children and families social work through critical reflection groups—Insights from Bourdieu. *British Journal of Social Work, 47*(4), 973–988. https://doi.org/10.1093/bjsw/bcw087

Sprang, G., Craig, C., & Clark, J. (2011). Secondary traumatic stress and burnout in child welfare workers: A comparative analysis of occupational distress across professional groups. *Child Welfare, 90*(6), 149–168.

Strolin, J. S., McCarthy, M., & Caringi, J. (2007). Causes and effects of child welfare workforce turnover: Current state of knowledge and future directions. *Journal of Public Child Welfare, 1*(2), 29–52. https://doi.org/10.1300/J479v01n02_03

Taylor, E. (2008). Transformative learning theory. *New Directions for Adult and Continuing Education, 2008*(119), 5–15. https://doi.org/10.1002/ace.301

Taylor, J., Schultz, M. J., & Noel, J. (2007). Other key players in the child welfare System. In P. Popple & F. Vecchiolla (Eds.), *Child welfare social work* (pp. 258–276). Boston, MA: Allyn & Bacon.

Tucker, A. R. (2009). Adventure-based group therapy to promote social skills in adolescents. *Social Work with Groups, 32*(4), 315–329.

Williams, N., & Glisson, C. (2013). Reducing turnover is not enough: The need for proficient organizational cultures to support positive youth outcomes in child welfare. *Children and Youth Services Review, 35*(11), 1871–1877.

Zlotnik, J. L., DePanfilis, D., Daining, C., & McDermott Lane, M. (2005). *Factors influencing retention of child welfare staff: A systematic review of research.* A report from the Institute for the Advancement of Social Work Research conducted in collaboration with University of Maryland School of Social Work Center for Families & Institute for Human Services Policy. Retrieved from http://www.social workpolicy.org/wp-content/uploads/2007/06/4-CW-SRRFinalFullReport.pdf

CHAPTER 11

TRANSFORMATIVE LEARNING IN TIMES OF ADVERSITY

Patrice B. Wunsch
Virginia Commonwealth University

Michael D. Webb
East Carolina University

Teresa J. Carter
Virginia Commonwealth University

ABSTRACT

Students in the health professions encounter many challenges during their educational experiences that require resilience to deal with adversity. What many professional learners do not yet realize is the extent to which adversity can occur during the years of practice, as well. The stories told in this chapter are from two experienced dental school educators. They reflect on the nature of disorienting dilemmas that can occur without warning to threaten professional identity and role while in practice. In learning to cope with the changes created by these situations, they discovered that resilience has to come from within, bolstered by supportive relationships and fostered by reflective, mind-

Transformative learning in Healthcare and Helping Professions Education, pages 221–236
Copyright © 2019 by Information Age Publishing
All rights of reproduction in any form reserved.

ful practices that allowed them to revise the meaning of their experiences and transform their perspectives to those of renewed purpose in life and career.

Life changing experiences can occur for students as well as for their educators. Learners in professional training often encounter difficult or challenging situations that require resilience in the face of adversity. What students may not realize is the extent to which the faculty members who teach and train them also encounter their own challenges in practice. Similar to unexpected events that may occur for professional trainees, life-changing events can occur without warning for professionals already in practice. These events have the potential to transform how they understand themselves and can cause them to question the very essence of what it means to be a professional. The ability to bounce back from challenging situations appears to be one indicator of the professional who can grow from adversity.

In this chapter, we share the reflections of two dental school educators who encountered unexpected events to which they needed to respond with resilience. They are the stories of transformative learning in response to adversity and they represent the continuum of possibilities for developing resilience as a health professional in practice. We introduce these stories as two separate vignettes then analyze them for the learning that occurred, building upon what has been written and researched about transformative learning, professional identity formation, and resilience.

THE ROLE CHANGE I NEVER ANTICIPATED: PATTY'S STORY

I entered the room and immediately recognized that something was wrong. After the door closed, I found myself seated face-to-face with my supervisor and two senior administrators in the dental school. My supervisor initiated the discussion by describing my performance as program director as inadequate and disappointing. Before she could continue, I interrupted to say that I had no idea of this since we had never discussed it, and my yearly evaluations did not reflect her assessment. We began to argue and I noticed how the senior administrators began to shift uncomfortably in their chairs. I was upset, and I could feel my face become red and my heart beat faster. I was about to continue defending my position when, suddenly, I sat back in my chair, took a deep breath, and exhaled slowly as what was really happening dawned on me. I said to myself, "Okay, this is a done deal."

I asked if the intent of this meeting was to terminate my employment. Everyone agreed that it was not, but they wanted me to step down from my current position of leadership and continue as a member of the faculty staff. This news was truly upsetting, but, finally, I was calm. I accepted the information and was grateful that I still had a job. After further conversation, I left the room utterly dazed, still confused, and upset. What had just happened?

Had the meeting occurred a few months earlier, I think I would have reacted differently. I would have continued to defend my position, becoming more entrenched in preserving what I had worked so hard to achieve. I would have been out to prove them wrong. In all likelihood, the conversation would have become more heated, with even fewer chances for an optimal outcome. At that moment, however, I closed my eyes, breathed deeply, and made a conscious decision to act differently.

Early in my career, I decided on academics over private dental practice due to the positive educational environment I encountered during my residency program in another state. What I now realize, after much reflection on this crucial day, was that my entire academic career had been filled with personal and professional challenges that I had simply ignored until now. Slowly, it began to dawn on me that I had encountered difficulty, first as a junior faculty member, then as a service chief, and, now, as the program director for an advanced dental specialty. I wondered how I could have ignored all the warning signs.

For weeks since that day, I have retraced my career in my mind, bringing events, places, and people back to the forefront in an effort to make some kind of sense of the situation. Removal from my leadership role, a position that I had earned, was a shock to my ego and my self-confidence. After completing my residency training, I had been encouraged to complete a fellowship in preparation for becoming a faculty member within the department. This fellowship position allowed me an opportunity for more clinical experience and a chance to hone my teaching skills. At the end of my fellowship year, a faculty position opened up at a hospital-based dental clinic, which I accepted. There I continued my clinical practice as well as my teaching role. After a short period, I was offered and accepted a leadership position by becoming the Chief of Dental Services. It seemed like everything was falling into place: I was excited about the position since I felt it was the next logical step for academic career advancement. I knew my background and experiences were primarily clinical, and I anticipated the responsibility of supervising community and academic staff dentists as well as clinical personnel with some "on-the-job" learning.

Until this time, I had always worked for someone else and never had to face the responsibility of reconciling budgets to ensure that the clinical and operating room revenues were sufficient to cover departmental costs. My inexperience in this area of financial management resulted in some executive decisions I made that did not go over very well with my staff. I later discovered that these decisions resulted in alienation with those who reported to me, leaving me feeling isolated and alone. I now see that my leadership style involved unilateral decision-making which did not allow us to work as a team. At the time, I felt powerless to figure out how to correct the damage created by my actions. While senior administrators were satisfied with the results of my leadership as Chief of Dental Services, I had nonetheless failed to create an atmosphere of teamwork and motivation within our group.

Eventually, I moved from the hospital-based clinic to a university-based residency program by becoming the program director for an advanced education dental specialty. My responsibility shifted to organizing an academic and clinical program for residents in compliance with standards set by the Commission on Dental Accreditation for the specialty. Early on, I discovered the delicate balance that occurs when working with faculty within and outside of the department, as well as clinical staff and residents in training. Even though I thought that I was managing everything well, I soon realized that I was managing more than I could handle. I started to have sleepless nights. I would awake in a panic, realizing that something was due the next day. Then I would get up and work through the night to complete the task. I did not take the opportunity to share the teaching responsibilities with other faculty and, eventually, I began to experience signs of burnout.

I found myself paying less attention to the residents and becoming short-tempered in many of my interactions with them. I complained so much to family and friends about my job that one day someone replied that I should stop acting like such a victim. It was not until much later that I began to understand what that comment meant. I continued to work as effectively as I could, always trying to do more, yet also complaining about work-related issues to anyone who would listen. One night, while complaining to my sister, she stopped me mid-sentence and recommended that I read a book that she thought would help change my perspective at work and in life. I took her recommendation and discovered the importance of being mindful and living in the present moment.

For much of my life and career, my focus was always on the future and my experiences from the past. I rarely focused on the present moment—that was quite evident by how I interacted with others. Instead of fully listening to someone as they talked, I would find myself first judging the usefulness of the conversation and then judging the person based on experiences with that individual or with someone who reminded me of that individual. If I did not like the person or did not find the conversation useful, I would find a way to move away from it as quickly as possible. Conversely, if I liked the person and the conversation were of use to me, I would think ahead about what to say to influence the conversation in a way that would position me more favorably. In other words, my ego was in charge, no one was getting to know my true self, and I was not truly interested in getting to know others. I was unconsciously moving through life allowing experiences to affect me emotionally which resulted in reactive behavior with negative results.

From the book I read, I discovered that mindfulness involves three key characteristics; the first is acceptance (Tolle, 2005), in which a person accepts what needs to be done and does it with a sense of peace and consciousness or surrendered action. When faced with the unfortunate experience of losing my leadership position in the dental school, I exhaled and released my anger. I could feel this enormous sense of relief that I was not allowing my ego to take over and defend itself in its usual reactive way of handling anything that challenges it. I was so grateful for learning how to be present enough to recognize how I unconsciously fall into the habit of allowing the ego-driven importance of time (the past and future) to guide me. By being present, I was able to surrender and accept what was happening at that moment.

In my study of mindfulness, I discovered that emotions can interfere with reasoning and therefore inhibit one's ability to make ethical decisions, so it is important to distance oneself from emotions to think clearly and objectively (Guillemin & Gillam, 2015). Practicing mindfulness helps in steering clear of emotional reactivity by enabling a person to become consciously aware. Mindfulness can be described as "paying attention on purpose, in the present moment, and nonjudgmentally to the unfolding of experience moment by moment" (Kabat-Zinn, 2003, p. 145). It involves the ability to have refined attentional skills and an open, nonevaluative attitude toward the different mental experiences that one encounters on a day-to-day basis (Malinowski & Lim, 2015). Brown and Ryan (2003) thought that "mindfulness captures a quality of consciousness that is characterized by clarity and vividness of current experience and functioning" when compared to the mindless state of automatic habits (p. 823). Cavanagh and colleagues (2014) claim that the practice of mindfulness and acceptance can be learned from self-help books, and Ciarrochi, Kashdan, and Harris (2013) relate mindfulness to foundational concepts associated with flourishing by describing it as a way to commit to action that improves and enriches life.

The second and third characteristics of mindfulness that I discovered are enjoyment and enthusiasm (Tolle, 2005). Once I accepted my situation after my change in leadership status, I began to focus on projects I rarely had time to work on previously. I discovered that by working diligently, without the background noise of my mind constantly thinking about past and future, I could enjoy my work again. I became enthusiastic about the work that I was doing and found that I no longer looked at the clock as much since my work was not dependent on time, but on my sense of accomplishment and fulfillment. I discovered that when a person works hard in the present moment, and does not dwell on things that have happened in the past or may happen in the future, doors will open to new possibilities as a result of dedication and hard work. I can now be much more productive because my interactions with others are more genuine. As a result, my faculty evaluations have become more favorable.

The tendency to slip into old habits is regrettably more frequent than I would like to admit, however; the ego is very strong and looks for every opportunity to take over, so I have realized that it is important to practice mindfulness on a regular basis. Throughout the day, I now take an occasional break from my routine to focus on how I inhale and exhale. Doing this brings my mind and activity back to the present moment. Other effective methods that I have found helpful include meditation and yoga, both of which focus on breathing and presence through conscious awareness. I now believe mindfulness practice has not only made me a more effective educator and clinician, but it may have saved my career.

PATTY'S REFLECTION
ON MINDFULNESS AS A RESILIENCY STRATEGY

My traumatic event led to a period of critical self-reflection. It began when I first realized that my life was out of control. This realization occurred months before that fateful meeting with the school's leadership. In a desperate attempt to get off the destructive rollercoaster created by unconscious habits, I entered a transformative process. According to Mezirow (1991), there are 10 phases of transformational learning. Transformative learning can begin with the event that disorients one's sense of self by leading to a period of self-reflection. The event prompted me to recognize how my leadership style and approach were negatively affecting me as well as those around me. Once I internalized how my pattern of behavior affected my life and my career, learning about mindful practice helped me to stop living an ego-driven life and begin to identify ways to rebuild my self-confidence as a faculty member whose contributions were still valued. I studied and practiced mindfulness and began to record my thoughts and feelings in a journal. After several months, when I assessed the results of my new course of action, I found that I had changed my perspective. I no longer felt responsible for the actions of the department or the actions of others. I was free to focus on my own role as a faculty member that included teaching, scholarship, and service. I was much happier and less stressed.

According to Langer (1989), the definition of mindlessness is clinging to the rules and laws by which one first attempts to understand the world; these can later lead to a falsified view of reality because of repetition, practice, and what psychologists call premature commitment (p. 21). As Langer notes, the grooves of mindlessness run deep because we know our scripts so well and thus become accustomed to routines; these can lead us into a narrow self-image, loss of control, learned helplessness, and stunted potential.

Mindful learning, on the other hand, involves the creation of new categories and an openness to new information with an implicit awareness of more than one perspective (p. 4). When writing about transformative learning, Mezirow (2012) refers to Langer's work on mindfulness when describing different levels of becoming aware of one's own thoughts (p. 76).

Mezirow (2012) defines transformative learning as the process by which we transform our taken-for-granted frames of reference (variously called meaning perspectives, habits of mind, or mindsets) to make them more open, inclusive and discriminating of experience, as well as reflective and emotionally capable of change (p. 76). The benefit to the individual of learning that is transformative, then, is to generate better actions and decisions, ones that can be justified to hold true for the individual. Because most of us have uncritically assimilated the perspectives of significant others as we grew up, we are largely unaware of how many of our beliefs are based on assumptions that no longer serve us well in the world. As Mezirow (2012) describes it,

> Transformation theory's focus is on how we learn to negotiate and act on our own purposes, values, feelings, and meanings rather that those we have uncritically assimilated from others—to gain greater control over our lives as socially responsible, clear-thinking decision makers. (p. 76)

When I neglected to pay attention to the signs and symptoms of stress within my work life, I was experiencing early signs of burnout. Rigid mindsets, narrow perspectives, the trap of old categories, and an outcome orientation all make burnout more likely (Langer, 1989, p. 146). Burnout sets in when two conditions prevail, according to Langer (1989): Certainties start to characterize the workday, and the demands of the job make workers lose a sense of control. It was not until my sister recognized the signs of my distress and suggested the book on mindfulness that I was ready to accept that there was a problem. According to Montero-Marin and colleagues (2015), mindfulness appears to be a better intervention for preventing the initial phases of burnout by reducing negative arousal states, and thereby reducing cognitive and emotional overload.

Practicing mindfulness prepared me for the uncomfortable encounter that occurred with the school's administrative leaders, which developed into a destabilizing and traumatic event and led me into a period of great self-reflection in the weeks and months that followed. During the meeting, if I had reacted strongly against the supervisor and administrators, the scenario most likely would have played out quite differently, and, potentially, with greater negative consequences for my career. The diligence gained from practice in mindfulness not only armed me with the strength to withstand adversity, it also provided me with the insight to know when to surrender by accepting the reality of the present moment.

WHEN THE UNEXPECTED HAPPENS TO A PATIENT: MIKE'S STORY

Catastrophic events that result in severe morbidity or mortality are rare in dentistry. When something like this does happen in a dental office, the practitioner is automatically deemed to be guilty of malpractice by the media, the community, and by other members of the profession. He or she is ostracized and has little support to help during this difficult time. The typical response from the profession is either "I am glad it wasn't me" or a nonpublic backing that is appreciated, but does not address the media trial that occurs long before any official action has been taken. This kind of event is life changing for all concerned, especially the patient's family and the dentist. Although several years have passed since this tragic event happened for a patient under my care, allowing me to make sense of the situation, my story of transformative learning began that fateful day.

Providing sedation or general anesthesia in the dental office carries some of the highest risk for adverse events. Dentists who deliver these services have extensive training in patient assessment, administration of sedative and anesthetic agents, and management of complications. They are trained in the technical aspects of treating complications, such as establishing an airway, administering reversal agents, and providing cardiopulmonary resuscitation. They are not, however, trained for the emotional impact that follows an adverse event that results in the death of a patient undergoing a dental procedure.

First and foremost, the practitioner has to face the patient's family. Telling a family that either an adverse event has occurred or that a patient has died is not something that we, as dentists, are prepared to do. Finding the right words to say and responding to a family's reaction is difficult at best. Then the dentist has to confront his or her own self-worth as a provider. The dentist will always ask, "Did I do everything I could have?" Finally, this type of event will affect the personal and professional life of the dentist from that day forward. Family support may be lacking as the reputation of the dentist is called into question and the eventual outcome of any state licensing board or court action will affect the dentist for the rest of a career. During this time, there is anxiety over the uncertainty of the future. "Will I be able to continue to practice, to support my family, to maintain my position in the community?" There was also uncertainty as to what to do, what to say to others, and how to continue with one's career and life. This kind of event falls into what Mezirow (1990, 1991) called a "disorienting dilemma," a catastrophic or life-changing experience that is dramatic and intense for which the individual is totally unprepared.

When this happened to me, legal counsel guided my initial actions. Outwardly, I did the things I had to do to answer investigations by the licensing board and the resulting legal action. However, I continued to review the events of the case in my mind and I kept asking myself, "Did I do everything I could have done?" I felt like the situation was controlling me, was taking over my life.

Eventually, while I could not change what had happened to my patient, or what might happen in the future, I realized that I needed to retake control of my situation so that I might begin to live again. I was finding no joy in life, no joy in my profession, no joy in my relationships. On reflection, these were symptoms of unrecognized depression, but instead of reaching out to others for help, I kept things in. I left the university under a cloud. I opened a private practice in town, incurring considerable debt for needed equipment and rental space for establishing my own practice. I hired staff with ongoing obligations to make payroll. The resulting financial problems only compounded my feelings of helplessness and despair. I was juggling creditors, and any cash reserves I had were gone. While outwardly I continued to display calm, I was emotionally at the end of my rope. I did not know what I was going to do. I was on the verge of bankruptcy and I was dissatisfied with the practice of dentistry. I found myself taking longer to get to work, getting frustrated with patients, and not paying attention to what needed to be done to maintain the practice. I guess you could say I hit rock bottom.

After a while, several things began to happen in my life at a time when I did not think things could get any worse. Fortunately for me, my wife remained by my side through this entire ordeal. One day she sat me down and told me that I was miserable and that I needed to do something to turn things around. She also said that whatever I decided to do, she would be with me. This was a significant event in my being able to envision a future that was not mired in the past.

When I told her that I wanted to return to academics, all she said was "fine, do it. Sell the practice and we will do what we need to do to move forward." That day was a big relief. There was still the uncertainty about the future but at least I knew that she and I would be working together to make our lives better. While this gave me some hope, the effects of that tragic day were continually resurfacing in my life. Initially, there was legal action from the family of the patient, then lulls in activity in which I did not hear anything anymore; suddenly, issues arose again that I needed to face. It seemed a never-ending treadmill of stops, starts, movement, and then no movement. The pace of legal activity was maddening—I just wanted to get it behind me, but I have since discovered that legal actions have a timeframe of their own.

Even after I sold my practice and was able to settle all my debt, I found that this event affected my ability to teach at certain dental schools and obtain licensure in some states. In addition to support from my wife and other family members, I was also fortunate to have the support of several close friends. I turned to my faith as a source of help and renewal. I spent time reflecting on what had happened, my role in it, and my life choice to become a dentist. This time made me value relationships even more and gave me some people to talk to about the event and the impact it had on my life. I also started focusing on the positive things rather than the negative things in my life. When I was initially unable to get a faculty position at a university, I looked on the positive side and figured that now I could be open to whatever other opportunity might come my way.

Even now, several years later, I feel the effects of that day. However, my coping is much better now. I take care of myself physically, emotionally, and spiritually. Eventually, my wife and I relocated to another state and another university that was glad to have my teaching skills and dental expertise. There are still long hours at work and a lot to do, but I make time to take care of myself. Working to build upon my relationships with family and friends, engaging in regular physical exercise, and participating in community and church volunteer activities have all helped me to achieve a good work–life balance, which makes me more effective in the care I provide patients and in the relationships I have with colleagues at work.

While I would never wish an experience like this on another practitioner in academic dentistry, it has been life changing in many ways, some of them positive and uplifting. I have learned about what it means to bounce back from adversity, to find reserves of strength you never realized that you had, and to value the most important people in my life. I transformed my perspective from one of hopelessness and despair into acceptance, grace, and thankfulness for the blessings that I have.

MIKE'S REFLECTION
ON THE IMPORTANCE OF RELATIONSHIPS

Early in his study of transformative learning, Mezirow (1990, 1991) believed that many people experience a 10-step process that includes a disorienting dilemma, self-examination, a critical assessment of assumptions, and eventually, exploration of new roles and relationships, as well as implementation of a new course of action. By trying on new roles and building competence and self-confidence in them, a person eventually integrates the new perspective into daily life. While some scholars have found that these phases can have variation within them (Coffman, 1991; Courtenay, Merriam, Reeves, & Baumgartner, 2000), I found that my own transformative learning experience followed the process initially described by Mezirow (1991, 2012) rather closely.

After the experience of losing my patient, I did not know what was going to happen to my career, my personal relationships, or how I was going to deal with the stigma of being associated with such an event. This led to a critical assessment of my assumptions. Was I "stuck" in my practice or did I want to do something else? Would I be able to do anything else? Could I return to academic practice and would I be able to find a position at another university? It was my wife who challenged me to not only assess these assumptions but to move forward in making a change. When she had the discussion with me about what *we* were going to do, it made me realize fully my dissatisfaction with private practice and that the change that needed to occur would be a shared experience. Her support was the turning point.

During his critical reviews of the literature in transformative learning, Taylor (1997) noted more references to the significance of relationships for their contribution to a perspective transformation than any other finding in the review (p. 53). Without this significant and supportive relationship at this time in my life, I do not believe the transformative process would have progressed to fruition. There were other relationships involved, but my relationship with my wife was the catalyst for change.

Once we made the decision that I would attempt to return to academics, the remaining steps in the process followed easily. Then it made sense to me that I could plan a course of action and proceed with the mechanics of finding an academic position. This I knew how to do. I looked at the advertisements in professional journals and websites, contacted colleagues and networked as best I could. At the same time, a more difficult task was selling the practice. However, since I had already made the decision to change, I learned as much as I could as quickly as I could and aggressively marketed the practice. With the practice sold, I was actually more attractive to academic institutions because I would be able to start a position without a delay. While some of the challenges associated with this difficult experience continue to this day, regaining my professional identity as an academic pediatric dentist again has allowed me to move forward with my transformative process.

TERRY'S THOUGHTS ON TRANSFORMATIVE LEARNING AND THE NEED FOR RESILIENCY

Rogers (2016), drawing upon the work of Walker and colleagues (2006), has described resilience as the capacity to endure ongoing hardship as well as the ability to recover from difficult situations. This definition certainly captures the nature of resilience needed to address unanticipated events that occurred for Patty and Mike in academic dental practice. Their ability to cope with these unexpected situations was not borne of an intentional strategy nor did it involve a specific educational intervention, although mindfulness practice has certainly gained attention as a deliberate method among healthcare professionals to respond to stresses and challenges in recent years (Kabat-Zinn, 2003; Kreitzer & Klatt, 2017; Rogers, 2016). Instead, both Patty and Mike were caught by the surprise of events, and dismayed and disoriented by them. Each of them had to work through the resulting discomfort by reflecting on what had happened and by drawing upon the resources that presented themselves at the time.

For Patty, it was the tacitly growing awareness that she was overwhelmed at work and unhappy in her managerial role. Her sister recognized it, and reached out to help. So when the opportunity presented itself to read a book on mindfulness a few months before the meeting with dental school administrators and her department chair, she had already taken the first steps to understand her situation and was beginning to learn the value of living in the present moment. The unexpected meeting crystallized the dilemma and brought her internal recognition full circle. Others had also realized that she was "in over her head," as developmental psychologist Robert Kegan (1994) describes it when exploring the mental demands of modern life.

For Mike, the traumatic event that occurred was even more dramatic: It was unparalleled in all his years of providing exceptional care for patients. It was unthinkable; unimaginable, yet it happened, and he was totally unprepared for the aftermath of legal and potentially career-ending fallout that occurred. Months and years of painful self-examination resulted, including a new start in private dental practice that still was not satisfying. It took a while before he recognized that he was being overcome by depression and despair. Mike's resilience appears to have arisen through the supportive relationships of family, friends, and church. He was slowly able to disentangle his sense of self-worth from the event and its aftermath. It required a loving spouse to challenge him to move forward with all the support and courage she could muster. When considered in light of transformative learning, the revisions to perspectives that resulted for both Patty and Mike represent a major shift, one described as a perspective transformation or a change in their frames of reference (Mezirow, 2000, 2012).

Learning Through Relationships

Mezirow (2012) describes a process of transformational learning as reflective discourse, or dialogue. Discourse involves a critical assessment of one's assumptions. It leads toward a clearer understanding by tapping collective experience to arrive at a tentative best judgment. Discourse, however, as Mezirow describes it, requires that the participants have the will and readiness to seek understanding and to reach some reasonable agreement. For this, both Patty and Mike relied on trusted individuals who were important to them; these relationships were free of distortions in power and influence and they knew that these special people in their lives had their best interests at heart. The nature of learning that occurred through these conversations created a shift, a movement from isolation and self-doubt to a feeling of comradery and confidence. Mezirow claims that feelings of trust, solidarity, security, and empathy are essential preconditions for free and full participation in the communicative dialogue he calls discourse. The learning experienced by Patty and Mike was facilitated and driven by the relational aspects of transformative learning.

Implications for Healthcare Professionals

Healthcare professionals in training, in practice, or in academia need to foster the ability to critically reflect on the assumptions embedded within their roles. These are often communicated to them by those who have a profound influence over both personal and professional development, including family members, parents, friends, mentors, teachers, and colleagues. As Kreber (2012), Kegan (1994, 2000), Cranton (2016), Dirkx (1998), and other scholars have noted, awareness of our own perceptions, thoughts, feelings, and actions are of fundamental importance as we attempt to address the challenges, responsibilities, and complexities associated with adult life.

Although the context of each of these traumatic events was quite different, they both required a revision in thinking before change could occur. These changes were not solely cognitive, but involved the influence of important relationships, strong emotions, intuitive powers, and deep insight into feelings. Each learned to become a more authentic person as a result, and became more capable of caring for themselves as well as caring for others. According to Jarvis (1992), authentic individuals choose to act as to "foster the growth and development of each other's being" (p. 113). Educators in an academic setting, practitioners working with patients and staff, or professional students can look at these experiences as examples of how to be resilient in the face of unexpected adversity. It is through mindfulness and conscious thought that individuals can develop the resilience necessary to handle the everyday stressors that occur in professional training or work. It is through the relationships that matter that the professional can discover the unvarnished truth, shared by someone who cares to help that person realize his or her value in the world.

CONCLUDING THOUGHTS ON TRANSFORMATIVE
LEARNING IN OVERCOMING ADVERSITY

Much is said and written about reflective practice. What does it mean to reflect, and to engage in the type of critical self-reflection that Mezirow (1990, 1998) writes about in describing learning that is transformative? Mezirow (2012) asserts that the distinction made by Argyris and Schön (1974) when describing single loop and double loop learning is central to the transformation of meaning perspectives (Mezirow, 2012, p. 326). Single loop learning is generally described as cause and effect learning; it involves detection of errors and corrections to thinking (Argyris & Schon, 1974). As Mezirow (2012) notes, such learning can enable us to correct distortions in beliefs and errors in solving problems. However, double loop learning that causes us to rethink the underlying assumptions of our actions can result in a more fundamental shift in the meaning an individual makes of experience since it causes us to question the very basis for our ideas, values, or beliefs. If underlying assumptions are faulty, then the individual must engage in a deeper, more traumatic or prolonged assessment of the very premises that undergird these assumptions. This is the nature of critical reflection described by Mezirow (1990, 1998) that can lead to transformation, changing the way individuals think and behave because it alters the very structure upon which perspectives and habits of mind are built.

The stories told by Patty and Mike reflect these deeper shifts in perspective. Each of them had to reflect on the role they had within academic dentistry and whether that role was still a good fit. For Patty, it was the realization that what her role had become was not the one she was best suited for, nor had it been the best for her personally for some time. This required a major readjustment in her own professional identity to step away from her previous leadership role. For Mike, acceptance of the painful loss of a patient required him to question his identity as a professional amid the upsetting consequences of legal action, departure from his university, and establishment of a private practice, which was still unsatisfying. He had to revisit the nature of his work as an academic dentist and educator to decide what type of work gave life meaning and was worth pursuing. The resulting professional identities for these two individuals that emerged from periods of introspection and critical self-reflection have become more resilient. They have learned what it means to bounce back from adversity rather than be conquered by it. The wisdom gained from such experiences has enabled them to grow in their professions and become better teachers and mentors for the students and residents they help prepare for their own professional challenges.

REFERENCES

Argyris, C., & Schön, D. A. (1974). *Theory in practice: Increasing professional effectiveness.* San Francisco, CA: Jossey-Bass.

Brown, K. W., & Ryan, R. M. (2003). The benefits of being present: Mindfulness and its role in psychological well-being. *Journal of Personality and Social Psychology, 84*(4), 822–848. https://doi.org/10.1037/0022-3514.84.4.822

Cavanagh, K., Strauss, C., Forder, L., & Jones, F. (2014). Can mindfulness and acceptance be learnt by self-help? A systematic review and meta-analysis of mindfulness and acceptance-based self-help interventions. *Clinical Psychological Review, 34*(2), 118–129. https://doi.org/10.1016/j.cpr.2014.01.001

Ciarrochi, J., Kashdan, T. B., & Harris, R. (2013). The foundations of flourishing. In T. B. Kashdan & J. Ciarrochi (Eds.), *Mindfulness, acceptance, and positive psychology* (pp. 1–29. Oakland, CA: Context.

Coffman, P. M. (1991). Inclusive language and perspective transformation. In *32nd annual adult education research conference proceedings* (pp. 49–55). Norman, OK: University of Oklahoma.

Courtenay, B. C., Merriam, S., Reeves, P., & Baumgartner, L. M. (2000). Perspective transformation over time: A 2-year follow-up study of HIV-positive adults. *Adult Education Quarterly, 50*(2), 102–119.

Cranton, P. (2016). *Understanding and promoting transformative learning* (3rd ed.). Sterling, VA: Stylus.

Dirkx, J. M. (1998). Transformative learning theory in the practice of adult education: An overview. *PAACE Journal of Lifelong Learning, 7,* 1–14.

Guillemin, M., & Gillam, L. (2015). Emotions, narrative, and ethical mindfulness. *Academic Medicine, 90*(6), 726–731.

Jarvis, P. (1992). *Paradoxes of learning: On becoming an individual in society.* San Francisco, CA: Jossey-Bass.

Kabat-Zinn, J. (2003). Mindfulness-based interventions in context: Past, present, and future. *Clinical Psychology: Science and Practice, 10*(2), 144–156. https://doi.org/10.1093/clipsy.bpg016

Kegan, R. (1994). *In over our heads: The mental demands of modern life.* Cambridge, MA: Harvard University Press.

Kegan, R. (2000). What form transforms? A constructivist-developmental approach to transformative learning. In J. Mezirow & Associates (Eds.), *Learning as transformation: Critical perspectives on a theory in progress* (pp. 35–69). San Fransciso, CA: Jossey-Bass.

Kreber, C. (2012). Critical reflection and transformative learning. In E. W. Taylor & P. Cranton (Eds.), *The handbook of transformative learning: Theory, research, and practice* (pp. 323–341). San Francisco, CA: Jossey-Bass.

Kreitzer, M. J., & Klatt, M. (2017). Educational innovations to foster resilience in the health professions. *Medical Teacher, 39*(2), 153–159. https://doi.org/10.1080/0142159X.2016.1248917

Langer, E. J. (1989). *Mindfulness.* Reading, MA: Addison-Wesley.

Malinowski, P., & Lim, H. J. (2015). Mindfulness at work: Positive affect, hope, and optimism mediate the relationship between dispositional mindfulness, work engagement, and well-being. *Mindfulness, 6*(6), 1250–1262. https://doi.org/10.1007/s12671-015-0388-5

Mezirow, J. (1990). How critical reflection triggers transformative learning. In J. Mezirow & Associates (Eds.), *Fostering critical reflection in adulthood* (pp. 1–20). San Francisco, CA: Jossey-Bass.

Mezirow, J. (1991). *Transformative dimensions of adult learning.* San Francisco, CA: Jossey-Bass.

Mezirow, J. (1998). On critical reflection. *Adult Education Quarterly, 48*(3), 185–198.

Mezirow, J. (2012). Learning to think like an adult: Core concepts of transformation theory. In E. W. Taylor & P. Cranton (Eds.), *The handbook of transformative learning: Theory, research, and practice* (pp. 73–95). San Francisco, CA: Jossey-Bass.

Montero-Marin, J., Tops, M., Manzanera, R., Piva Demarzo, M. M., Alvarez de Mon, M., & Garcia-Campayo, J. (2015). Mindfulness, resilience, and burnout subtypes in primary care physicians: The mediating role of positive and negative affect. *Frontiers in Psychology, 6*, 1895. https://doi.org/10.3389/fpsyg.2015.01895

Rogers, D. (2016). Which educational interventions improve healthcare professionals' resilience? *Medical Teacher, 38*(12), 1236–1241. https://doi.org/10.1080/0142159X.2016.1210111

Taylor, E. W. (1997). Building upon the theoretical debate: A critical review of the empirical studies of Mezirow's transformative learning theory. *Adult Education Quarterly, 48*(1), 34–59.

Tolle, E. (2005). *A new earth: Awakening to your life's purpose.* New York, NY: Penguin Books.

Walker, C., Gleaves, A., & Grey, J. (2006). Can students within higher education learn to be resilient and, educationally speaking, does it matter? *Educational Studies, 32*(3), 251–264. https://doi.org/10.1080/03055690600631184

CHAPTER 12

BUILDING RESILIENCE IN HEALTHCARE PROFESSIONAL TRAINEES

Wendy L. Ward
University of Arkansas for Medical Sciences

Carrie J. Boden
Texas State University

Ashley Castleberry
University of Texas at Austin

ABSTRACT

This chapter presented a series of vignettes of healthcare professional trainees whose experience of stress resulted in transformative learning and behavioral change. We analyzed the vignettes according to theories of transformative learning and offered ways trainees and their educators can apply these concepts to stress management and resiliency training efforts.

Healthcare professional (HCP) trainees often experience stress during training and are at high risk for stress and burnout. Today's health

Transformative Learning in Healthcare and Helping Professions Education, pages 237–259
Copyright © 2019 by Information Age Publishing
237

professionals need to develop a professional identity that includes self-care along with proficiency in resiliency skills. However, this experience of stress alone is not sufficient for the transformational learning needed to change behaviors in how they learn to cope.

Transformative learning is a "deep, structural shift in basic premises of thought, feelings, and actions" (Transformative Learning: Centre for Community Activism, n.d., para. 1). This chapter presents the literature on stress and burnout in healthcare professionals' training and practice, followed by a series of vignettes as examples of lived experiences of HCP trainees. The vignettes illustrate the diverse sources of stress along with multiple strategies for promoting individual resilience, followed by an analysis of transformative learning theory within the context of these vignettes. Finally, we offer suggestions for how educators can create experiences that serve as catalysts for transformative learning. The chapter concludes with a discussion that synthesizes how transformative learning relates to professional identity formation by addressing the priority of self-care during HCP training and how this process can be facilitated by educators.

BURNOUT AND STRESS AMONG HEALTHCARE PROFESSIONALS

Today's healthcare professionals are at high risk for stress and burnout (Shatté, Perlman, Smith, & Lynch, 2017) and this is a matter of national concern (Dyrbye et al., 2013; Shanafelt et al., 2015). In fact, a significant number of HCPs across a wide variety of professions are experiencing stress. Among them are physicians (Shanafelt et al., 2012), nurses (Branch & Klinkenberg, 2015; Rees, Breen, Cusack, & Hegney, 2015), physician assistants (Benson et al., 2016), pharmacists (Mott, Doucette, Gaither, Pedersen, & Schommer, 2004), audiologists (Severn, Searchfield, & Huggard, 2012), respiratory care practitioners (Shelledy, Mikles, May, & Youtsey, 1992), and others.

Stress levels are rising as a result of the instability in the healthcare system and its reform (Shatté et al., 2017), increased clinical workloads (Tayfur & Arslan, 2013), longer work hours (Ozyurt, Hayran, & Sur, 2006), frenzied clinical care environments (Linzer et al., 2017), and administrative burdens from duplicative documentation, electronic health record processes, and the paperwork associated with coding and billing (Linzer et al., 2017; Shanafelt et al., 2012; Van Dyke & Seger, 2013). HCPs grapple with patients' serious health issues and feel the weight of their responsibilities for patient safety and health outcomes (Helfrich et al., 2017; Welp, Meier, & Manser, 2015). The prolonged periods of stress experienced by HCPs can lead to burnout (Leiter & Maslach, 2009) and other mental health issues (Zwack &

Schweitzer, 2013), including depression (Kuhn & Flanagan, 2017), suicidal thinking (Shatté et al., 2017), anxiety (Harker, Pidgeon, Klaassen, & King, 2016; Rees et al., 2015;), and substance abuse, including smoking and alcohol use (Kreitzer & Klatt, 2017). These trends are true across inpatient, outpatient, and primary care settings (Moss, Good, Gozal, Kleinpell, & Sessler, 2016; Van Bogaert et al., 2013), contributing to the current crisis in the healthcare system as a whole.

Preparing HCP trainees to be resilient in the face of these stressors is now a critical aspect of professional training. In fact, trainees themselves are at particular risk for stress—they must cope with all the same clinical stressors, but also are under pressures academically to perform to the high standards expected of their professions. Stress can negatively impact academic performance, increase fatigue which impacts studying, and increase test-related anxiety (Crego, Carrillo-Diaz, Armfield, & Romero, 2016). Trainees must be prepared for the work-related stress present in the healthcare system by building skills of stress management, self-reflection, and self-care (Fares, Tabosh, Saadeddin, Mouhayyar, & Aridi, 2016).

VIGNETTES OF EXPERIENCE

The University of Arkansas provides an interprofessional curriculum for healthcare professional trainees to learn collaborative practice skills through active learning methods. We offer these stories, drawn from the authors' recollections of actual encounters with learners in the health professions, as composite vignettes to illustrate the highly individualized and diverse sources of stress present within the professional education and work-based practice environments in which HCPs train. In each case, a pseudonym has been used and certain details changed to protect the learner's identity; however, the stories are based upon actual experiences that students have shared with us during recent years.

Sarah's Story

Sarah was a student in the physician assistant program. In high school, she was on the track team and in her undergraduate years, she continued running as a hobby. She enjoyed the emotional benefits of running—having time to think and process and leave the stressful world of grades and studying behind. She made high As and was pleased to be accepted into the competitive physician assistant program. However, in the first year, she discovered that all of the trainees in her program were as bright as she was and also that the course work was very challenging. She began to spend more of her time studying and less time doing things she loved, such as running.

As time went on, she was surprised to discover she was gaining weight and feeling run down and overwhelmed by the demands of her program. Finally, Sarah met with her primary care physician to determine the cause and found she had high blood pressure. As a young adult, she was shocked to have high blood pressure. More than that, negative findings from a variety of tests suggested her constellation of symptoms seemed to be a result of stress. The physician prescribed an antihypertensive and low impact physical activity. She was so upset she went home and cried.

Once spent, she began to write in her journal. She wrote about the stress of advanced training, which was more difficult than anything Sarah had ever attempted. She described her fear that the other trainees would perform better than she would on tests, and of how hard it is to excel in a group of bright trainees. Finally, she wrote angrily about the physician's comments about low impact activity—she was a RUNNER. She was indignant! But as she reflected on the swirl of feelings—frustration, disappointment, lowered self-esteem, and anger—she had to decide to either leave the physician assistant program or to find a way to cope with the stress and academic pressure. It seemed hopeless, and in the absence of knowing what to do, she decided to do something she enjoyed. She recalled that running helped her clear her head. She went for her first run in over a year. Slower than before, for sure, but she again felt the effects—her spirit lifted, her mood brightened, and she had the space to reflect while her feet pounded the pavement methodically. She began running again.

The absence of running was something Sarah had not even considered as a factor, but over the first few weeks, she tracked in her journal the increasing cardiovascular endurance as running became easier. She was proud of the greater distances she was able to travel. She added new routes in parks and trails near the river. She began to realize the importance running had in her mood, her ability to handle stress, and her overall health. It wasn't easy; she would get busy and put off a run. But as she began to recognize her feelings of stress climbing, it was not long before she rescheduled her run. Her health improved dramatically, too. As she ran, she reflected on the need to take care of herself so that she would be in a position to take care of others as a physician assistant in training.

Susan's Story

Susan was a third-year pharmacy student who was assigned to Reflection Rounds (RR). This was a required element of her training as part of a class on professionalism and self-awareness. She did not want to go. She had been told attendance was mandatory in a variety of activities, but the degree of participation was up to the individual—some listened, others actively engaged in the discussion. Susan had a nationally-normed test later that week. She wanted, and felt she needed, every minute to study. As the co-facilitators began the first of four RRs, they requested that pagers and other electronic devices be turned off. Susan ignored the request and left her laptop open with her study materials in view, intending to listen half-heartedly and scan her study material. She was worried about doing well on this test since a lot was riding on it.

After reviewing the purpose of RR and an overview of how a session would proceed, the facilitators opened the floor for someone to discuss a topic. An awkward silence occurred but the facilitators were patient and remained silent. Finally, a student tentatively began telling a story about her experience in chronic pain clinic earlier that day. A patient had confided in her that he did not like the pain physician—wanting his physician to care about him, to see him as a person, to be empathic about his chronic pain, and to not assume he wanted opioid medication.

Other students began to share how hard it is to work with pain patients: the frustration and feelings of failure they experienced because they cannot make the pain go away, blaming of the patient who they concluded must be overreacting to small pain experiences, the desire to distance themselves from patients who were clearly suffering in pain, and more. Susan thought—boring—and started studying harder and tuned out the conversation. The facilitators noticed Susan's behavior and one politely requested that she put away her laptop and be present by actively listening to the student speaking. Susan exploded—"This activity is a joke; it is a waste of time to talk about our feelings! We need to focus on learning the assessment and treatment protocols and we especially need to STUDY FOR OUR TEST TOMORROW!" She stormed out.

Several other students agreed though no one else left. The conversation turned toward academic pressure, the hectic schedule, the reduced sleep, and the impact on stress levels. After the session, the facilitators talked to the training director. It was agreed that according to school policy, unprofessional behavior would be documented for this student as a formal complaint in her file. When Susan was informed, she was devastated. Formal complaints were rare and would surely impact her recommendation letters and thus her chances of placing in the top residency positions after graduation. Worse still, the decision had been vetted across the leadership of the program and it was agreed to by all. As an option, they provided her with an alternative to having a formal complaint documented in her record—however unappealing—training in RR facilitation and assisting with co-facilitating the next year's group.

Susan arrived early for her disciplinary hearing and was respectful when entering the room. She was scared that the report would go in her file and was determined to grit her teeth and get through RR training and implementation next year to avoid that possibility. She was respectful and polite. Later, during the RR facilitator training, she was surprised to learn about the theory and evidence behind RR and its outcomes. This was more science-based than she thought! She practiced and learned how to facilitate, even how to deal with disrupters such as herself. She co-facilitated several cohorts the following year and joined an optional research group that obtained feedback from facilitators and students to make the program even better the next year, including the opportunity to present a poster at a conference on their study results. In the end, she felt she might enact RR with her own students down the line.

Joseph's Story

Joseph was training as a speech and language pathologist. In his first year, his program provided a series of experiences designed to improve awareness of the health and wellness services and programs that are provided by his institution. One such service that he was required to experience was a meditation group that met daily at 7:00 a.m. Joseph was nervous about this particular experience. He had enjoyed visiting the fitness center (free for students) and was planning to attend regularly. But the meditation class—he thought that stuff was just crazy! Meditation is just for spiritual healers and yoga nuts, he thought. Spending time quietly sitting did not seem to be a good use of time. Boring, really. Were they going to make him say "Om"? Yuck.

So, Joseph was a reluctant attendee to the class. He sat down and looked around. The people seemed normal enough, and the instructor was about his age. He began to think that it might not just be boring, but also might be difficult to focus on breathing and to clear his mind of thoughts. What did it matter anyway, there was no hard research on the benefits of this stuff. Resigned, he sat in one of the chairs and looked at the instructor. The instructor explained that before starting some important information about meditation would be shared. He indicated that meditation in and of itself is not difficult. It is not necessary to quiet your mind but, instead, to distance yourself from its thoughts. The metaphor used was of airplanes at a busy airport. You can ride a plane and follow one train of thought or you can simply watch the thoughts come and go. You don't escape your thoughts; you are just no longer at the mercy of anxious, worried, or angry thoughts.

The instructor explained that it does not take years of practice to gain benefits from meditation, and that many people find reduced stress, more empathy, better memory, and a sense of calm from even one or a few sessions. He also mentioned that meditation was not necessarily a spiritual or religious practice; it simply promotes calm. Meditation is not mystical—no visions, no magical revelations. Simply calm, peacefulness, happiness, and gratitude. In fact, Joseph discovered that research has found reduced blood pressure, more restful sleep, and the ability to change negative behavior patterns can all result from participation in meditation. Deepak Chopra first started meditation to stop smoking (Chopra & Tanzi, 2018). He hadn't known that! There is even a lot of research on reducing the risk or the return of cancer. He discovered that meditation is used by sports enthusiasts to heighten enjoyment and performance in their chosen sport. This spoke to his interests in physical fitness. Maybe meditation is not so crazy after all.

Joseph settled in for the first session, which was in a chair and not on the floor. At first he was not sure if he was doing it right, but he followed the simple instructions and came to a place of calm. When he found his thoughts distracting to himself, he simply returned to a focus on his breath or the instructor's words. There was no mantra or repeated phrases like "Om." It was simple and straightforward, not mystical and weird. Ten minutes later he actually felt better—clearer thinking, relaxed, and with a sense of calm. He thought he might attend another, even though one session was all that was mandatory. Over time, Joseph became a regular attendee and found that these meditation practices helped with a wide variety of things—test taking anxiety, sports performance, general stress, even just to take a break in the middle of a hectic day.

David's Story

David was a fourth-year student in medical school. He was becoming withdrawn and his advisor asked to meet with him. After some resistance, he indicated to the advisor that he was very discouraged. He was racking up a large medical school bill and the letters reminding him of the need for eventual payment were weighing heavily on him, especially now that his wife was pregnant. He was feeling unable to provide for his family and, instead, he was bringing them into serious debt. To complicate the situation, he was feeling less and less excited about what he was doing. The work was hard; much of the training involved the use of technological devices, electronic health records, and insurance paperwork that he completed under the supervision of a resident. It was less people-oriented than he expected. He was not sure that medical training was for him, but felt trapped by the debt and the time he had invested already so he felt unable to quit. Plus, he was doing very well—excelling on tests and clinical practice assessments. In short, he was becoming depressed and withdrawn. He described it as a "black hole" where he could peer out and see what was going on around him—clinical work, classroom experiences, fellow students, but he never felt really connected.

After allowing him to share his feelings, the advisor asked him to think back to what brought him to medical school in the beginning. He talked about his father's cancer illness and seeing the compassionate care received from care team members before his death. He remembered also his adolescent medicine physician who was kind and thoughtful and always had time to talk when he came in for a physical. His early experiences were also fun and enjoyable—shadowing at a community pediatrics clinic, volunteering at a health fair, and such.

The advisor asked him what specialty he was considering after medical school. He admitted that he couldn't decide—feeling uncommitted to medical school made it difficult to choose a specialty. They reviewed options slowly, one at a time. The advisor pointed out his early interest in compassionate care and patient-centered practice. After much discussion, palliative care, internal medicine, and family practice were on his short list. He started to show interest and became more animated in the discussion, which was building a positive expectancy about next steps and the transition to residency. She also provided him with information about reducing student debt—working in institutions that were government-supported or charitable organizations for 10 years, which often qualified for small payments during that time and then removal of the remaining debt. She mentioned the names of those sites she knew that qualified for the loan forgiveness program and were linked to his interests. He was thrilled! Low payments for 10 years, working in a field he would enjoy (more people centered, less technical), and then finally the remaining debt removed! He left feeling much lighter and more positive about his training. Out of all the clinical experiences, he began to look for those that were patient focused and involved empathy and support. He became known for his rapport with patients and family members, and his ability to manage emotionally difficult situations. The advisor talked with him before he left for residency in Family Medicine and his mood was bright. He was excited about the next steps in his training and about his future in medicine.

Andrea's Story

Andrea was a 25-year-old nursing student in her first year of training, a nontraditional student with young children at home and a strong desire to better herself and provide for her children. Andrea worked a full-time job at night while attending classes and clinical rotations during the day. She chose nursing because of her deep desire to care for others—her own mother who suffers from Type II diabetes with sores on her feet that will not heal, her children (two with asthma and one with learning difficulties), and her patients. She was particularly interested in pediatric nursing.

Andrea had been feeling very run down lately and more dejected of spirit. She was not only a single parent, caretaker for her medically-ill mother and children, but also her sought-after pediatric clinical rotations had exposed her to an unexpected degree of human tragedy. These included sweet children who were dying from incurable diseases, impaired children from motor vehicle, farming, or other accidents (brain, spinal cord, and loss of limb injuries), and children harmed physically or by neglect, typically by parents or other family caregivers. She found it weakening to her spirit. Rotations in her desired specialty were more draining, more disheartening, and not gratifying. That was not to say there were not moments of joy among the sorrow, moments where she clearly made a difference in a child's care or a parent's grief, and moments where she made a child more comfortable to ease her passing. These were deeply satisfying moments, but few in a larger experience of emotional and physical drain.

In one of her classes, the instructor discussed a concept called "compassion fatigue." Somewhat similar to medicine's preferred "burnout" term, compassion fatigue refers to the constant giving of emotional support and medical care to others, which over time can be draining to the body and spirit. As the instructor spoke, she wondered if she was already experiencing this condition and began to question her ability to manage a pediatric nursing career long term.

She began to talk to her advisor about her experiences, recanting case after case of injured, ill, or dying children on top of her own caregiver tasks for her mother and her own children. Her advisor asked a few questions that deepened her thinking on these issues. "Are you sure that pediatric nursing is where you want to be practicing?" She thought through the other options and their pros and cons, both from an intellectual interest level and also for their potential emotional drain. She wondered whether they would be as deeply satisfying. Her response in the end was a resounding "yes." The instructor then asked what strategies she thought would help restore her positive energy and compassion capacity so that she could withstand the emotional and physical drain long term in order to care for pediatric patients.

After much discussion over several meetings, and personal reflection in the interim, Andrea resolved to try several things to see which were sustainable in her current busy lifestyle, and also which had the most benefit. She tried journaling her thoughts at the end of the day. She processed the heartaching situations she encountered, and mourned the innocent children lost to disease or injury. She reveled in the situations where she made a difference—children became healthier, children became more comfortable, parents felt supported, and the miraculous improvements where she felt God had intervened. She marked those pages for review on days when she felt lower. This exercise would take from 5 to 30 minutes, allowed her to process the events of the day and her resulting feelings, and enabled her to refocus when needed on the moments where her compassionate care and nursing expertise made a difference. She found this a helpful exercise and decided to maintain this activity over time.

She next resolved to try a half a day a week away from caregiving for others or studying. She chose to do whatever she wanted—go for a walk, shop for herself, crochet, read, sit in reflective prayer. Protecting this time was difficult for her. She often let activities with her children, needs with her mother, or studying get in the way. She began to see that on weeks when she had this time, even just a couple of hours, she felt less down-trodden and was more positive and compassionate with her mother, children, and patients. When she let other activities encroach on this time, she became more tired, less happy, and less responsive to the needs of others. It suddenly occurred to her that giving that time to herself made her more able to give to the others in her care. Eventually, she began to see it as the "gas" that made herself go. Rather than getting in the way of giving to others, she found that making time for herself actually made her better able to give to others. She resolved to continue her "me time" indefinitely.

Cynthia's Story

Cynthia was studying to be a dietician. She had always thought that healthy eating improved the functioning of the body—improved cognition, heightened physical performance, and improved resistance to disease. She was committed to healthy eating and modeled this behavior with her fellow students. Cynthia went to school full time and had a part-time work-study position in the hospital cafeteria. She was working on redesigning cooking practices to be more in line with healthy eating so that employees, patients, and family members would be eating healthier while in the hospital environment. She was delighted—her position felt right in line with her own career goals and aspirations.

However, as Cynthia progressed in her training and worked hard at her part-time job, she became tired. She was staying up very late studying after work ended and getting up early to review material before classes the next day. She loved everything she was learning, and, at first, the long days were interesting, stimulating, and enjoyable. But over time, she became more and more tired. She started craving unhealthy foods, sometimes drank caffeinated beverages to stay awake to study, and her performance seemed to be slipping. She had gotten a lower grade on a test despite studying heavily for it. She was slower on her work-related projects than she liked. Her thinking seemed to be slower and slower.

One day, she was yawning in a class, and her professor asked to speak to her afterward. She and the professor sat down to talk through how she was doing. Cynthia talked at length about her passion for her chosen field, her excitement to be in school working toward her dream, and the thrill that her work-study assignment was another opportunity to learn and use her emerging expertise in dietetics. At the end of that long discussion, the instructor reflected that she seemed to be happy and doing well. Cynthia burst into tears. She then began to share the toll taken by the classes, working, and long hours studying. She listed her symptoms of fatigue, slower thought processing, and concern about her perception that her work and academic performance were beginning to deteriorate despite her best efforts. The professor provided supportive encouragement and reflected that she was still one of the top performers in the class. Yet, the professor agreed that her symptoms were fairly pronounced, and asked had she thought about what might help? Cynthia had not really come up with any solutions, feeling her commitment to her training and her need for the work-study job dictated her current schedule.

So she and the professor engaged in a problem-solving activity. Together, they listed all the potential changes she could make and what impact they might have. It was a long list—go to part-time status, take a loan in order to stop working, engage in more physical activity, sleep more, take a vacation. There were pros and cons for each of these. Given the school schedule, the earliest vacation she could take was 2 months away. That seemed to be a good idea and she made some plans to travel to see her parents. However, she also felt that a more immediate step was needed. She did not want to go part-time and slow down her training, nor did she want to take on debt by leaving what was an enjoyable work-study position in her field of interest.

The issue of getting more sleep, however, was a topic that she and her professor discussed at length. The professor provided some information about typical sleep needs (7 to 8 hours a night, with more sleep than normal when stress is higher or illness is present) and appropriate sleep habits (consistent sleep and wake schedule, and a quiet, dark sleep environment), as well as a calming bedtime routine. They also discussed the impact of sleep deprivation—physical fatigue, slower cognitive processing, increased error rates, poor memory.

Cynthia realized that she was typically getting 4 hours of sleep and accumulating a "sleep debt" even if she slept in a bit on her one day off. She began to see the correlation between sleep and performance. After much discussion, she resolved to keep to a consistent bedtime, truncating her study hours to 2 hours on the weekdays and 4 on each weekend. She took an online module on maximizing study time so she would get the most out of it. She developed a 30-minute bedtime routine of reading a fiction book and sipping decaffeinated tea. She made sure to study on the couch and only sleep while in bed, and she made sure the lights and radio were off and her phone was charging in the other room so texts and calls at night would not disturb her sleep. She allowed herself to nap on the weekends anytime she felt tired to catch up on her sleep.

After a few weeks she noticed she rarely needed a nap. She was awakening refreshed and rested. And she was managing to study what she needed to perform well in the time she had allotted. She was surprised to realize that more sleep and less studying time actually led to heightened performance because her cognitive processing was more efficient, her memory improved, and her fatigue was gone. She resolved to continue these behaviors as lifestyle changes from here going forward.

THE TRANSFORMATIVE LEARNING PROCESS

These experiences shared in the stories of Sarah, Susan, Joseph, David, Andrea, and Cynthia are powerful. They bring to life the stressful journey that HCP trainees take to prepare themselves for a career of giving to others. They also capture the diversity in sources of stress, highlight the need for stress management skill-building experiences, and illustrate the individual potential pathways to resilience. However, simply experiencing stress during training is not sufficient for transformative learning to occur.

Frequently, transformative learning involves a crisis or "disorienting dilemma," followed by critical self-reflection that leads to challenges in assumptions, and ends in a process of attitudinal, cognitive, and behavioral changes (Foshee et al., 2017). In these vignettes, the end result was change suggestive of a professional identity that includes self-care. In some situations, transformative learning is a gradual accumulation of changes in the way a person thinks, believes, and challenges previously unchallenged assumptions. Both paths can lead to a professional identity that evolves over time to become one that is more resilient and capable of positive responses to stressful situations and lifestyles.

To better understand the potential for transformative learning, one needs to examine the learning process carefully. Stressful experiences can be a potential catalyst for change (Cranton, 2002). MacKeracher (2012) emphasizes the role of experience in transformative learning and the personal meaning that individuals create to make sense of those experiences. However, experiences alone will not result in the development of resiliency skills nor a professional identity that includes self-care, along with the care of others. The experience of stress can be beneficial, however. The positive benefits from stress, termed "eustress," include positive feelings that result from being engaged and challenged in new directions (Lazarus, 1966). Eustress often prompts feelings of meaning in work, work satisfaction, and career vigor (Nelson & Cooper, 2005). However, the experience of stress can also be negative: the negative consequences from stress, termed "distress," include inability to adapt to stressors and, occasionally, maladaptive behaviors such as aggression, withdrawal, smoking and alcohol overuse, and more (Russ et al., 2012). Distress creates a dilemma that catalyzes inward attention and concern, and outward action to find a way through it.

Events that cause distress are often described as acute personal crises (Mezirow, 1978). They can happen when individuals who enter the healthcare professions in order to care for others feel the strain and drain of giving of themselves. The dilemma involves how to care for oneself while also remaining a "giver" of care to others. The generation of cognitive dissonance and the experience of emotional reaction (anger, sadness, or fear) are often a result of this dilemma; the intensity can be great enough to be disorienting (Mezirow, 1978; Roberts, 2006). Such experiences can create a complex love–hate relationship for the profession in which HCPs are training (Robertson, 1996), and trainees may question whether they should be in the field at all (O'Sullivan, 1999). Thankfully, for most trainees, this is not the end of the story.

IMPLICATIONS FOR HEALTHCARE PROFESSIONALS IN TRAINING

Each of the vignettes showed a trainee who experienced stress from different sources, which led to distressing emotional reactions and a realization that the trainee must make sense of what was happening. Whether the cause was financial burden, compassion fatigue, national testing, or the physical and emotional effects of stress, all of them came to a place of anger (Sarah and Susan), fear (David and Cynthia), sadness (Andrea), or even surprise (Joseph). Each experience was intense enough to focus attention on the trainee and what was happening to try to make sense of the experience (Mezirow, 1978). While thoughts and emotions both play a role in transformative learning, some scholars feel that emotion provides the strongest impetus to critically reflect on one's situation and the need for change (Taylor, 1998). Educators can also help to facilitate this process in trainees and should therefore be aware of the process and their role in helping students develop.

In this space of disorientation, self-examination begins and self-reflection becomes necessary due to the intensity of emotional reactions. Making meaning of these events is a learning process. To do this, one must be reflective and engage in reflective discourse (Dirkx, 1998) through conversation with others. During this communicative learning, trainees discuss and work toward critical analysis of the assumptions which underlie their feelings and behaviors (Mezirow, 1997).

Transformative Learning in the Vignettes

All of the trainees' stories indicated self-reflection in the context of their distress. They talked with others who knew them well, seeking not only support, but also exploring meaning as they conveyed their feelings in words. In some cases, the dialogue that occurred was self-talk, cognitive ruminations or writing in a journal as students worked to find the meaning within their experiences. As they discussed, rediscussed, and gained confidence in their interpretations, they were able to draw meaningful conclusions about their experiences. In this way, the trainees could explore the source of stress, their feelings related to that stress, and their understanding of themselves and their professional career choices that lay beneath the feelings. This active participation in reflective discourse is critical to the transformative learning process. Through discourse, they attached meaning to their experiences and validated what was being shared with them (Cranton, 2002; Mezirow, 1997). MacKeracher (2012) refers to this process as naming the change, but there also appears to be such a fundamental critical reflection on assumptions that an emerging readiness for change has been created (Mezirow, 1997).

Self-reflection and reflective discourse can lead to identifying new ways of behaving. Such reflection can include planning for new behaviors, building competence and self-confidence, acquiring knowledge or skill needed to implement the new behaviors, trying out new behaviors, and identifying any positive benefits and habits that facilitate a healthy lifestyle (Cranton, 2002). Healthy lifestyle change can include behaving, talking, and thinking in a way that is congruent with the new emerging professional identity that includes self-care (Cranton, 2006a).

As the trainees derived meaning from their experiences and reframed their understanding of what it is to be a healthcare provider to include the need for proactive prevention or intervention to facilitate self-care, they then "named" their change. They began exploring options for new behaviors based on an emerging perspective. Whether they considered re-engaging in a familiar behavior like running, or incorporating a new behavior like meditation, they noticed the incongruity between their new professional identity as a care provider and their current behavior that involved self-neglect. They began to take small steps, which were reinforced with reduced stress and congruent with new understandings of a developing professional identity.

Sarah began to run again, starting slowly and building up her pace and distance. In a series of information-gathering steps, David explored financial options with charitable organizations, which both provided opportunities to reduce his debt and also facilitated a return to patient-centered interactions, which he found most fulfilling. Joseph started with one meditation class and over time developed a meditation practice. Susan began with training as an RR facilitator, and developed her interest and skill in reflection as a facilitator of student groups. Cynthia slept with higher quality and duration one night and determined the positive benefits which led to the development of ongoing, good sleep habits. Andrea identified the need to replenish her energy with self-directed activities. With small steps, she began to find time for herself that allowed her the increasing capacity to give again to others—her children, family, and patients. Cranton (2002) describes transformative learning as a perspective transformation that yields three changes—changes in understanding oneself (the sources of stress and its impact on oneself), changes in one's belief system (in this case, the beliefs about what a HCP needs), and behavioral changes (changes toward a healthier lifestyle). Foshee and colleagues (2017) report that transformative learning has been successfully initiated by educators via structured educational interventions with learners.

Implications for Educators

Some scholars have asserted that transformative learning should be a central goal for educators (Cranton & King, 2003), and others believe that educators need skills in teaching for transformation (Slavich & Zimbardo, 2012). Educators can help learners to recognize these "disorienting dilemmas" by exposing the limitations of learners' current knowledge or approaches. Cranton and King found that these need not be punitive or negative, but thought-provoking experiences that invite learners to consider the case for change (Apte, 2009). This can be facilitated through active learning activities such as problem-based learning or by providing feedback strategically, inviting the student to experience the emotions of a situation, rather than simply reading about them, for maximum impact. Teachers need to develop skill in how they help trainees use thoughts and feelings to prompt critical reflection. Educators also need skills in facilitating through defensiveness and resistance that are likely to accompany intentional efforts toward change (Apte, 2009).

Trainees can remain unaware of the sources of their stress by engaging in denial, fixating on the process of attempting to understand what is happening, or by not coming up with any alternative lifestyle behaviors to try (Cranton, 2006a). Educators need to actively design educational events that facilitate the distress needed to spur critical self-reflection. Program design should include an understanding of learning needs as well as preparation for a variety of learning styles (Apte, 2009). This can include learner-centered teaching strategies such as flipped classrooms, student teaching experiences, group-based learning experiences, and other peer-led learning (Weimer, 2012). Learning activities that facilitate critical reflection are particularly important for trainees and educators alike, including writing in blogs, reflective journaling, artistic work, mindfulness practices in the classroom, and teaching journals for educators (Cranton, 2006b).

Educators also need to facilitate reflective discourse in their conversations with learners. In several of the vignettes, trainees sought instructors to discuss their concerns. Assisting trainees in identifying underlying assumptions and reframing them can be helpful. David asked for options to address his mounting debt. Andrea sought support and her teacher shared her own history of dealing with compassion fatigue. Thus, educators can provide experiences that identify alternative behaviors, such as training in RR or a class that provides meditation exposure. They can also model these healthy lifestyle behaviors so that when trainees are under distress and are looking for alternatives, these options are readily available. Dirkx (1997, 1998) describes how both emotions and thoughts help us learn about ourselves, our relationships with others, and how we make sense of all aspects of our experiences, both objective and subjective.

As educators, we need to approach teaching in an intentional way by possessing a strong self-awareness of who we are as teachers (including strengths and weaknesses) and reflecting on our learning activities and the discussions that we have with our learners (Brookfield, 1995; Cranton, 2006a). Furthermore, the development of a teacher–student relationship that fosters openness, questioning, emotional connection, and reflective discourse is critical for educators to be able to facilitate the transformative learning process (Cranton, 2006a). Educators must be attuned to learners' individual and collective worlds (Apte, 2009) to learn together and foster each other's growth (Jarvis, 1992). Asking for feedback from trainees—their qualitative and quantitative feedback along with reflections upon their learning activities—is an important part of that intentional teaching process (Cranton, 2006b). Even within the constraints of a mandatory curriculum and large class sizes, thought-provoking and deeply personal learning experiences can be created that catalyze transformative learning (Cranton & Carusetta, 2004).

Discussion

It is critical for HCP trainees to build and practice skills in stress management, not only to be resilient during training, but also in practice settings as they develop their professional identities. This chapter has analyzed vignettes that specifically address physical, emotional, spiritual, social, and intellectual well-being and the potential for transformative learning as a result of difficult experiences. These examples are not meant to be an exhaustive list of strategies to promote personal wellness or reduce burnout, but, rather, they illustrate a process that can be applied to other stressful experiences during HCP training. These pathways to resilience can result in development of a resilient professional identity as a result of transformative learning.

Trainees need to have skills in stress management to be adequately prepared for professional practice where environments will often be more stressful and have higher consequences for actions than training environments. Furthermore, the culture in which HCPs transition as professionals may or may not value self-care. Trainees need to be prepared for this with skills on how to persevere in self-care despite these challenges. Additionally, they should be empowered to advocate for cultural change in new workplace environments where self-care is not practiced or esteemed. Although culture change requires a long time and senior leadership involvement to develop, trainees can promote this in order to begin gradual workplace changes. Experience with transformative learning in their training can prepare them to overcome these challenges.

While much of the responsibility for efforts to engage in effective self-care strategies falls to trainees, educators can provide instruction regarding transformative learning to facilitate self-reflection, and model positive self-care wellness practices and resilience skills. Visibly modeling self-care behaviors includes scheduling time in the work day for reflection or prayer, using time off as real time away from work, eating healthy foods, getting appropriate amounts of sleep, maintaining appropriate work boundaries through such strategies as out of office notices, taking vacation and sick time, not responding to emails at odd hours, and more. Other ideas for modeling self-care practices include leading walking meetings, participating in team-building physical activities, and reflecting on one's practice often. Educators can foster a culture of transformative learning in their learning environments that includes open communication between trainers and trainees so that conversations which could traditionally be viewed as "uncomfortable" become engaging, productive, and inspiring. Educators may even disclose personal experiences that resulted in their own transformative learning and professional identity formation, as appropriate, to explicitly model this skill to trainees.

POSSIBILITIES FOR FUTURE RESEARCH AND WORKPLACE INITIATIVES

Very little research has examined the relationship between components of wellness and resiliency and the practice of transformative learning. More research is needed to fully explore the impact of educational methods and interventions on the transformative learning process as experienced by HCP trainees. Because stress and burnout rates are widespread, interventions should not be limited to individual, personal levels of change, but also to changes at the programmatic and institutional levels. Some of these conversations might include changing requirements for trainees on shift length, sleep needs, time off, and advocating support for these from accrediting bodies and institutional leadership in the health professions. Discussions on needed changes to support an emphasis on self-care should not stop with trainees; interventions should be made in the existing workforce, as well.

Future training efforts include an opportunity to focus on resiliency training through transformative learning in interprofessional education. As highlighted in the vignettes of trainees from multiple professions, issues of stress and the need for self-care affect all professionals. The newest revision to the Institute for Healthcare Improvement's framework to describe an approach to optimize health system performance is known as the Quadruple Aim. The original framework, called the Triple Aim, focused on (a) improving the patient experience of care, (b) improving the health of populations, and (c) reducing the per capita cost of healthcare (Institute for Healthcare Improvement, 2009). This model was widely adopted by many agencies and institutions to better care for patients. In 2014, some suggested that the Triple Aim should actually be a Quadruple Aim to include a fourth dimension to address provider satisfaction since burnout can jeopardize achievement of the Triple Aim (Bodenheimer & Sinsky, 2014). Ultimately, the well-being of providers is necessary to guarantee success of the Triple Aim (West, 2016). A formal interprofessional curriculum can be designed to help trainees from multiple professions learn about these important concepts of self-care and transformative learning together. We need best practices for development and implementation of such programs across HCP training institutions.

The transformative learning process is not intuitive to all trainees or even to educators. While the steps of critical self-reflection and subsequent action needed for behavioral change may seem obvious from these vignettes, the transformative learning process is sometimes more difficult to implement when a trainee is in the midst of a crisis. Prior awareness of transformative learning and how it occurs can help the person to identify the need for reflection during the crisis and facilitate the steps of change. Having a teacher, mentor, or friend who can help walk through the transformative learning process is also of value. Therefore, educators need to know more about transformative learning and how to help trainees navigate reflection on their issues and develop a plan of action.

Since some stressors are inherent to the healthcare field and are not always modifiable, individual coping skills development will continue to be needed (Jesse, Abouljoud, & Eshelman, 2015). We need to prepare HCP trainees to effectively manage this challenging workplace environment so that we do not lose high quality, well-trained health professionals who are unable to cope and become burned out. This development, for both trainees and professionals already in the current workforce, can be accomplished through an understanding of how change occurs through transformative learning. By explicitly teaching for transformation, educators serve as facilitators of a process that unfolds inside and outside the walls of a classroom or an institution. Transformative learning can help to facilitate resiliency and professional identity development in trainees with careful attention to the nature of growth through adversity.

AUTHORS' NOTE

Individual identifiers in the vignettes have been changed to protect the trainees' identities. Our use of these vignettes and the experiences they represent honors the career choices of these trainees and their peers, and expresses our desire for educators to recognize the need for resiliency skill development to support transformative learning after stressful experiences during training.

REFERENCES

Apte, J. (2009). Facilitating transformative learning: A framework for practice. *Australian Journal of Adult Learning, 49*(1), 168–189. Retrieved from http://files.eric.ed.gov/fulltext/EJ864437.pdf

Benson, M. A., Peterson, T., Salazar, L., Morris, W., Hall, R., Howletter, B., & Phelps, P. (2016). Burnout in rural physician assistants: An initial study. *The Journal of Physician Assistant Education, 27*(2), 81–83.

Bodenheimer, T., & Sinsky, C. (2014). From triple to quadruple aim: Care of the patient requires care of the provider. *Annals of Family Medicine, 12*(6), 573–576. https://doi.org/10.1370/afm.1713

Branch, C., & Klinkenberg, D. (2015). Compassion fatigue among pediatric healthcare providers. *American Journal of Maternal Child Nursing, 40*(3), 160–166.

Brookfield, S. (1995). *Becoming a critically reflective teacher.* San Francisco, CA: Jossey-Bass.

Chopra, D., & Tanzi, R. E. (2018). *The healing self: A revolutionary new plan to supercharge your immunity and stay well for life.* New York, NY: Harmony.

Cranton, P. (2002). Teaching for transformation. *New Directions for Adult and Continuing Education, 2002*(93), 63–71.

Cranton, P. (2006a). *Understanding and promoting transformative learning: A guide for educators of adults* (2nd ed.). San Francisco, CA: Jossey-Bass.

Cranton, P. (2006b). Fostering authentic relationships in the transformative classroom. *New Directions for Adult and Continuing Education,* Spring(109), 5–13. https://doi.org/10.1002/ace.203

Cranton, P., & Carusetta, E. (2004). Perspectives on authenticity. *Adult Education Quarterly, 55*(1), 5–22. https://doi.org/10.1177/0741713604268894

Cranton, P., & King, K. (2003). Transformative learning as a professional development goal. *New Directions for Adult and Continuing Education, 2003*(98), 31–37.

Crego, A., Carrillo-Diaz, M., Armfield, J. M., & Romero, M. (2016). Stress and academic performance in dental students: The role of coping strategies and examination-related self-efficacy. *Journal of Dental Education, 80*(2), 165–172.

Dirkx, J. (1997). Nurturing soul in adult learning. *New Directions for Adult and Continuing Education,* Summer(74), 79–88.

Dirkx, J. (1998). Transformative learning theory in the practice of adult education: An overview. *PAACE Journal of Lifelong Learning, 7*, 1–14.

Dyrbye, L. N., Varkey, P., Boone, S. L., Satele, D. V., Sloan, J. A., & Shanafelt, T. D. (2013). Physician satisfaction and burnout at different career stages. Mayo Clinic Proceedings, *88*(12), 1358–1367. https://doi.org/10.1016/j.mayocp. 2013.07.016

Fares, J., Tabosh, H. A., Saadeddin, Z., Mouhayyar, C. E., & Aridi, H. (2016). Stress, burnout and coping strategies in preclinical medical students. *North American Journal of Medical Sciences, 8*(2), 75–81. https://doi.org/10.4103/ 1947-2714.177299

Foshee, C., Mehdi, A., Bierer, S., Traboulsi, E., Isaacson, J., Spencer, S.,...Burkey, B. (2017). A professionalism curricular model to promote transformative learning among residents. *Journal of Graduate Medical Education, 9*(3), 351–356. https://doi.org/ 10.4300/JGME-D-16-00421.1

Harker, R., Pidgeon, A. M., Klaassen, F., & King, S. (2016). Exploring resilience and mindfulness as preventative factors for psychological distress burnout and secondary traumatic stress among human service professionals. *Work, 54*(3), 631–637. https://doi.org/10.3233/WOR-162311

Helfrich, C. D., Simonetti, J. A., Clinton, W. L., Wood, G. B., Taylor, L., Schectman,..., & Nelson, K. M. (2017, July). The association of team-specific workload and staffing with odds of burnout among VA primary care team members. *Journal of General Internal Medicine, 32*(7), 760–766. doi:10.1007/ s11606-017-4011-4

Institute for Healthcare Improvement. (2009). The triple aim: Optimizing health, care, and cost. *Healthcare Executive, 24*(1), 64–66.

Jarvis, P. (1992). *Paradoxes of learning: On becoming an individual in society.* San Francisco, CA: Jossey-Bass.

Jesse, M. T., Abouljoud, M., & Eshelman, A. (2015). Determinants of burnout among transplant surgeons: A national survey in the United States. *American Journal of Transplantation, 15*(3), 772–778. https://doi.org/10.1111/ajt.13056

Kreitzer, M. J., & Klatt, M. (2017). Educational innovations to foster resilience in the health professions. *Medical Teacher, 39*(2), 153–159. https://doi.org/10.1080 /0142159X.2016.1248917

Kuhn, C. M., & Flanagan, E. M. (2017). Self-care as a professional imperative: Physician burnout, depression, and suicide. *Canadian Journal of Anesthesia, 64*(2), 158–168. https://doi.org/10.1007/s12630-016-0781-0

Lazarus, R. S. (1966). *Psychological stress and the coping process.* New York, NY: McGraw-Hill.

Leiter, M., & Maslach, C. (2009). Nurse turnover: The mediating role of burnout. *Journal of Nursing Management, 17,* 331–339. https://doi.org/10.1111/j.1365-2834.2009.01004.x

Linzer, M., Poplau, S., Brown, R., Grossman, E., Varkey, A., Yale, S.,...Barbouche, M. (2017). Do work condition interventions affect quality and errors in primary care? Results from the healthy work place study. *Journal of General Internal Medicine, 32*(1), 56–61. https://doi.org/10.1007/s11606-016-3856-2

MacKeracher, D. (2012). The role of experience in transformative learning. In E. W. Taylor & P. Cranton (Eds.), *The handbook of transformative learning: Theory, research, and practice* (pp. 342–354). San Francisco, CA: Jossey-Bass.

Mezirow, J. (1978). Perspective transformation. *Adult Education, 28*(2), 100–110.

Mezirow, J. (1997). Transformative learning: Theory to practice. *New Directions for Adult and Continuing Education, 1997*(74), 5–12.

Moss, M., Good, V. S., Gozal, D., Kleinpell, R., & Sessler, C. N. (2016). An official Critical Care Societies Collaborative statement—Burnout syndrome in critical care health-care professionals: A call for action. *CHEST, 150*(1), 17–26. https://doi.org/10.1016/j.chest.2016.02.649

Mott, D. A., Doucette, W. R., Gaither, C. A., Pedersen, C. A., & Schommer, J. C. (2004). Pharmacists' attitudes toward worklife: Results from a national survey of pharmacists. *Journal of the American Pharmacists Association, 44*(3), 326–336.

Nelson, D., & Cooper, C. (2005). Stress and health: A positive direction. *Stress and Health, 21*(2), 73–75.

O'Sullivan, E. (1999). *Transformative learning: Educational vision for the 21st Century.* Toronto, CA: University of Toronto Press.

Ozyurt, A., Hayran, O., & Sur, H. (2006). Predictors of burnout and job satisfaction among Turkish physicians. *The Quarterly Journal of Medicine, 99,* 161–169.

Rees, C. S., Breen, L. J., Cusack, L., & Hegney, D. (2015). Understanding individual resilience in the workplace: The international collaboration of workforce resilience model. *Frontiers in Psychology, 6,* 73. https://doi.org/10.3389/fpsyg.2015.00073

Roberts, N. (2006). Disorienting dilemmas: Their effects on learners, impact on performance, and implications for adult educators. In M. S. Plakhotnik & S. M. Nielsen (Eds.), *Proceedings of the Fifth Annual College of Education Research Conference: Urban and International Education Section* (pp. 100–105). Miami, FL: Florida International University. Retrieved from https://digitalcommons.fiu.edu/cgi/viewcontent.cgi?referer=https://us.search.yahoo.com/&httpsredir=1&article=1249&context=sferc

Robertson, D. (1996). Facilitating transformative learning: Attending to the dynamics of the educational helping relationship. *Adult Education, 47*(1), 41–53.

Russ, T. C., Stamatakis, E., Hamer, M., Starr, J. M., Kivimäki, M., & Batty, G. D. (2012). Association between psychological distress and mortality: Individual participant pooled analysis of 10 prospective cohort studies. *British Medical Journal, 345,* e4933. https://doi.org/10.1136/bmj.e4933

Severn, M. S., Searchfield, G. D., & Huggard, P. (2012). Occupational stress amongst audiologists: Compassion satisfaction, compassion fatigue, and burnout. *International Journal of Audiology, 51*(1), 3–9. https://doi.org/10.3109/14992027.2011.602366

Shanafelt, T. D., Boone, S., Tan, L., Lotte, N. D., Sotile, W., Satele, D., . . . Oreskovich, M. R. (2012). Burnout and satisfaction with work-life balance among US physicians relative to the general US population. *Archives of Internal Medicine, 172*(18), 1377–1385. https://doi.org/10.1001/archinternmed.2012.3199

Shanafelt, T. D., Hasan, O., Dyrbye, L. N., Sinsky, C., Satele, D., Sloan, J., & West, C. P. (2015). Changes in burnout and satisfaction with work-life balance in physicians and the general US working population between 2011 and 2014. *Mayo Clinic Proceedings, 90*(12), 1600–1613. https://doi.org/10.1016/j.mayocp.2015.08.023

Shatté, A., Perlman, A., Smith, B., & Lynch, W. D. (2017). The positive effect of resilience on stress and business outcomes in difficult work environments. *Journal of Occupational & Environmental Medicine, 59*(2), 135–140. https://doi.org/10.1097/JOM.0000000000000914

Shelledy, D. C., Mikles, S. P., May, D. F., & Youtsey, J. W. (1992). Analysis of job satisfaction, burnout, and intent of respiratory care practitioners to leave the field or the job. *Respiratory Care, 37*(1), 46–60.

Slavich, G., & Zimbardo, P. (2012). Transformational teaching: Theoretical underpinnings, basic principles, and core methods. *Educational Psychological Review, 24*(4), 569–608.

Tayfur, O., & Arslan, M. (2013). The role of lack of reciprocity, supervisory support, workload and work-family conflict on exhaustion. *Evidence from Physicians, Psychology, Health & Medicine, 18*(5), 564–575. https://doi.org/10.1080/13548506.2012.756535

Taylor, E. W. (1998). *The theory and practice of transformative learning: A critical review.* Information Series No. 374. Columbus, OH: Clearinghouse on Adult, Career, and Vocational Education, Center on Education and Training for Employment, College of Education, The Ohio State University. Retrieved from ERIC database. (ED423422)

Transformative Learning: Centre for Community Activism. (n.d.). *About the Transformative Learning Centre (1993–2016): The TLC approach to transformative learning: Grounded hope.* Retrieved from https://www.oisc.utoronto.ca/tlcca/About_The_TLC.html

Van Bogaert, P., Clarke, S., Wouters, K., Franck, E., Willems, R., & Mondelaers, M. (2013). Impact of unit-level nurse practice environment, workload and burnout on nurse-reported outcomes in psychiatric hospitals: A multilevel modeling approach. *International Journal of Nursing Studies, 50*(3), 357–365. https://doi.org/10.1016/j.ijnurstu.2012.05.006

Van Dyke, A., & Seger, A. M. (2013). Finding, keeping, and revitalizing the meaning in family medicine. *International Journal of Psychiatry in Medicine, 45*(4), 323–331. https://doi.org/10.2190/PM.45.4.c

Weimer, M. (2012). Learner-centered teaching and transformative learning. In E. W. Taylor & P. Cranton (Eds.), *The handbook of transformative learning: Theory, research, and practice* (pp. 439–454). San Francisco, CA: Jossey-Bass.

Welp, A., Meier, L. L., & Manser, T. (2015). Emotional exhaustion and workload predict clinician-rated and objective patient safety. *Frontiers in Psychology, 5,* 1573. https://doi.org/10.3389/fpsyg.2014.01573

West, C. P. (2016). Physician well-being: Expanding the triple aim. *Journal of General Internal Medicine, 31*(5), 458–459. https://doi.org/10.1007/s11606-016-3641-2

Zwack, J., & Schweitzer, J. (2013). If every fifth physician is affected by burnout, what about the other four? Resilience strategies of experienced physicians. *Academic Medicine, 88*(3), 1–8. https://doi.org/10.1097/ACM.0b013e318281696b

CHAPTER 13

FLOURISHING IN THE WORKPLACE

Enhance Professional Resilience and Promote Well-Being With Appreciative Inquiry

Marion Nesbit
Lesley University

Teresa J. Carter
Virginia Commonwealth University

ABSTRACT

Beginning with Cooperrider's groundbreaking research into what gives life to human systems in the mid-1980s, Appreciative Inquiry has enabled organizations and the people within them to shift their focus away from a problem-solving orientation toward realization of individual strengths and patterns of success by envisioning a desired future. Simultaneous discoveries in positive psychology and positive organizational scholarship not only redirected thinking away from a deficit-based model of health toward one of well-being, but also reoriented negative thinking in organizational contexts toward constructive

Transformative Learning in Healthcare and Helping Professions Education, pages 261–282
Copyright © 2019 by Information Age Publishing
All rights of reproduction in any form reserved.

perspectives and expectations. Whole system interventions, such as Appreciative Inquiry, present an alternative paradigm for individual and organizational change to enable professionals to create healthier, more effective and sustainable workplaces. This chapter explores the historical development of these three streams of inquiry—positive psychology, positive organizational scholarship, and Appreciative Inquiry—to support the development of resilient professional identities and the potential for transformative learning and change.

What if professionals in practice and in training found that the questions they asked of each other were growth-oriented, positive, and energizing, inquiring about exceptional outcomes and life-affirming experiences instead of the difficulties encountered in the workplace? How might the language of these conversations differ from the usual problem orientation and root-cause analysis used to improve what is not working that dominates many institutions? What benefits might these conversations have for individuals, their practice settings, and the satisfaction and sense of accomplishment that they express in their work?

For years, institutions have traditionally emphasized problem-oriented analysis in attempts to bring about change, often with mixed results (Burnes, 2006; Chin & Benne, 1969; Piderit, 2009). Educators and administrators within helping and healthcare settings are among those who have responded to institutional problems by establishing committees and work groups to gather data, explore options, and recommend solutions to "fix" whatever is wrong within the system. Nevertheless, some of these efforts result in a never-ending investigatory cycle that fails to produce lasting change, since the unintended consequences of one corrective action often generate additional problems that need to be solved (Burke, 2008). For many, these types of inquiries have drained energy, enthusiasm, and resources, lowering the resilience of individuals and dampening the potential for an organizational culture based on optimism and hope.

Lack of success with traditional approaches to address problems within an institution spawned the rise of many "whole system" efforts to generate positive change during the latter part of the 20th century (Bunker & Alban, 1997), work that continues today (Cameron & Quinn, 2011; Grieten, Lambrechts, Bouwen, Huybrechts, & Cooperrider, 2018; Stavros & Torres, 2018; Watkins, Dewar, & Kennedy, 2016). These approaches to organizational change attempt to gather people from all parts of the system in one place and time to examine their collective history and envision an ideal future (Bunker & Alban, 1997; Weisbord, 1987, 2004). Future Search conferences introduced by Weisbord and Janoff (2000) were one such initiative that proved to be successful in moving an organization in a positive direction to achieve strategic change. This interest in creating a positive future for people and organizations has been supported by two areas of research that have emerged in parallel with interest in whole system change during the past 20 years: Seligman's (2002, 2008) seminal studies in positive psychology and the work of Cameron, Dutton, and Quinn (2003) in positive organizational scholarship. The counter-narrative posed by these two streams of scholarly inquiry has captured the imagination of those who are interested in reversing the problem-based, gap analysis focus of most change initiatives.

With deliberate attempts to shift the emphasis from what is not working toward a vision of a more positive future, a different kind of conversation has found its way into the corridors of workplaces and educational institutions (Cameron et al., 2003; May et al., 2011; Watkins et al., 2016). The resulting dialogue is more affirming of individuals and what they do on a day-to-day basis, allowing people to build upon their strengths and experience a sense of well-being. Scholars who have studied change initiatives that emphasize the power of positive questions, such as Appreciative Inquiry, have discovered outcomes that promote resilience in both individuals and institutions, reduce burnout, and restore the vitality of those who give so much of their time to the care of others (Cooperrider & Sekerka, 2006; May et al., 2011).

In this chapter, we explore the nature of positive change for professionals in training, as well as those engaged in practice environments, through use of Appreciative Inquiry (Cooperrider, 1986, 2012; Cooperrider & Srivastva, 1987; Cooperrider & Whitney, 2005). We begin by providing background on the history of positive psychology (Seligman, 1999; Seligman & Csíkszentmihályi, 2000; Seligman, Steen, Park, & Peterson, 2005). We present concepts such as *learned optimism* (Seligman, 1990); *flow*, the psychology of optimal experience (Csíkszentmihályi, 1990); and *authentic happiness* (Seligman, 2002). We introduce the concept of *flourishing* (Seligman, 2011), a holistic perspective best described by the acronym PERMA, that encompasses positive emotions (Johnson & Fredrickson, 2005), engagement, positive relationships, meaning and purpose in life, and accomplishment in using one's strengths and talents for personal and organizational success (Peterson & Seligman, 2004; Seligman, 2011). All of these constructs emerged through empirical research and study into aspects of positive psychology. Then we introduce strategies and interventions specifically developed to measure and promote them.

Next, we describe the emergence of positive organizational scholarship at the University of Michigan through studies of positive outcomes, processes, and attributes of organizations and their members (Cameron et al., 2003). Since the introduction of Appreciative Inquiry in Cooperrider's (1986) groundbreaking dissertation research at the Weatherhead School of Management at Case Western Reserve University, a synergistic, interdisciplinary relationship between these three streams of inquiry has developed. An intentional strategy to focus on what gives life to human systems,

Appreciative Inquiry is based on the central principle that individuals and organizations move in the direction of the questions they ask and what they study. Affirmative questions lead to more positive organizational responses (Cooperrider & Srivastva, 1987).

In the decades since its introduction, Appreciative Inquiry has been used by healthcare and helping professionals to promote innovative ideas in teaching and practice settings (Richer, Ritchie, & Marchionni, 2009). These have included efforts to build capacity in nursing practice and patient care (Havens, Wood, & Leeman, 2006; Watkins et al., 2016), support quality improvement and transformative change in healthcare settings (Carter et al., 2007), build connections between students and role models in academic settings (Butani & Plant, 2016), learn about professionalism through faculty stories (Quaintance, Arnold, & Thompson, 2010), and enhance teaching of individuals and groups within medical education (Sandars & Murdoch-Eaton, 2017), among others. Scholars have noted that this approach to positive organizational change has been adopted successfully to enable people and the organizations in which they work become more resilient and better able to flourish (Whitney & Fredrickson, 2015).

In 2007, the University of Virginia (UVA) Schools of Medicine and Nursing, along with the university's medical center and physicians' practice group, founded the Center for Appreciative Practice by focusing Appreciative Inquiry efforts within the institution on a single question: "What do we look like when we're at our best?" (University of Virginia School of Nursing, 2018). May and her colleagues (2011) describe Appreciative Inquiry as both a philosophy and methodology for positive change:

> It is founded on the simple assumption that human systems—teams, organizations, and people—move in the direction of what they study, what they focus on, and what they talk about regularly. The essence of Appreciative Inquiry, then, is the study of what "gives life" to organizations, teams, and people when they are at their best. Appreciative Inquiry does not assume that any person or organization is always at its best. Appreciative Inquiry does posit— and both research and experience show—that people learn and organizations change most readily when they focus on, study, and engage in dialogue about strengths, patterns of success, and who they are at their best. (p. 3)

In this chapter, we provide examples of how Appreciative Inquiry works for individuals and their institutions through the published literature in healthcare. Positively worded questions challenge others to consider how this shift in focus from problem-solving to question-posing might enable them to realize greater strengths to flourish in rapidly changing environments. The field of positive psychology and the development of positive organizational scholarship provide a research basis for this creative approach to individual and organizational change.

WHAT IS POSITIVE PSYCHOLOGY?

The field of positive psychology was introduced by psychologist Martin Seligman in mid-1998 at the American Psychological Association's national conference during his presidential address (Seligman, 1999). Considered the "father" of positive psychology, Seligman sought to transform the discipline from its predominant medical model of pathology and problem remediation that had existed since World War II to focus on making the lives of all people more fulfilling and productive (p. 559). His aim was to create a strengths-based emphasis to help individuals find happiness and pleasure, achieve a sense of belonging through social engagement, and find meaning in work to live life to the fullest and experience well-being. Concerned that psychology was neglecting to continue its pre-war focus on individual strengths, Seligman's goal was to emphasize "the most positive qualities of an individual: optimism, courage, work ethic, future-mindedness, interpersonal skill, the capacity for pleasure and insight, and social responsibility" (p. 559). Consequently, while other forms of psychology helped individuals alleviate problems, positive psychology added value by focusing on human potential to help individuals imagine a lifetime of well-being, create future vision, and move forward purposefully to achieve that vision. Seligman's (1990) book *Learned Optimism*, focused on the power of individuals to cultivate a mental attitude and personal narrative that reflected positive thinking and expectations. It offered a life-changing alternative to learned helplessness, behaviors associated with depressed individuals who behave dependently according to edicts and wishes of those with perceived power (Garber & Seligman, 1980; Peterson, Maier, & Seligman, 1993).

From Learned Helplessness to Learned Optimism

It may seem unusual that a field that recognizes positive personal control and human agency began in a classical conditioning animal laboratory by examining the relationship between electrical shock stimuli and dogs' subsequent behavior. In Seligman's laboratory, the dogs who were not recipients of shocks took action to jump a small barrier, whereas most dogs who experienced aversive shock stimuli did not try to escape stimuli, even if avoidable. The dogs who did not try to jump the barrier to escape the anticipated pain of a shock exhibited learned helplessness (Peterson et al., 1993). However, they also noticed with great curiosity that one third of the shocked dogs did, in fact, try to escape from subsequent pain by jumping the barrier. These researchers realized that it was not the shock that kept dogs from moving away from aversive stimuli; it was perceived lack of control over their situation. Careful scientists, Seligman and his colleagues replicated their findings and moved to human subjects, this time using sound as an aversive stimulus to see if they could replicate the animal studies with humans. When similar results from replications were incontrovertible, Seligman (1990) decided to switch direction and apply his learned helplessness insights to help others by studying depression.

Situated at the University of Pennsylvania, Seligman sought out Beck (2011), an established psychiatrist who was in the process of modifying his psychoanalytic presuppositions that mental illness stemmed from childhood issues toward an appreciation of adult patterns of cognition and behavior. Seligman discovered that Beck had moved toward a patient-participatory stance in patient interactions that was based on dialogue to foster personal growth. Gaining insights into what predisposed some individuals to become depressed, Beck (2011) not only revolutionized the treatment of clinical depression, but also the process of therapy by creating a Cognitive Behavioral Therapy (CBT) approach to care. Beck's professional transformation paralleled Seligman's insights from experimental psychology on the nature of resilience found within studies of learned helplessness (Seligman, 1990; Peterson et al., 1993). Their interests in depression, though different in course, positioned Beck as a mentor and co-pioneer in re-visioning treatment (Seligman, 1990).

Seligman's path went beyond individuals' receiving therapy, however, toward the realm of human possibility to live meaningfully in the present and future. In his efforts to bring public awareness to the field, he began to realize that in addition to the upside of an individual's assuming power and agency to uphold well-being and create better circumstances in life, there was a downside of promoting self-absorption (Seligman, 1990). He took note of the historical changes that had occurred in society following World War II and the Korean War in which a sense of common purpose and shared beliefs that promoted community welfare had devolved to a focus on lifestyle and the purchase of consumer goods. Seligman (1990) noticed the repercussions of this felt loss of community and recognized that "the strengths of the maximal self to shift the balance from self to expand the commitment to the commons" (p. 287) could facilitate learned optimism. He realized that individuals possessed the personal power to move beyond dependency and codependency to find meaning in actions that could foster community, benefit others, and strengthen morals as well as develop healthy physical habits. He proceeded to explore the concept of authentic happiness (Seligman, 2002) and discovered through his research that happiness and meaning in life require connection with others and, moreover, "belonging to and serving something that you believe is bigger than the self" (Seligman, 2011, p. 12).

The Concept of Flow

Seligman developed a collegial relationship with a like-minded colleague, Hungarian-born psychologist Mihály Csíkszentmihályi, whose contribution to positive psychology paralleled Seligman's shift from learned helplessness to learned optimism. In developing the concept of flow from his research into optimal experience, Csíkszentmihályi (1990) described a thoroughly engaging mental state in which individuals are so absorbed in work activity that they lose all sense of time, becoming fully focused, energized, and maximally engaged in accomplishment. The two scholars shared research approaches with a common positive attitude and belief in the importance of finding meaning in work. They sought the possibilities inherent in applying their findings to understanding and designing positive institutions that would cultivate a culture of well-being. Their collaborations led to coauthoring of the "manifesto" of positive psychology (Seligman & Csíkszentmihályi, 2000) by drawing on independent discoveries that focused on attaining flow and achieving positive emotions to counteract stress, burnout, and depression. They refocused psychology on motivational concepts of constructive energy and behavior toward optimal human functioning. Their work provided a strong research basis for the underlying principles of what gives life to human systems in an Appreciative Inquiry (Cooperrider, 1986; Cooperrider & Srivastva, 1987) and contributed to the power of positive energy in positive organizational scholarship.

The Ability to Flourish

Seligman (2002) explored the concept of authentic happiness by conducting empirical research during his time at the University of Pennsylvania and determined, in addition to pleasure and flow factors, happiness involved finding meaning in life, not solely for oneself but beyond one's own parameters through connections with others. In his book, *Flourish*, Seligman (2011) committed to exploring "what makes life worth living" (p. 1), stating "the content itself [of positive psychology]—happiness, flow, meaning, love, gratitude, accomplishment, growth, better relationships—constitutes human flourishing" (p. 2). Seligman's inclusion of gratitude here is worth noting for its connection to positive organizations and its causal links to positive outcomes, including mood and prosocial behavior (Emmons, 2003, p. 85).

How an individual sees the world, chooses to behave, and explains his or her behavioral and lifestyle choices matters. Seligman (1990) posited that an individual's explanatory style contributes to how that individual lives out life and, in so doing, affects the lives of others. He suggested explanatory style "can produce depression in response to every day setbacks or pro-duce resilience even in the face of tragedy" (p. 116). Having the courage to thrive and flourish in face of life's daily challenges is a choice. By engaging in a process of cognitive self-mediation using intervening ideas, one can move into a different, more forward-oriented behavioral pattern that, in turn, can be incorporated into a revised explanatory style and create the opportunity for authentic happiness.

Progress in Research and Study in Positive Psychology

In 2005, Seligman, Steen, Park, and Peterson authored a report on prog-ress in the field of positive psychology. Ever since the 1998 call to action, Seligman and his colleagues at the University of Pennsylvania had sought to reorient psychology as a discipline that embraced "a more complete and balanced scientific understanding of the human experience—the peaks, the valleys, and everything in between" (Seligman et al., 2005, p. 410). Their work in the emerging science of positive psychology was careful to draw upon established, rigorous methods with randomized, placebo-controlled designs to create an evidence-based practice (p. 410). Seligman and his re-search colleagues (2005) found strong agreement between the strengths profiles of U.S. adults and adolescents. The results of these studies led them to posit that "strengths of the heart," such as zest (approaching life with excitement and energy), gratitude, hope, and love were more robustly asso-ciated with life satisfaction than cerebral strengths such as curiosity or love of learning (p. 412). They also sought to move research findings into the public domain by publishing statistical results and describing strategies and interventions to promote authentic happiness.

In a large-scale, randomized controlled trial, Seligman and his col-leagues (2005) designed a study using internet-based recruitment to ex-plore the effectiveness of short-term interventions in generating positive emotions, engagement, and meaning in life for the study participants (p. 416). Among the interventions was a "gratitude visit" in which study participants wrote a letter of gratitude to someone who had been especially kind, but whom they had not previously thanked for their kindness. They were then asked to deliver the letter in person to the individual within a week's time. In the "three good things in life" exercise, study participants wrote down three things that went especially well for them each day dur-ing a week's time and then provided an explanation for each one. Another intervention was the "you at your best" exercise in which study participants wrote about a time when they were at their best. They then reflected on the personal strengths displayed in the narrative and described how they had used these strengths each day for a week. In the "using signature strengths in a new way" exercise, study participants completed the online inventory of character strengths (University of Pennsylvania, 2018a) and received feedback on their top five signature strengths. They were instructed to use one of these strengths in a new or different way on a daily basis for a week. Finally, in the "identifying signature strengths" exercise, study participants were simply asked to complete the survey which would identify their top five strengths and to use them more often over a week's time (Seligman et al., 2005, p. 416).

Seligman et al.'s (2005) analysis of results showed that using signature strengths in a new way and the three good things exercises increased happiness and decreased depressive symptoms for 6 months. The gratitude visit was shown to cause large positive changes for 1 month. The other exercises were found to yield positive effects on happiness and decreases in depressive symptoms, but the effects were transient once the interventions ended. The researchers also found that when study participants continued to participate in the exercises beyond 1 week, they extended their positive effects. Not surprisingly, researchers suggested that lack of continued use of the positive interventions by incorporating them into lifestyle changes and practices resulted in a loss of their beneficial effects.

In studying character development and well-being, Seligman found a like-minded positive psychology colleague in the late Chris Peterson, a leading scholar in the field known also for his work on character and flow. Together, they linked character strengths with positive psychology, and Peterson and colleagues developed the Character Strengths Inventory at the Values in Action (VIA) project, where the survey was launched (Peterson & Seligman, 2004). Since then, considerable international research has been conducted with the six million global participants. The survey (VIA Institute on Character, 2018) is a Web-accessible survey involving questions that determine the rank order of 24-character strengths, organized according to six virtues: wisdom, courage, humanity, justice, temperance, and transcendence. The top five strengths identified for an individual respondent are considered "signature strengths," those that are essential to the person and how he or she lives in the world. Peterson and Seligman (2004) strove to clarify the definition of character and make results useful for the individual personally and professionally. They saw character strengths, particularly the signature strengths, as the unique hallmark of an individual and central to professional identity, recognizable as the essential or authentic self: "This is the real me."

Among the attributes of signature strengths are their consistency over time and wide use across multiple life domains and situations, the feeling of excitement that an individual has when using them, especially at first, and the ease with which these strengths are initially learned and then used continuously in new ways to enact the strength over time. Peterson and Seligman (2004) believed that individuals express a yearning to act in accordance with the strength, and experience a feeling of inevitability in using the strength, as if the person cannot be stopped from doing so. Using the strength is energizing, rather than exhausting, driven by intrinsic motivation and the creation and pursuit of projects that involve using the strength (VIA Institute on Character, 2018).

In 2009, Seligman and his positive psychology colleagues were tapped to provide a large-scale intervention for the U.S. Department of Defense by working with the Army to improve soldiers' and their families' personal health and well-being (University of Pennsylvania, 2018b). Recognizing the increased stress associated with deployments and the rise of post-traumatic stress syndrome and its effects on judgment and decision-making, Army leadership sought an individual level of intervention across ranks, rather than at the systems level. In the newly created Comprehensive Soldier and Family Fitness program, they envisioned a prevention model to build self-awareness, comprehension, and appreciation of strengths and attributes that contribute to resiliency "to create a force of 'optimally fit' individuals who can overcome stress-producing events and grow from these experiences" (University of Pennsylvania, 2018c).

Emotions and the Elements of Well-Being

Seligman (2011) proposed five elements of a construct called well-being in what came to be known as PERMA, an acronym for positive emotion, engagement, relationships, meaning, and accomplishment. Each element meets criteria by containing three properties: "it contributes to well-being," "many people pursue it for its own sake," and "it is defined and measured independently of the other elements" (p. 16). These terms and definitions make up the PERMA model of well-being to contribute to human flourishing:

- Positive emotion, defined as the pleasant life, feeling good, happiness, and life satisfaction;
- Engagement, being completely absorbed in activities by matching one's skills to work expectations so that one is consumed in the very flow of the experience itself;
- Relationships that are positive, authentically connected to others so that one loves and is loved and cares for others by showing kindness, respect, and compassion;
- Meaning, defined as living a purposeful existence, not only for oneself but also by contributing something, small or large, that makes a difference to others; and

- Accomplishment, gaining a sense of achievement and success that can be pursued for its own sake (pp. 16–21).

Seligman (2008) also reported research findings demonstrating health benefits for individuals who expressed positive emotion, including many applicable to healthcare professionals and their patients: alleviating depression, enhancing creative thinking, diagnosing conditions more quickly and accurately, improving response to cardiovascular surgery, adhering to medical treatment protocols post-heart transplant surgery, and healing times that were faster, as well as lowering risk of frailty onset, protecting against stroke, and lowering mortality rates (pp. 5–7). Similarly, Lyubomirsky, King, and Diener (2005) found that happy individuals are healthier and experience success in multiple environments, including home, work, and friendships. Based on their findings, Lyubomirsky and colleagues developed a conceptual model to illustrate that positive affect contributes to success. Interestingly, rather than success leading to happiness, the findings indicated that happiness leads to success.

Other scholars, including Fredrickson (2001, 2003), contributed to the study of positive emotions and their beneficial effects. Labeling herself an emotion scientist, Fredrickson (2001) advanced a "broaden and build" theory to see what happens when people increase their positive emotions. From numerous research studies, she learned that if individuals could keep a 3:1 ratio of three positive thoughts to one negative, it made a difference between flourishing and losing their vitality. Fredrickson (2003) hypothesized that positive emotions produce optimal individual functioning, not only in the present moment when experienced, but also over the long term as well: "positive emotions appear to *broaden* people's momentary thought-action repertoires and *build* their enduring personal resources" (p. 166, emphasis in original). Fredrickson also found that positive emotions are unique in their capacity to regulate the negative emotional arousal that occurs when fear, anxiety, anger, and even sadness produce increases in heart rate, vasoconstriction, and blood pressure (p. 168). Positive emotions, then, contribute to upward spirals in well-being to "transform individuals into more resilient, socially integrated, and capable versions of themselves" (p. 169) by improving their ability to cope and by increasing the likelihood that they will continue to function well and flourish in the future. With interest in the organizational dimensions of positive psychology, researchers at the University of Michigan began to shift the focus from an individual unit of analysis to a collective one to study a positive approach to well-being in organizational life.

POSITIVE ORGANIZATIONAL
SCHOLARSHIP AND APPRECIATIVE INQUIRY

According to Cameron et al. (2003), the emerging discipline of positive organizational scholarship (POS) draws upon a full range of organizational theories to understand positive states in organizational contexts. It is an attempt
to examine phenomena that include positive outcomes, processes, and attributes of organizations and their members in the study of human potential
(p. 4). Words such as excellence, thriving, flourishing, abundance, resilience,
altruism, meaningfulness, high quality relationships, and virtuousness can all
be considered enablers of organizational effectiveness as well as motivations
and outcomes of an emphasis on human potential in organizational studies
(p. 5). Such study includes how organizational practices enable individuals
to achieve meaningful work and maximize individual talents and strengths
in service of organizational goals. Positive organizational scholarship seeks
to "develop rigorous, systematic, and theory-based foundations for positive
phenomena. POS requires careful definitions of terms, a rationale for prescriptions and recommendations, consistency with scientific procedures in
drawing conclusions, and grounding in previous related work" (p. 6).

Positive organizational scholarship is closely allied with organization development (OD), a facilitator-led field of practice and inquiry (Beckhard, 1997;
Harrison, 1994; Schein, 1988, 1999) that strives to increase effectiveness and
enhance organizational learning. OD practitioners work either as internal
consultants (employees of the organization) or external consultants (hired
from outside firms) to collaborate with institutional leaders to address issues
of organizational culture and climate, work processes, team effectiveness,
and productivity (Block, 2011; Weisbord, 1987, 2004). Positive organizational
scholarship can serve as an underlying framework to guide OD practitioners
as they determine best practices and interventions to achieve their aims. The
unconditionally positive approach of Appreciative Inquiry is in sharp contrast to Kurt Lewin's (1947) action research methods used by OD facilitators to "unfreeze" the organization as a system with information about the
seriousness or severity of its problems prior to initiation of a change effort
(Burnes, 2006; Weisbord, 1987, 2004). While action research methods have
a long and respected tradition in consulting practice, organizations change
much too rapidly today for the time-intensive data-gathering and analysis that
has traditionally informed most OD initiatives (Weisbord, 1987, 2004).

Embracing Appreciative Inquiry as a Change Strategy

Whole system interventions, such as Appreciative Inquiry, derive from
a totally different paradigm about how people and organizations change

(Fry, 2014). The Appreciative Inquiry approach to change depends upon four basic beliefs: first, people, both individually and collectively, have unique gifts, skills, and contributions to make; second, organizations are human social systems with unlimited relational capacity that can be expressed through their words; third, the images that individuals hold of the future are socially created and can be used to guide actions; and fourth, through inquiry and dialogue, people can shift their focus away from problem analysis to generate worthwhile ideals and possibilities for the future (Whitney & Trosten-Bloom, 2010, p. 2). The focus on unconditionally positive questions that ask about peak experiences when organization members perceived themselves to be at their best has an entirely different motivational effect to generate a future reality that mirrors the best of present and past successes (Fry, 2014).

Most importantly, more than 30 years of inquiry with positive questions have shown that Appreciative Inquiry works and can bring about transformative change for organizations, as well the individuals working within them (Cooperrider & Whitney, 2005; Fry, 2014; Stavros & Torres, 2018; Whitney & Trosten-Bloom, 2010). How does Appreciative Inquiry work? Appreciative Inquiry involves establishing the topics of interest and four basic phases of inquiry that are conducted sequentially. These are referred to as the 4-D cycle, which stands for Discovery, Dream, Design, and Destiny (Cooperrider & Whitney, 2005).

Choosing Appreciative Topics

Topics for the inquiry arise from the desires of a group to explore the nature of experience in depth to discover its positive potential for strategic change. As Carter et al. (2007) suggest, topics arise from discussions of issues and opportunities with key stakeholders prior to the inquiry event, whether it is a 2-day Appreciative Inquiry summit or a series of shorter sessions held over multiple days or weeks. Three to five topics of interest are then reframed as constructive opportunities to align with strategic goals for the team, department, or organization (p. 195). Appreciative topics, also called affirmative topics, include examples such as these that have been used in a healthcare context:

- the need to create a communication system that will best meet the need of patients for personalized access and the needs of healthcare providers for managing responses (Carter et al., 2007),
- the need to build upon exemplary practice to create a better sign-out process for resident physician handoffs at the end of a hospital

shift to improve patient care and reduce medical errors (Helms et al., 2011),

- the need to develop a new strategic plan within a School of Nursing (Harmon, Fontaine, Plews-Ogan, & Williams, 2012), and
- the need to do a better job of transmitting the values associated with professionalism to medical students (Quaintance et al., 2010).

Whatever the organizational context, the need for strategic change drives the choice of appreciative topics and establishes the purpose of the Appreciative Inquiry intervention. The answers to the inquiry, discovered through phases of the 4-D cycle, yield the positive core—what the institution does when it is at its very best (Whitney & Trosten-Bloom, 2010). It follows that implementation will not be driven by executive mandate or even consultant recommendations. Instead, it becomes a collectively-held ideal in which individuals have invested their hopes, desires, and dreams for the future. Since the desired outcome has been inspired and designed by organization members, it represents what they are most interested in creating to build upon existing strengths and motivations for success. Organization members become the ones who enact and sustain the desirable future they have envisioned. The paradigm of how change occurs within a human system has shifted a full 180 degrees.

Surfacing the Ideal Through Discovery

Discovery is the initial, energizing query that surfaces individual and collective motivations by tapping into the meaning of positive experiences: "It is an extensive, cooperative search to understand the 'best of what is and what has been'" (Whitney & Trosten-Bloom, 2010, p. 7). This search asks about peak experiences when things were working really well, when people felt good about the work accomplished, or when someone or a group was able to tap into personal or collective strengths to benefit others. Discovery is the heart and soul of Appreciative Inquiry as individuals interview each other for stories about their most rewarding moments. Individuals who come from multiple levels and stakeholder groups within the organization, with different roles and responsibilities, conduct the interviews with each other in "improbable pairs," since they are unlikely to have interacted as peers previously within the organizational hierarchy. They use well-crafted, positively-worded questions that have been designed by a planning group to elicit full and complete descriptions of peak experiences on the appreciative topic.

In the example below, written by May et al. (2011) for use at the University of Virginia's Medical Center, interview questions asked about the skills and work environment qualities needed to ensure that everyone who helped families and patients deal with loss was fully prepared and able to do so. Participants were asked to recall their own experiences, and those of others they had observed, for the qualities, attributes, and conditions that provided the best experiences of support and comfort during the most difficult of times:

> Think of a time when someone was relying on you to help him or her with a serious loss...Alternatively, think of a time when you faced a loss and someone did or said something that comforted you.
>
> > What was done by you or for you that proved to be helpful? Be as specific as you can.
> > What lessons can you take from this experience?
> > If you were providing support for someone else, without being modest, what allowed you to provide this support? If someone else was there for you, what strengths did that person bring that allowed him or her to help you?
> > Who else does this really well? What is it that allows this person to be there for others so exceptionally? (May et al., 2011, p. 32)

Discovery asks individuals to share their stories of exceptional experiences in depth and with personal relevance. After the interviews, small groups consisting of multiple interview pairs meet to share stories and elaborate upon what they see as themes discovered through collective experience. These are then collated and analyzed for common themes from all the participants.

Envisioning the Dream of What Might Be

The Dream phase allows participants in the inquiry to envision the ideal future imaginable, using the strengths and skills of individuals in the best possible work environment. In a continuation of the example of loss, it is a look into the future to imagine what the healthcare setting would be like if everyone involved performed exceptionally well when providing support and care for families and patients. May and her colleagues (2011) offer these questions to explore the Dream phase of an Appreciative Inquiry on this topic:

> Imagine that you have been magically transported several years into the future and this type of support is available for patients whenever they need it.
>
> - What changes have been made in the way patients are cared for during difficult times?
> - What has happened to allow this to occur?
> - What difference has it made for patients? (p. 32)

The Dream phase allows participants in the Appreciative Inquiry to anchor the future into their minds today, imagining what could be within their own organizational environment and what changes are needed to enable this anticipatory reality (Fry, 2014). Dream transforms memory of the best that is and has been into an ideal future of real possibility. As Whitney and Trosten-Bloom (2010) note, the Dream phase is both practical and generative:

> It amplifies the positive core and challenges the status quo... Typically conducted in large-group forums, Dream activities result in alignment around creative images of the organization's most positive potentials and strategic opportunities, innovative strategic visions, and an elevated sense of purpose. (p. 8)

Designing a Future to Realize the Ideal

The third phase of an Appreciative Inquiry, Design, involves writing a set of provocative propositions: concrete statements that describe an ideal of what the organization should be. These are created either in a large group forum or by smaller groups or teams. Appreciative Inquiry participants build upon the Discovery and Dream phases to draft affirmatively worded statements about the desired organizational qualities that will be the future. These create a bold image of the positive core by describing what the organization will be like in all of its strategies, systems, decisions, and the successful collaborations within it. In this manner, participants co-construct the image of the future in all of their systems and processes.

Empowering and Sustaining a Destiny

Destiny is the final phase of the cycle, one that is essential to the success of Appreciative Inquiry. It provides organizational members who have taken part in the process a chance to step forward in an open forum to make personal and organizational commitments to take actions that will support the learning and innovation needed to make the envisioned future a reality (Whitney & Trosten-Bloom, 2010). It is literally "where the rubber meets the road." The activities accomplished in the Destiny phase are multifaceted, involving large group commitments to action steps and also specific actions outlined by small groups and teams. Destiny creates the path forward and becomes the realization of the Dream through specific plans and concrete changes that people are committed to make in their daily work. As a result, the organization has generated the momentum to put into place an array of changes with full support of the organization's members. These range from management practices, measurement and evaluation systems, customer service systems, work processes, and the needed structural elements to ensure that the positive core—the best of what this organization can be—becomes its future (Whitney & Trosten-Bloom, 2010, p. 9).

CHALLENGES TO ORGANIZATIONAL IMPLEMENTATION

All whole system interventions, such as Appreciative Inquiry, seek to involve as many organizational members as possible from as diverse, broad, and deep a swath of roles and responsibilities as time and facilities will allow. In a department or team, it may be possible to be all inclusive. However, it is literally impossible to involve everyone in a large organization or institutional system to carry out an Appreciative Inquiry for many reasons. In healthcare, the nature of the work means that many work functions operate on a 24/7 basis. Attendees need to be strategically chosen to come from different levels and functions within the organization, and certainly not all from senior management ranks. Many are likely to be informal leaders within their teams or departments, individuals who have the personal power to influence and share what they have learned, but who are not among the managerial team.

What about all the others who did not take part in creating the Dream? How do they learn to live it out, and how does the organization capture their commitment to the process? This is the challenge of whole system interventions in which the excitement and enthusiasm of those who participated needs to influence the rest. Many strategies exist for engaging others who were not present; among them is professional video-recording of parts of the Appreciative Inquiry events so that the recordings can be shared and displayed throughout the organization and discussed in department meetings. Organizational forums can be held to disseminate the ideas developed by describing the process. Most importantly, others will see the influence of the Appreciative Inquiry experience in day-to-day interactions, meetings, and hallway discussions.

What occurred in the Appreciative Inquiry has altered the vision for future direction in the team, department, or organization as a whole. Over time, this new reality influences the agendas for meetings, the conversations among colleagues, and the goals and objectives of organizational units. "Trickle-down" commitment in whole system interventions is not necessarily as rapid a process as a 2-day Appreciative Inquiry summit, but it does happen as those who were there consistently display and enact the new vision over time. The path forward becomes clear, others catch the enthusiasm, and, eventually, they will travel together to realize the desired future.

Watkins and her colleagues (2016) studied Appreciative Inquiry as an intervention to change nursing practice in in-patient settings through an integrative review of publications between 1990 and 2015 retrieved from multiple databases. They concluded that Appreciative Inquiry does offer sound potential for nurse practice development and change, but not without full cognizance of the pivotal components as described by Cooperrider and Whitney (2005). They make two key points: First, Appreciative Inquiry should have expert facilitation to guide and lead the process. The dynamics of large group forums and alternating small group processing are complex. Managing a process that involves multiple stakeholders requires necessary pre-work in setting appreciative topics that are appropriate. Guiding a small planning group to create unconditionally positive questions for the inquiry requires experience, and facilitators need sufficient expertise in group dynamics and deep understanding of the change mechanisms that operate in human systems.

Second, groups and organizations considering the use of Appreciative Inquiry should guard against having a pre-set agenda that attempts to mold participant experiences to fit a previously established set of outcomes (Watkins et al., 2016). Appreciative Inquiry is an emergent process that requires a leap of faith from organizational leaders and trust in the inherent strengths and talents of individuals to generate an idealized future that will be good for all. This kind of leadership is empowering. Leaders learn to place their trust in those who so eloquently expressed their loftiest ideals of what they and the organization can achieve when they are at their best. Appreciative Inquiry can serve to enhance well-being, support individual and group excellence, promote resilience, and allow everyone the opportunity to flourish. The result of this change can be transformative for individuals and the organization as a whole (Carter et al., 2007; Cooperrider, 2012).

CONCLUDING THOUGHTS

Building resilient professional identities does not occur in isolation as an individual endeavor. What happens within the institutional or practice setting matters. Whether day-to-day occurrences are framed as problems to be solved, opportunities for growth and development, or blessings to be appreciated makes a difference in the overall culture and work climate. Every helping or healthcare professional is part of multiple communities of practice; collectively, these form broad landscapes of professional endeavor, all of which serve to reinforce what is learned and socially acquired as the "right" way to think, feel, and act (Wenger-Trayner & Wenger-Trayner, 2015) in providing care for patients and clients as well as self. As students and trainees are enculturated into these professional communities, they acquire the tacit environmental attitudes of their work settings and the beliefs that others have about what they do. How much more satisfying might this work be if everyone involved applied basic ideals of positive psychology and organizational scholarship by using the approach in Appreciative Inquiry to flourish in the workplace to achieve well-being?

AUTHORS' NOTE

Permission to use the two questions that appear in this chapter from *Appreciative Inquiry in Healthcare* (2011) was granted by Crown Custom Publishing.

REFERENCES

Beck, J. (2011). *Cognitive behavior therapy: Basics and beyond* (2nd ed.). New York, NY: Guilford.

Beckhard, R. (1997). Who needs us? Some hard thoughts about a moving target—the future. In D. F. Van Eynde, J. C. Hoy, & C. C. Van Eynde (Eds.), *Organization development classics: The practice and theory of change—The best of the OD Practitioner* (pp. 11–25). San Francisco, CA: Jossey-Bass.

Block, P. (2011). *Flawless consulting: A guide to getting your expertise used* (3rd ed.). San Francisco, CA: Pfeiffer.

Bunker, B. B., & Alban, B. T. (1997). *Large group interventions: Engaging the whole system for rapid change.* San Francisco, CA: Jossey-Bass.

Burke, W. W. (2008). *Organization change: Theory and practice* (2nd ed.). Los Angeles, CA: SAGE.

Burnes, B. (2006). Kurt Lewin and the planned approach to change: A reappraisal. In J. V. Gallos (Ed.), *Organization development: A Jossey-Bass reader* (pp. 133–157). San Francisco, CA: Jossey-Bass.

Butani, L., & Plant, J. (2016). Building connections with role models using an Appreciative Inquiry approach. *Academic Pediatrics, 16*(4), 411–412.

Cameron, K. S., Dutton, J. E., & Quinn, R. E. (2003). Foundations of positive organizational scholarship. In K. S. Cameron, J. E. Dutton, & R. E. Quinn (Eds.), *Positive organizational scholarship: Foundations of a new discipline* (pp. 3–13). San Francisco, CA: Berrett-Koehler.

Cameron, K. S., & Quinn, R. E. (2011). *Diagnosing and changing organizational culture: Based on the competing values framework.* San Francisco, CA: Jossey-Bass.

Carter, C. A., Ruhe, M. C., Weyer, S., Litaker, D., Fry, R. E., & Stange, K. C. (2007). An Appreciative Inquiry approach to practice improvement and transformative change in health care settings. *Quality Management in Health Care, 16*(3), 194–204.

Chin, R., & Benne, K. D. (1969). General strategies for effecting changes in human systems. In W. G. Bennis, K. D. Benne, & R. Chin (Eds.), *The planning of change* (2nd ed.; pp. 32–59). New York, NY: Holt, Rinehart, & Winston.

Cooperrider, D. L. (1986). *Appreciative Inquiry: Toward a methodology for understanding and enhancing organizational innovation (theory, social, participation).* ProQuest Dissertations Publishing. No. 8611485

Cooperrider, D. L. (2012). The concentration effect of strengths: How the whole system "AI" summit brings out the best in human enterprise. *Organization Dynamics, 41*(2), 106–117. https://doi.org/10.1016/J.orgdyn.2012.01.004

Cooperrider, D. L., & Sekerka, L. E. (2006). Toward a theory of positive organizational change. In J. V. Gallos (Ed.), *Organization development: A Jossey-Bass reader* (pp. 223–238). San Francisco, CA: John Wiley.

Cooperrider, D. L., & Srivastva, S. (1987). Appreciative Inquiry in organizational life. *Research in Organisational Change and Development, 1*, 129–169.

Cooperrider, D. L., & Whitney, D. (2005). *Appreciative Inquiry: A positive revolution in change.* San Francisco, CA: Berrett-Koehler.

Csíkszentmihályi, M. (1990). *Flow: The psychology of optimal experience.* New York, NY: Harper.

Emmons, R. A. (2003). Acts of gratitude in organizations. In K. S. Cameron, J. E. Dutton, & R. E. Quinn (Eds.), *Positive organizational scholarship: Foundations of a new discipline* (pp. 81–93). San Francisco, CA: Berrett-Koehler.

Fredrickson, B. L. (2001). The role of positive emotions in positive psychology: The broaden and build theory of positive emotions. *American Psychologist, 56*(3), 218–226.

Fredrickson, B. L. (2003). Positive emotions and upward spirals in organizations. In K. S. Cameron, J. E. Dutton, & R. E. Quinn (Eds.), *Positive organizational scholarship: Foundations of a new discipline* (pp. 163–175. San Francisco, CA: Berrett-Koehler.

Fry, R. (2014). Appreciative Inquiry. In D. Coghlan & M. Brydon-Miller (Eds.), *The SAGE encyclopedia of action research* (pp. 45–48). Thousand Oaks, CA: SAGE. http://doi.org/10.4135/9781446294406

Garber, J., & Seligman, M. E. P. (1980). *Human helplessness: Theory and application.* New York, NY: Academic Press.

Grieten, S., Lambrechts, F., Bouwen, R., Huybrechts, J., Fry, R., & Cooperrider, D. (2018). Inquiring into Appreciative Inquiry: A conversation with David Cooperider and Ronald Fry. *Journal of Management Inquiry, 27*(1), 101–114. https://doi.org/10.1177/1056492616688087

Harmon, R. B., Fontaine, D., Plews-Ogan, M., & Williams, A. (2012). Achieving transformational change: Using Appreciative Inquiry for strategic planning in a School of Nursing. *Journal of Professional Nursing, 28*(2), 119–124. https://doi.org/10.1016/j.profnurs.2011.11.007

Harrison, M. I. (1994). *Diagnosing organizations: Methods, models, and processes* (2nd ed.). Thousand Oaks, CA: SAGE.

Havens, D. S., Wood, S. O., & Leeman, J. (2006). Improving nursing practice and patient care: Building capacity with Appreciative Inquiry. *Journal of Nursing Administration, 36*(10), 463–470.

Helms, A. S., Perez, M. S., Baltz, J., Donowitz, G., Hoke, G., Bass, E. J., & Plews-Ogan, M. L. (2011). Use of an Appreciative Inquiry approach to improve resident sign-out in an era of multiple shift changes. *Journal of General Internal Medicine, 27*(3), 287–291. https://doi.org/10.1007/s11606-011-1885-4

Johnson, K. J., & Fredrickson, B. L. (2005). We all look the same to me: Positive emotions eliminate the own-race bias in face recognition. *Psychological Science, 16*(11), 875–881.

Lewin, K. (1947). Frontiers in group dynamics: II. Channels of group life; Social planning and action research. *Human Relations, 1*(2), 143–153.

Lyubomirsky, S., King, L., & Diener, E. (2005). The benefits of frequent positive affect: Does happiness lead to success? *Psychological Bulletin, 131*(6), 803–855. http://dx.doi.org/10.1037/0033-2909.131.6.803

May, N., Becker, D., Frankel, R., Haizlip, J., Harmon, R., Plews-Ogan, M., . . . Whitney, D. (2011). *Appreciative Inquiry in healthcare: Positive questions to bring out the best.* Brunswick, OH: Crown.

Peterson, C., Maier, S. F., & Seligman, M. E. P. (1993). *Learned helplessness: A theory for the age of personal control.* New York, NY: Oxford University Press.

Peterson, C., & Seligman, M. E. P. (2004). *Character strengths and virtues: A handbook and classification.* New York, NY: Oxford University Press.

Piderit, S. K. (2009). Rethinking resistance and recognizing ambivalence: A multidimensional view of attitudes toward an organizational change. In W. W. Burke, D. G. Lake, & J. W. Paine (Eds.), *Organization change* (pp. 418–437). San Francisco, CA: John Wiley.

Quaintance, J. L., Arnold, L., & Thompson, G. S. (2010). What students learn about professionalism from faculty stories: An "Appreciative Inquiry" approach. *Academic Medicine, 85*(1), 118–123. https://doi.org/10.1097/ACM.0b013e3181c42acd

Richer, M., Ritchie, J., & Marchionni, C. (2009). "If we can't do more, let's do it differently!": Using Appreciative Inquiry to promote innovative ideas for better health care work environment. *Journal of Nursing Management, 17*(8), 947–955.

Sandars, J., & Murdoch-Eaton, D. (2017). Appreciative inquiry in medical education. *Medical Teacher, 39*(2), 123–127. https://doi.org/10.1080/014215 9X.2017.1245852

Schein, E. H. (1988). *Process consultation, Vol. 1: Its role in organization development.* Reading, MA: Addison-Wesley.

Schein, E. H. (1999). *Process consultation revisited: Building the helping relationship.* Reading, MA: Addison-Wesley.

Seligman, M. E. P. (1990). *Learned optimism.* New York, NY: Knopf.

Seligman, M. E. P. (1999). The president's address. 1998 APA Annual Report of the American Psychological Association. *American Psychologist, 54*(8), 559–562. https://doi.org/10.1037/0003-066X.54.8.537

Seligman, M. E. P. (2002). *Authentic happiness: Using the new positive psychology to realize your potential for lasting fulfillment.* New York, NY: Free Press.

Seligman, M. E. P. (2008). Positive health. *Applied Psychology: An International Review, 57*(s1), 3–18.

Seligman, M. E. P. (2011). *Flourish: A visionary new understanding of happiness and well-being.* New York, NY: Free Press.

Seligman, M. E. P., & Csíkszentmihályi, M. (2000). Positive psychology: An introduction. *American Psychologist, 55*(1), 5–14.

Seligman, M. E. P., Steen, T. A., Park, N., & Peterson, C. (2005). Positive psychology progress: Empirical validation of interventions. *American Psychologist, 60*(5), 410–421. https://doi.org/10.1037/0003-066X.60.5.410

Stavros, J., & Torres, C. (2018). *Conversations worth having.* Oakland, CA: Berrett-Koehler.

University of Pennsylvania. (2018a). *Authentic happiness*. Retrieved from https://www. authentichappiness.sas.upenn.edu/home

University of Pennsylvania. (2018b). *Resilience training for the Army*. Retrieved from https://ppc.sas.upenn.edu/services/resilience-training-army

University of Pennsylvania. (2018c). *Resilience training for the U.S. Army: Comprehensive Soldier and Family Fitness Program*. Retrieved from https://www.authentichappiness.sas.upenn.edu/learn/soldiers

University of Virginia School of Nursing. (2018). *Center for Appreciative Practice*. Retrieved from https://www.nursing.virginia.edu/centers-initiatives/center-for-appreciative-practice/

Values in Action Institute on Character. (2018). *Character strengths survey*. Retrieved from https://www.viacharacter.org/www/Character-Strengths

Watkins, S., Dewar, B., & Kennedy, C. (2016). Appreciative Inquiry as an intervention to change nursing practice in in-patient settings: An integrative review. *International Journal of Nursing Studies, 60*, 179–190. https://doi.org/10.1016/j.ijnurstu.2016.04.017

Weisbord, M. R. (1987). *Productive workplaces: Organizing and managing for dignity, meaning, and community*. San Francisco, CA: Jossey-Bass.

Weisbord, M. R. (2004). *Productive workplaces revisited: Dignity, meaning, and community in the 21st Century* (updated ed.). San Francisco, CA: Jossey-Bass.

Weisbord, M. R., & Janoff, S. (2000). *Future search: An action guide to finding common ground in organizations and communities* (2nd ed.). San Francisco, CA: Berrett-Koehler.

Wenger-Trayner, E., & Wenger-Trayner, B. (2015). Learning in a landscape of practice: A framework. In E. Wenger-Trayner, M. Fenton-O'Creevy, S. Hutchinson, C. Kubiak, & B. Wenger-Trayner (Eds.), *Learning in landscapes of practice: Boundaries, identity, and knowledgeability in practice-based learning* (pp. 13–29). New York, NY: Routledge.

Whitney, D., & Fredrickson, B. L. (2015). Appreciative inquiry meets positive psychology: A dialogue between Diana Whitney and Barbara Fredrickson about organizational change, transformation and innovation. *AI Practitioner, 17*(3), 18–26. https://dx.doi.org/10.12781/978-1-907549-24-3-3

Whitney, D., & Trosten-Bloom, A. (2010). *The power of Appreciative Inquiry: A practical guide to positive change* (2nd ed.). San Francisco, CA: Berrett-Koehler.

PART IV

CARING FOR SELF AND OTHERS

CHAPTER 14

HOW A NEW HEART
TRANSFORMED MINE

Mary L. Falk
Virginia Commonwealth University

ABSTRACT

This chapter describes an autoethnographic account of personal transformation in my role as a cardiac surgery critical care nurse who is also a faculty
member responsible for teaching undergraduate baccalaureate nursing students. An unexpected and extended encounter with a heart transplant patient and his family led me to a fresh realization of the purpose of my calling
and transformed my perspective of what it means to give of oneself in the care
of another, and the personal rewards of doing so. As a result, I have learned
how to use the relationships fostered through patient care to revitalize the
passion I once held for the work I do to help nurses and those in training
understand how to remain resilient in this demanding health profession.

HOW A NEW HEART TRANSFORMED MINE

As my brain begins to wake up, my eyes open and I realize it is still dark
outside. My mind hasn't fully registered what I am supposed to be doing

Transformative Learning in Healthcare and Helping Professions Education, pages 285–300
Copyright © 2019 by Information Age Publishing

today, but then the feeling of heaviness in my legs reminds me. I look at my cell phone on my bedside table and the time reads 4:00 a.m. I sigh because I don't need to wake up for another hour and a half, but I know that I won't fall back asleep before then. My mind begins to wander and I start fretting.

I got home at 8:30 p.m. last night from working a shift in the cardiac surgery intensive care unit (CSICU) and spent about 30 minutes shoveling down a dinner before showering and getting right into bed. My body felt like a quarterback on a Monday. As I lay in bed now, I start to think about the patients I took care of yesterday. In the intensive care unit (ICU), a nurse is either "singled" with a patient deemed sick enough to require one to one nursing care, or paired with two patients who are still sick enough to need ICU care, but not so sick that a nurse needs to be in the room with them every single minute of the shift. The reality is that short staffing often means that patients are paired before they are truly ready to be, and both the nurses and the patients end up feeling the consequences.

My patient assignment yesterday was the dreaded "heavy pair," meaning two patients who require total care and are also still fairly medically unstable. John (a pseudonym) was a 39-year-old male who was post-op day one of an abdominal aortic aneurysm repair. He had severe substance abuse issues, including the use of alcohol and cocaine, and his surgeon wanted him to stay intubated because the anesthesia team had determined that he had a difficult airway. We also wanted his blood pressure to be more under control. Anna (a pseudonym) had been in and out of the ICU for the past 2 months after originally coming in with a perforated esophagus requiring an esophagectomy. She weighs 375 pounds and is unable to really move herself at all because of poor conditioning that has been made worse by numerous surgical complications. These led to more surgery and more ICU time. She has only one vasoactive drip to control her blood pressure now, but is described in handoff between nurses as needy because she is now awake and requires someone to help her with everything, from pillow readjustments to television channel changes, and she uses the call bell liberally.

ICU nurses prioritize patient care by assessing which patient is most sick, and they work to take care of the needs of the sickest patient first. John was much sicker than Anna and, as such, I spent the first hour of my shift at his bedside, slowly decreasing his sedation to assess his neurological status while titrating his numerous other vasoactive drips to keep his blood pressure and heart rate within ranges specified by his surgical team. The team of ICU doctors had relayed to the night shift nurse, who subsequently told me, to start weaning his sedation to the point where we could safely remove his endotracheal tube later on in the day. As we weaned his sedation and John started to wake up, he began to try to pull at the numerous lines and tubes that entered his body at various points. Because of this, the night shift nurse had applied wrist restraints to both of his upper extremities so that he could not pull any of his numerous invasive lines out, which could cause enormous harm to him. As part of my morning assessment, I checked his restraints and everything was correctly in place. John's sedation was at a point where he responded to my commands like "squeeze my hand," but he was still fairly out of it, which is right where I wanted him at this time of day. I made sure everything that was critical had been done—vital signs were stable on his vasoactive drips and morning labs had been drawn before leaving him to go check in and complete a more in-depth assessment of Anna.

After sending in John's morning lab work, I went into Anna's room. The first thing she said was "Where have you been? Eating bon bons?" and laughed heartily to herself as her eyes remained glued to a crime show on the television. I did my best to not show her my annoyance with this type of comment. It can be so frustrating when patients do not realize how busy we are, assuming she is the only patient in the hospital under our care. I gave her my best half smile and my stock answer to patients in her position: "Sorry, I was with another patient who is still very sick. It's good news that you aren't the one requiring as much attention anymore; that means you're getting better!" Anna then proceeded to direct me on the various things she wanted done immediately—a warm washcloth for her face, Chapstick for her lips, and, "Could I find that special lotion they had in the step-down unit?" I kept my face neutral as I followed her directions, but my mind is next door in John's room. His substance abuse history makes me nervous about extubating him (taking out his breathing tube), and apparently he has gone through bad withdrawal in the past after other major surgeries. But here I am, washing a woman's face because she is too weak, but mostly too unwilling, to do it herself.

Suddenly, I smell something awful. Without taking her eyes off of the crime show on the television, Anna announces that she has had a bowel movement. I know she is fully capable of using a bedpan, but when I mention that we could have placed one under her, she responds with, "Oh, that's too much work, rolling on and off that thing every time." I plaster the neutral look on my face that I have mastered over the years and call the care partner to come help me get her cleaned up. As the care partner enters the room, I hear the ventilator alarm go off next door. I tell the care partner I will be right back, assuming John has just moved his head slightly or taken a few extra breaths now that his sedation is being weaned down.

As I walk into John's room, I am horrified to see the endotracheal tube laying on his chest. His left hand is reaching up to the central line in his neck, and the restraint on his left wrist is on, but completely loosened from the bed. I dash into the room to tighten the restraint so that he doesn't pull his central line out, and to stabilize his airway. He takes a swing right at my face and I lean back to avoid the punch like some sort of ninja nurse. As I call out for help, I can't help but think to myself, "How on earth did this happen? His restraint was tight when I left ten minutes ago!" and I feel a sinking pit in my stomach. This would not have ever happened if I did not have a second patient who required such total care and I could have stayed in his room. Another nurse comes into the room and helps me get the equipment I need to stabilize John's airway while we call our ICU resident to re-intubate him if he cannot adequately breathe on his own. The ICU resident comes in and asks "How did this happen?" He isn't even trying to sound accusatory—he just wants information—but I still take it personally because this is *my patient*. I tell him that I literally left the room less than 10 minutes ago, and the patient is apparently a Houdini who somehow pulled hard enough to loosen the restraint to the point where he could reach his breathing tube. The resident just nods and says "Yeah, I heard this guy went wild when he had surgery a year ago." The other nurse and I continue to make sure John's oxygen levels are stable without the breathing tube, and to reorient him to the situation. The good news is that John seems to be maintaining his own airway and we don't need to put the breathing tube back in. The bad news is that John is now angry, confused, and apparently has superhuman strength. I ask the resident if we can switch him to a sedative drug called Precedex that can be used without intubating the patient. He readily agrees and I start the drug as fast as possible. After a few tense minutes, John begins to calm down and he is medically stabilized again. The resident and other nurse leave the room and I am left to continue monitoring him while now faced with a mountain of extra documentation because of the unplanned extubation.

I sit down at the computer in the room to start documenting in the chart everything that has just happened, and then I hear the call bell going off next door. It hits me that Anna has been sitting in her own stool while we have been stabilizing John. I feel horrible, knowing that the care partner would not have been able to clean her up by herself—the patient is simply too big—and all of the other nurses are tied up with their own busy assignments. I feel uncomfortable leaving John, knowing what just happened the first time I did, but I have no choice and I walk wearily to Anna's room, glancing at the clock as I go out. It is only 9:00 a.m., but so it continues all day, going back and forth, trying to put out fire after fire, just trying to make it to change of shift.

Suddenly, I am transported back to the space I am actually in, my bed, at home, with my husband sound asleep beside me. I look at my cell phone again and it is now 4:45 a.m. For the last 45 minutes, I have fretted about the day I had yesterday and everything that went wrong. My alarm has not even gone off for today, but I already feel anxious because I know what is coming. Patients seem to be getting sicker, and staffing seems to become thinner with each passing year. My legs are heavy from 13 hours on my feet yesterday, but I decide to get out of bed before my alarm goes off so that my husband does not wake up early. I start to make coffee and sit down while it brews. I feel tired and cannot help but think about how far away 8:00 p.m. seems.

BURNOUT IN THE NURSING PROFESSION

I became a nurse because I feel it is an enormous privilege to be entrusted to care for people in the time of their greatest need, but my mind and my body are tired. With each passing shift it is becoming harder for me to get up when my alarm goes off. The flame within me that used to burn so brightly seems to be diminishing. I have felt envious of my friends and family with normal 9 to 5 jobs that do not appear to me to present the same level of stress that accompanies working in a Level 1 trauma center intensive care unit. Weekly, I hear of more nurses leaving the bedside and taking easier jobs in outpatient clinics or going back to school for advanced degrees that will take them away from the bedside. I am guilty of this myself. I left full-time bedside nursing and became a full-time clinical faculty member in academic nursing because while I truly love to teach, I also knew that I would be dealing less with situations like the one just described. A piece of my heart belongs in bedside nursing though, so I maintain a per diem (as needed) position in the CSICU, and still work several shifts a month as a bedside nurse on the weekends.

The reduction of the flame that drives people into nursing, and other caregiving professions, has been recognized as a phenomenon known as compassion fatigue. Compassion fatigue as a form of burnout unique to people in the caregiver role was first written about by a nurse named Carla Joinson (1992). Joinson described how the very attributes that draw people into nursing, namely a desire to help others, are those that contribute to the development of compassion fatigue. According to Joinson, by consistently placing the needs of others before their own, some nurses seem to lose their ability to nurture.

Experiencing Compassion Fatigue

The term compassion fatigue was adopted as a way to describe secondary post-traumatic stress disorder, or STSD (Figley, 1995). Coetzee and Klopper (2010) define STSD as

a state of exhaustion and dysfunction (biologically, psychologically, and socially) . . . that results from prolonged exposure to secondary stress (compassion stress), where the person experiences a lack of relief from the burden of responsibility of the sufferer and the suffering and an inability to reduce the effects of the compassion stress. (p. 238)

The symptoms of compassion fatigue can be physical, emotional, or work-related issues. Physically, nurses can experience sleep disturbances (too much or too little), headaches, fatigue, digestive issues, and even stress-induced chest pain. Emotional symptoms can manifest as anxiety or depression. Feelings of dread and lack of empathy can affect work performance and lead to increased call outs from scheduled work shifts (Lombardo & Eyre, 2011).

These manifestations of compassion fatigue are prevalent among all types of nurses, and studies have shown no statistically significant variables among years of nursing experience, specialty, gender, education, country of training, ethnicity, age, hours worked per week, or marital status (Abendroth & Flannery, 2006). Compassion fatigue, as a special type of burnout, may be contributing to high turnover rates in registered nurse (RN) positions in U.S. hospitals. The American Association of Colleges of Nursing (2014) has reported that the average RN turnover rate is 13.9% and that the average vacancy rate is 16.1%. They also report that 37% of newly licensed RNs feel ready to change jobs after just one year, and that 13% of them actually do so. Other studies have shown that 40% of staff nurses score in the high range on the Maslach Burnout Inventory for job-related burnout, and patient dissatisfaction increases when nurses are more burned out (Vahey, Aiken, Sloane, Clarke, & Vargas, 2004). Alarmingly, some studies have shown that in units with poor nurse staffing, a major contributor to burnout, hospital-acquired infections are more likely to occur (Cimiotti, Aiken, Sloane, & Wu, 2012).

Dealing With Compassion Fatigue

As compassion fatigue has become more widely recognized as a serious problem affecting nurses and other people working in the helping professions, research has been carried out on how to combat it. In 2015, Gillman and colleagues published a large systematic review of 20 studies that provided insight into effective strategies to promote resilience and combat compassion fatigue among oncology nurses. While these studies focused only on oncology nurses, the results may be applicable to others working in the helping professions.

Gillman et al.'s (2015) systematic review found several strategies that have helped develop resilience in caregivers. First, individuals who sought work–life balance and allowed time for self-care reported lower levels of stress and burnout (p. 164). Second, organizations that fostered relationships among staff, and who subsequently participated in meaningful reflection with each other, saw decreased levels of burnout. It is believed that through meaningful reflection and storytelling, people are able to unburden stress levels while also finding meaning and purpose in difficult situations. These actions subsequently build resilience in individuals who are then more able to effectively cope with the stressors presented in their daily work lives (p. 166).

Today's hospitalized patients are more complex than ever before (Brimmer, 2012). The increasing wealth of knowledge about human physiology has led to an explosion of technological and scientific capabilities that are keeping patients alive longer than ever before (Brimmer, 2012). Chronic diseases, such as heart failure and chronic obstructive pulmonary disease (COPD), can now be managed with medical therapies that are ever-evolving and always improving. In 2016, the World Health Organization (WHO) stated that the world prevalence of obesity has more than doubled between 1980 and 2014. Furthermore, 1.9 billion adults worldwide are overweight, with 600 million of those adults considered obese. The prevalence of chronic disease is worsening as the obesity epidemic continues to grow (WHO, 2016).

What does all of this mean for the bedside nurse? The more complex the patient, the more needs the patient will have. Patients with diagnoses that would have meant certain death 20 years ago are now being kept alive in intensive care units. The patients who would have been deemed sick enough for the ICU in the past are now being cared for on progressive or general care units because the ICU beds are reserved for patients who would not have survived past the emergency department or operating room in previous years. Patients who used to be admitted to general care units are now sent home and managed as outpatients. As patients become sicker, their physical needs increase and, coincidently, their emotional needs also grow as they and their loved ones cope with their illnesses. While these complex patients are seen by large interdisciplinary teams, it is the bedside nurse who remains at their side throughout day and night.

ICU patients often rely on the bedside nurse for every need imaginable and these nurses can leave work feeling mentally, emotionally, and physically drained. From managing hemodynamic drips and sedation, to ensuring that patients are kept clean after an incontinent episode so that the patient maintains dignity, the bedside nurse provides for every physical need. It is estimated that the average bedside nurse lifts 1.8 tons *per shift* (Howard, 2010). The bedside nurse must be mentally sharp so that any errors made within the complex web of the interdisciplinary care team do not actually reach the patient and cause harm. I teach my nursing students my motto of "nursing assessment drives physician intervention" to impress upon them the importance of astute nursing assessment which guides patient care to optimize patient outcomes.

Realizing My Own Burnout

One does not perform these intimate actions in robotic silence at the bedside, and conversations between bedside nurses and patients and their loved ones can become quite personal. For more than 15 years, nurses have been ranked by the American public as the most trusted of professions (American Nurses Association, 2016). Patients and families intuitively trust the bedside nurse, and as a result, they tend to open up to them in a way that may differ from how they interact with other healthcare professionals.

Over time, while talking with my patients and their families, I began to develop my own unconscious strategy that helped me come back to the bedside each day regardless of the nature of stressors from the day before. As I assessed each patient, I would ask personal questions to get to know the patient as someone more than another person in a hospital gown. As someone only a few years into my own marriage, my favorite question to ask older couples was how long they have been married, and then to probe into the secrets of a successful relationship. I have grown to greatly value the advice I hear from people who have lived longer than I have, and the knowledge I have gained from these conversations at the bedside has changed the way I live my life.

This type of intimate time at the bedside can sometimes lead to the development of emotional connections between patients, their loved ones, and the nurse. Often, it is the nurse who then takes on the burden of carrying the emotional baggage that surrounds a hospitalization for a patient and the patient's support system. This emotional baggage can be heavy, and for some nurses, it contributes to the development of compassion fatigue. For me, whenever a patient I had bonded with did not do well, I struggled to compartmentalize my work life so that I would not replay my work day over and over in my head. Gradually, I realized how burned out I had become. Even though I recognized what was happening to me, and acknowledged that I was not effectively taking care of myself so that I could help others, I seemed unable to build enough resilience to continue giving 100% of myself every day. Going into my work shifts, all I cared about was surviving and preserving myself until 12 to 13 hours had passed and I could go home. I felt myself go from engaged clinician trying to take care of the physical, emotional, mental, and spiritual needs of my patients and their loved ones to a nurse just trying to get tasks done so that my patients would progress through their hospitalizations successfully and be discharged. Eventually, I stopped trying to get to know my patients beyond what was pertinent to their hospitalization because the weight of everything had just become too much for me. I was exhausted, and I stopped giving my all because I had nothing left to give.

THE TRANSFORMATION

And then one Sunday afternoon, I was floated (nursing lingo for when a nurse is pulled from the home unit to another unit for staffing resource purposes) to the cardiothoracic surgery progressive care unit for the last 4 hours of my day. Annoyed at having been floated, a notoriously unpopular activity among bedside nurses, I began by getting reports on the three patients I would be taking care of until my shift ended. One of the patients I was assigned to was a patient named Chris (a pseudonym) who had had a total artificial heart (TAH) implanted about a month prior. I remembered Chris, and his wife Maggie (pseudonym), from the time when he was in my own unit. Surgically, things had gone about as well as possible, but Chris and Maggie had developed a reputation for not being the easiest couple to work with in the unit. Chris's reaction to waking up with a TAH was typical for these patients. He was depressed, occasionally snappy, and had a very flat affect about the prospect of his life now connected to a machine weighing several hundred pounds that was doing the work of his own failed native heart while he waited for a heart transplant to become available. Maggie was anxious about every detail, and did not hide her frustration with the entire situation from the staff.

I went into Chris's room to reintroduce myself to him and Maggie. Even though I had briefly cared for them during their time in the CSICU, many patients do not remember a lot about their ICU nurses because of the nature of their critical illnesses. Chris and Maggie were polite, and I performed a basic assessment on Chris before going to check in on my other patients. When I went back to Chris's room to give him evening medications, something struck me about the connection between him and his wife. Something unexplainable was there, and I took a moment to ask them the question I had used so much in the past, but had recently stopped asking. "How long have you been married?" "It will be 33 years on March 11th," Maggie answered. I stopped in my tracks. "Really? March 11th is my wedding anniversary, too."

Suddenly, I felt overwhelmed, and it hit me that *this could be me*. As I turned my head to look at them, in my mind, I did not see them; instead, I saw my husband and myself. Almost immediately, I felt for them in a way that I had not felt for a patient in a very long time as my burnout had been worsening. It struck me that this situation, which had become so routine for me, is not routine at all. Having your heart taken out of your body, replacing it with a plastic pump which then connects to the notorious "big blue" TAH machine is not normal. Having a six foot hose come out of your abdomen and tether you to a machine that weighs several hundred pounds is not normal. Relying on a machine to keep you alive, while you hope for an organ transplant every day, is not normal. Because all of this had become routine in my work life and I was just trying to make it through my shifts, I forgot that all of this is not at all normal.

However, having a wedding anniversary, on the other hand, is normal, and I felt blindsided, and a sense of disappointment in myself by the realization of how much I had changed as a nurse as I struggled with my dwindling resilience and increasing level of burnout. Knowing that my other patients were okay, I sat down and started to talk with Chris and Maggie. I asked them about their family, learned that they have three children, and that they had actually come from another state to have the TAH implanted in Chris. His cardiology team at home told him that there were no other options available to him there and he would die if he did not go to a facility that could perform the TAH surgery and provide the necessary postoperative care. So, Chris was put on a medical jet and brought to my hospital where he received the TAH the next day. Maggie drove 9 hours to get to my state and ended up renting an apartment about 20 minutes from the hospital. Then the waiting game started.

By the time I began to get to know Chris and Maggie, they had already been in the hospital waiting for a heart transplant for 4 months. While I work on an as needed basis as a bedside nurse in the CSICU now, part of my job as a full-time clinical faculty member in the School of Nursing is to teach undergraduate nursing students on the cardiothoracic surgery progressive care unit where Chris was now living. After my brief 4-hour stint taking care of him when I was floated, I made it a point to start checking in on him whenever I was on that unit with the students. As the weather started to improve, Chris mentioned to me that he was desperate for a breath of outside, fresh air, and he said he was starting to feel like a caged animal inside of the hospital all of the time. As an avid outdoor lover, it struck me as almost inhumane to keep someone inside for so long. After talking with the unit leadership, it was decided that I could take Chris and his TAH outside to an outdoor landing in the hospital that had the necessary electrical and medical air outlets to keep the device working.

So, I began looking for opportunities when I could take a break from my responsibilities in the School of Nursing to take Chris and Maggie to the outdoor landing, which usually ended up being biweekly. We would sit outside and just talk while Chris soaked up as much vitamin D as he could. I learned all about their life together, what their children were up to, and where their extended family lived. Over time, when their children or extended family visited, I got to meet them, too, and eventually came to know their entire family.

With the first indication of warmer spring days approaching, March 11, our mutual wedding anniversary, loomed closer. My husband started mentioning ideas to celebrate our own third anniversary date, but I could not stop thinking about how Chris and Maggie would be celebrating more years together than the length of time that I had been alive, and how he was stuck in the hospital. So one day, while outside with Chris, I asked Chris if he had any interest in planning a surprise anniversary dinner for his wife, with me as coordinator. He immediately jumped on board with the idea and we got to work.

Over the next few weeks, Chris and I covertly poured over menus from top area restaurants. We discussed timing of the dinner, and how to keep it a surprise from Maggie. I went out and bought multiple anniversary cards for him to choose from, keeping the runner-up for my own use. Our mission must have been obvious to Maggie. For instance, there was the time I dropped by at 8:00 p.m. on a Sunday after my own shift in the CSICU "just to see how they were doing," when I was really trying to touch base with Chris about some details of the upcoming dinner. Eventually, we settled on an incredible local Italian place and selected the menu. Chris readily expressed that he wanted to meet my husband, whom he had heard so much about by now.

When the day of the anniversary arrived, I made sure that everything was in order. I gathered up my best dishes, glassware, and table settings from home, and my husband and I picked up the Italian meal from the restaurant. Arriving at the hospital, we initially planned to set everything up outside, but the early spring weather had dissipated, so we did our best to transform a hospital conference room into a restaurant. My husband, who was part of the plot, turned on a playlist, customized to Chris and Maggie's favorite music, and I went to Chris's room to "go for a walk before I left for vacation for a week." As we walked down the hall towards the conference room, I wondered if Maggie began to suspect anything. I typically am not the best at keeping secrets, and I am certain my demeanor was suspicious in some way.

As we got closer to the conference room, the music playing become obvious, and Maggie gave me a puzzled look. I returned her look with my best smile, and as I turned the TAH into the conference room so that she realized what was going on, tears came into her eyes. She looked at Chris and me and said "Are you kidding me?" All I could do was smile back while she took in my best effort to transform a dull hospital conference room into an intimate Italian restaurant.

For the next few hours, Chris and Maggie enjoyed a three course meal, served by my husband and me. Chris jokingly called out "Oh garçon!" every time they needed a refill or were ready for the next course. Chris and Maggie asked my husband and me to join them for dessert and we ended up sitting there talking until almost midnight that evening. When we eventually left, Maggie hugged me and thanked me for "making her feel normal for the first time in months."

As I went home that night, I could not stop ruminating on how so much of life is left up to chance. Only 3 years into my own marriage, I wondered where the next 30 would take us. Chris and Maggie certainly never expected to end up in a city they did not know, relying on an artificial heart to keep Chris alive. Waiting for time to pass can make life feel tedious, but I realized that life is brief and precarious.

After returning home from our vacation and getting back into classes with my nursing students after spring break, I resumed my biweekly outside outings with Chris and Maggie for the next several months. To say that they were exercising patience would be an understatement. At this point, Chris had been in the hospital for almost eight months. Every time we went outside, I gained insight into the world of how it feels to take a deep breath every time someone walks into your hospital room because that person might be bringing you the news that a matched transplant has become available. I had a firsthand view to see what it was like to go from being an independent person to being dependent on a plugged-in machine. I thought about what it might be like in a world in which you cannot sleep in the same bed as your wife of 33 years, and realized how that can become a strain on your relationship.

The time I spent talking to Chris and Maggie about their lives and their ordeal taught me more than I can ever put into words. As I reflected on their situation, and mine, I began to perceive life very differently and realized that I had undergone a major shift in my perspective, one that had unfolded over the months of my growing relationship with Chris and Maggie. I now saw life as nothing more than a game of cards, and you never know which hand you might draw. My perception of time had changed radically. No longer something to be used or counted, I saw it as limited, valuable beyond measure, and irreplaceable. I realized that time is the most precious commodity that we have, and every heartbeat should not be taken for granted.

The precious time that I was privileged to spend with Chris and Maggie softened my heart. The spark that had initially driven me into nursing, which had burned out, began to flicker again. For me, having such an intimate glimpse into someone else's heart, more than medically, meant that I was reminded of the privilege nurses are granted in being entrusted with patient care. In the language of Mezirow (1990, 1991) and others who have written eloquently about transformative learning (Clark, 1993; Cranton, 2016), I had experienced the dramatic shift in perspective that Mezirow (1978) first labeled a perspective transformation.

While hospitals become increasingly technological, and the complexity of patients increases, reminding myself that I am there as a person to take care of another person matters more than anything to me now. Chris and Maggie gave me this gift. In their review of the transformative learning literature, Taylor and Snyder (2012) mention the significant role of relationships in the process of transformation, asserting that insight into this phenomenon is growing with additional research into the importance of relationships in facilitating the transformative process. As we shared experiences and opened ourselves up to each other, this family unit began to feel like part of mine.

Chris and Maggie reminded me that I am taking care of so much more than someone connected to multiple machines in the ICU. I am taking care of a human life, a person who has goals, passions, and a family who care about him. No matter what the circumstances, I have realized that this can be said about all patients, understanding that part of our job as clinicians is to remind ourselves of this incredible gift we have to share so that when work becomes tough, we can find resilience through our caring for another person.

Ironically, the literature on resilience has identified this aspect of caring as well. The care that engenders compassion fatigue can also become the care that restores, a concept in the literature called compassion satisfaction (Fahey & Glasofer, 2016). These scholars define compassion satisfaction as the affirming and positive experiences related to nursing care. As noted by Fahey and Glasofer (2016), "compassion satisfaction and compassion fatigue are theoretical opposites, suggesting that as compassion satisfaction increases, compassion fatigue decreases" (p. 32).

What I have discovered that makes the difference is the balance between giving and receiving. If all we do as caregivers is give, we soon become depleted. But if we are open to learning from others, to sharing their personal histories and stories in a meaningful way, then we also become open to receiving what they have to offer us. I have come to understand that it is not the giving that diminishes us, it is lack of willingness to receive the care that others are willing to show us if we let them. Not every patient will be someone from whom we can receive such restorative care, but those who are able to provide this to us offer us a gift as special as the one our profession aims to provide for the patient.

Chris's artificial heart softened mine, but the day his transplant came, my heart was transformed. Hearing the news from Chris's wife that a heart had become available, I felt a renewed energy within myself that reminded me that difficult days in the hospital are not for naught. While resources become thinner, and patients become increasingly complex, causing caregivers' stress levels to rise, I am reminded that there is a human being on the other side of this complexity who is relying on me. I am reminded that my job matters. And it took someone else's new heart to transform mine in a way so that I did not lose sight of what I was doing and where I was going with my life. Chris and Maggie gave me that insight, and I will never be the same nurse as before since I have learned to receive as well as give care.

DISCOVERING THE POWER OF AUTOETHNOGRAPHY

The story presented here is my true story. It is a researcher's account of her own lived experience while engaged in patient care within a unique cultural setting. While John, Anna, Chris, and Maggie are all pseudonyms for individuals who are part of my story, they represent composite depictions of the actual patients and family members involved; I have attempted to preserve their confidentiality by altering sufficient details to avoid their resemblance to actual living patients and family members. The events that occurred during this transformative experience, however, are real: the surprise wedding anniversary dinner and the events associated with my care of these patients happened pretty much as told.

Traditionally, qualitative research in nursing has involved the researcher taking a more objective, rather than subjective, stance as an observer of others' actions and interpreter of their experiences (Peterson, 2015). The power of autoethnography, however, lies in its ability to draw the reader in through the use of a subjective, first-person account of experience, one that is grounded in a particular cultural context, time, and place so that readers might identify with my experience in some way. As Peterson (2015) notes, as a research methodology, the purpose of autoethnography is to enable reflection on experience in new ways:

> [A]utoethnography gives nurses the opportunity to tell stories that would otherwise not be heard. It involves a courageous laying bare of the self to gain new cultural understandings and it offers the potential for nurses to learn from the experiences and reflections of other nurses. (p. 226)

By examining my own experience and reflecting upon its personal meaning, I uncovered the truth about the burnout I was experiencing, even after only a few years in intensive care nursing. In describing the value of autoethnography for medical education research, Farrell, Bourgeois-Law, Regehr, and Ajjawi (2015) see this research methodology as the ability to engage in self-reflective narration of one's own cultural biography. In their words, the purpose of autoethnography is to

> move beyond simple autobiography through the inclusion of other voices and the analytical examination of the relationships between self and others. Autoethnography has achieved its goal if it results in new insights and improvements in teaching practices, and if it promotes broader reflection amongst readers about their own teaching and learning environments. (p. 974)

Not only have I learned how to gain strength and resilience from some of the special relationships that present themselves during patient care, but I have the ability to share what I have learned with the nurses that I teach, and that, I think, will make all the difference in the years to come.

REFERENCES

Abendroth, M., & Flannery, J. (2006). Predicting the risk of compassion fatigue. *Journal of Hospice & Palliative Nursing, 8*(6), 346–356.

American Association of Colleges of Nursing. (2014). *Nursing shortage* (Fact sheet). Retrieved from http://www.aacn.nche.edu/media-relations/fact-sheets/nursing-shortage

American Nurses Association. (2016). *Nurses rank #1 most trusted profession for 15th year in a row* (Press release). Retrieved from https://www.nursingworld.org/news/news-releases/2016/nurses-rank-1-most-trusted-profession-for-15th-year-in-a-row/

Brimmer, K. (2012). AHA: Americans living longer but getting sicker. *Healthcare Finance.* Retrieved from http://www.healthcarefinancenews.com/news/aha-americans-living-longer-getting-sicker

Cimiotti, J., Aiken, L., Sloane, D., & Wu, S. (2012). Nurse staffing, burnout, and health care–associated infection. *American Journal of Infection Control, 40*(6), 486–490.

Clark, M. C. (1993). Transformational learning. *New directions for adult and continuing education,* 57, 47–56. Hoboken, NJ: Wiley. https://doi.org/10.1002/ace.36719935707

Coetzee, S. K., & Klopper, H. C. (2010). Compassion fatigue within nursing practice: A concept analysis. *Nursing & Health Sciences, 12*(2), 235–243.

Cranton, P. (2016). *Understanding and promoting transformative learning: A guide to theory and practice* (3rd ed.). San Francisco, CA: Jossey-Bass.

Fahey, D. M., & Glasofer, A. (2016). An inverse relationship: Compassion satisfaction, compassion fatigue, and critical care nurses. *Nursing in Critical Care, 11*(5), 30–35.

Farrell, L., Bourgeois-Law, G., Regehr, G., & Ajjawi, R. (2015). Autoethnography: Introducing "I" into medical education research. *Medical Education, 49*(10), 974–982. https://doi.org/10.1111/medu.12761

Figley, C. R. (1995). *Compassion fatigue: Coping with secondary traumatic stress disorder in those who treat the traumatized.* New York, NY: Brunner-Mazel.

Gillman, L., Adams, J., Kovac, R., Kilcullen, A., House, A., & Doyle, C. (2015). Strategies to promote coping and resilience in oncology and palliative care nurses caring for adult patients with malignancy: A comprehensive systematic review. *JBI Database of Systematic Reviews and Implementation Reports, 13*(5), 131–204. doi:10.11124/jbisrir-2015-1898

Howard, N. (2010). Patient handling: Fact vs. fiction. *American Nurse Today, 5*(7), 32–34.

Joinson, C. (1992). Coping with compassion fatigue. *Nursing, 22*(4), 116–121.

Lombardo, B., & Eyre, C. (2011). Compassion fatigue: A nurse's primer. *The Online Journal of Issues in Nursing, 16*(1). Manuscript 3. doi: 10.3912/OJIN.Vol16No01Man03

Mezirow, J. (1978). Perspective transformation. *Adult Education, 28*(2), 100–110.

Mezirow, J. (1990). How critical reflection triggers transformative learning. In J. Mezirow & Associates (Eds.), *Fostering critical reflection in adulthood* (pp. 1–20). San Francisco, CA: Jossey-Bass.

Mezirow, J. (1991). *Transformative dimensions of adult learning.* San Francisco, CA: Jossey-Bass.

Peterson, A. L. (2015). A case for the use of autoethnography in nursing research. *Journal of Advanced Nursing, 71*(1), 226–233. doi:10.1111/jan.12501

Taylor, E. W., & Snyder, M. J. (2012). A critical review of the research on transformative learning theory, 2006–2010. In E. W. Taylor & P. Cranton (Eds.), *The handbook of transformative learning: Theory, research, and practice* (pp. 37–54). San Francisco, CA: Jossey-Bass.

Vahey, D. C., Aiken, L. H., Sloane, D. M., Clarke, S. P., & Vargas, D. (2004). Nurse burnout and patient satisfaction. *Medical Care, 42*(2), II57–II66.

World Health Organization. (2016). *Obesity and overweight* (Fact Sheet). Retrieved from http://www.who.int/mediacentre/factsheets/fs311/en/

CHAPTER 15

A CASE FOR SELF-CARE

Changing Luxury to Necessity

Amanda J. Minor
Salve Regina University

ABSTRACT

Helping professionals, particularly those who work as counselors and therapists, are at risk for burnout and compassion fatigue due to the situations they encounter in daily practice. Secondary traumatic stress and vicarious trauma are commonplace reactions in which counselors internalize the traumatic experiences of individuals they seek to help, whether their clients are perpetrators of abuse or survivors of it. Professional counselors and therapists can experience emotional exhaustion, depersonalization, depression, anxiety, and a host of symptoms that make them less able to function optimally in their roles. Self-care, then, becomes a necessity to build resilience, rather than a luxury. This chapter presents strategies for regaining personal wellness with attention to the care of oneself and the rationale for doing so.

Individuals in professional helping careers, including mental health workers, educators, health care professionals, and others encounter various amounts of pressure in their day-to-day routine. Research shows if these

Transformative Learning in Healthcare and Helping Professions Education, pages 301–321
Copyright © 2019 by Information Age Publishing
All rights of reproduction in any form reserved.

individuals do not participate in self-care there may be adverse effects to mental and physical health as well as to personal relationships (Christopher, Christopher, Dunnagan, & Schure, 2006; Maslach, Schaufeli, & Leiter, 2001; Newell & Nelson-Gardell, 2014; Wise, Hersch, & Gibson, 2012). This chapter will discuss concepts such as secondary traumatic stress (STS) and vicarious trauma. The primary purpose is to make an argument for why self-care is not merely important but, rather, fundamental to sustaining an appropriate level of care for our clients and ourselves.

As a counselor educator and professional counselor, I will discuss what the literature says about self-care and its ability to help with resilience. It can be common for counselors and therapists to put their own needs after the needs of others, specifically if they were not taught about the necessity for self-care during formal education (Young & Cashwell, 2017). As a profession, counselors learn that putting personal needs aside is often necessary when in acute work situations; however, this can lead to neglect of the self in the long-term. Norcross and Guy (2007) provide an example of this within psychotherapy:

> We oftimes feel hypocritical or duplicitous—suggesting to others that they work less, exercise more, renew themselves...while we do not take our own advice. How often do we sit with patients, encouraging them to "relax and take a vacation," while calculating in our own case our lost therapy revenue and airfare and concluding that we can't afford to take the time away from the office right now. (p. 7)

It can be argued that we neglect our basic needs when we neglect self-care. The act of discovery related to self-care and how transformative learning can foster and sustain resilience is extremely important in the evermore demanding world of professional mental health care. A conversation about self-care must occur if counselors are to truly understand and be successful in our professional identity as helpers.

SECONDARY TRAUMATIC STRESS

Individuals in the mental health helping fields have a higher likelihood of working in stressful environments that often involve seeing or hearing about acute and sustained trauma. From the perspective of knowledge as socially constructed, harrowing or stressful client stories, specifically when frequent, can not only bring back memories from one's own experience, but also have the high likelihood to create new, traumatic memories (Killian, 2008). Continuous unattended exposure to these instances in the work environment can cause professional burnout characterized by a lowered quality of care (Salyers et al., 2014); physical and mental health issues such as exhaustion, depersonalization, depression, or anxiety (Killian, 2008); lowered self-efficacy, detachment, and feelings of cynicism towards clients (Gündüz, 2012); and emotional exhaustion (Maslach, Jackson, & Leiter, 1996). Crowe (2015) suggests three questions for health care workers related to burnout: "Do you care less about work or dread going to work? Are you anxious, irritable, or snappy with your colleagues? Do you feel disengaged, or have a loss of passion for what you were once passionate about?" (p. 192). At one point or another, the answer to these questions from most counselors and therapists is undoubtedly yes.

Sustained stress, burnout, or a particularly triggering experience can create an increased level of trauma response. This response can result in STS which occurs when a professional counselor or therapist is in close contact with another traumatized person. Figley (1995), whose research focused on the nursing profession, reflected that compassion fatigue, which some consider synonymous with STS (Ivicic & Motta, 2017; Jenkins & Baird, 2002), can occur when one witnesses or has knowledge of trauma as it has impacted another person. Figley suggested that the syndrome of compassion fatigue is a blend of the symptoms of STS and professional burnout, and Newell and Nelson-Gardell (2014) state that it is the overall emotional and psychological fatigue due to the chronic use of empathy. Coetzee and Klopper (2010) describe compassion fatigue as occurring when the need for compassionate energy exceeds the energy that one can exert. Coetzee and Klopper's description has a visceral feel for me, perhaps because I have felt it in my work as a counselor with women and children who are survivors of abuse.

In their 2002 article, Jenkins and Baird state that STS is identical to posttraumatic stress disorder (PTSD). Another variation commonly discussed in mental health care literature is vicarious trauma (Baird & Jenkins, 2003; McCann & Pearlman, 1990; Sommer, 2008), which is described as the spread of trauma reactions from the person being treated to the counselor.

Within the mental health counseling and therapy field, a better understanding of what STS is and does to practitioners is vital. Symptoms of STS can be present for professional counselors and therapists who are responsible for protecting confidentiality related to clients' stories of isolation, loneliness, trauma, loss, and abuse. When confidentiality must be broken, mental health workers often have little support within an overburdened and underfunded system. While not all counselors and therapists will react in this way to exposure to client trauma, awareness and proactive action is critical. Within this chapter, I will use the term STS unless an author has specifically used a different term to refer to secondary traumatic stress and the experience of vicarious trauma.

Professional counselors are under constant threat of being impacted by the traumatic experiences of clients. According to Joinson (1992), when faced with compassion fatigue, caretakers can have occurrences comparable to flashbacks with repeated exposure to similar experiences, which ultimately leave the provider with feelings of helplessness that manifest into withdrawal, apathy, or cynicism. The effect of this type of re-traumatization can be serious for those who experience it. From the perspective of a counselor, this experience also leaves clients without the needed action steps from their mental health care provider. There has been a fair amount of research that suggests, given the prevalence of impairment due to issues such as burnout, STS, and vicarious trauma, not participating in self-care can pose an ethical concern (Barnett, Baker, Elman, & Schoener, 2007; Newell & Nelson-Gardell, 2014; Norcross & Guy, 2007; Sommer, 2008; Wise et al., 2012).

The impact of stress and trauma on those within mental health care is evident. A study of 88 psychologists, social workers, mental health counselors, and creative arts therapists indicated a relatively high rate of secondary trauma (Ivicic & Motta, 2017). Baird and Jenkins (2003) showed various levels of burnout in counselors working with trauma survivors who experienced sexual violence. Schauben and Frazier (1995) found that sexual violence counselors experienced heightened trauma symptoms, and Sommer and Cox (2005, 2006) reported physical and emotional reactions in professional counselors who worked with those affected or who had inflicted sexual violence on others.

In nonsexual violence situations, Hodgkinson and Shepard (1994) found social workers who had responded to large-scale catastrophes had statistically significant levels of cognitive disturbances and depressive symptoms. Wee and Myers' (2002) survey of counselors who had worked with survivors of the 1995 Oklahoma City bombings found similar results. Multiple studies indicate higher levels of secondary trauma for novice counselors (Lyndall & Bicknell, 2001; Sheehy Carmel & Friedlander, 2009). Sommer (2008) discussed additional studies that detailed mental health workers' hypervigilance to keep themselves and those they loved safe after experiencing vicarious trauma from working with clients who were traumatized. These studies speak to the need for training programs to purposefully discuss the significant impact of STS and vicarious trauma with students going into mental health care fields (Newell & Nelson-Gardell, 2014; Sommer, 2008). They also indicate the necessity for continuous education and practice related to the need for strategies, resources, and skills to avoid and recognize the signs of STS-like syndromes. It is evident something must be done to lessen these reactions to client trauma within the mental health field. The need for better self-care is abundantly clear, yet for some, it is not a priority.

SELF-CARE

While a multitude of articles on self-care and related topics exist, there has been little empirical research conducted to date (Dorociak, Rupert, Dryant, & Zahniser, 2017). Mayorga, Devries, and Wardle (2015) adopted the original definition of self-care as designated by the World Health Organization (WHO) in 2009 by describing its multifaceted nature. In this definition, self-care encompasses physical, psychological, emotional, and spiritual elements to include all behaviors that promote health and disease prevention (Mayorga et al., 2015, p. 21). In 2017, Dorociak et al. created a 21-item professional self-care scale (PSCS) for practicing psychologists. Within the scale, the authors define professional self-care as "a multidimensional, multifaceted process of purposeful engagement in strategies that promote healthy functioning and enhance well-being" (p. 326). Saakvitne and Pearlman (1996) also provide a definition of self-care as a way to promote and foster healthy functioning with their self-care assessment in a workbook for professional helpers who deal with vicarious trauma. Ultimately, it is impossible for professional counselors to banish or eliminate stress. However, mental health professionals can work towards sustained resilience to protect themselves and their clients.

With the connection between burnout and STS-related symptoms, it seems obvious that a discussion of self-care would be advantageous to include within the various fields of mental health care. However, this does not always occur. Within the 2014 Code of Ethics for the American Counseling Association, there is a specific standard that closely follows the WHO's (2009) definition of self-care: "counselors engage in self-care activities to maintain and promote their own emotional, physical, mental, and spiritual well-being to best meet their professional responsibilities" (American Counseling Association, 2014, p. 8).

While other mental health-focused organizations discuss the need for avoiding clinician impairment and promoting client well-being within their ethical codes (American Psychological Association, 2010; National Association of Social Workers, 2008), they do not explicitly mention self-care. Newell and Nelson-Gardell (2014) question why specific standards related to self-care are not encapsulated within the social work code of ethics (as well as in the standard curriculum) based on the recognition in multiple sources that identify self-care as critical to the longevity of those who work in the helping field. It is possible, as is the case in education, that students focus and discuss appropriate dispositions but not critical elements such as self-care related to longevity in the field.

The newly created PSCS is one of, if not the only, empirically-based scales assessing specific professional self-care (Dorociak et al., 2017), and it is currently limited within the mental health field for use by psychologists. The

PSCS includes subscales which assess five dimensions of professional self-care: professional support, professional development, life balance, cognitive awareness, and daily balance. Professional support elements include supportive coworkers and their actions to provide support from work life. Professional development signifies participation in work activities that are pleasurable, such as professional organizations and conferences. It also includes staying up-to-date on professional knowledge and standards. The life balance subscale refers to the ability to have a personal identity outside of work. This domain emphasizes both social support and work–life balance. Cognitive awareness represents mental and emotional wellness, as well as proactive maintenance and management of emotional needs and challenges. Finally, daily balance focuses more on day-to-day strategies to foster awareness and resource gathering.

Dorociak and colleagues (2017) note that within the creation of the PSCS measure, prompts related to physical health and activities did not independently comprise a salient dimension. However, the instrument developers believe these behaviors vary greatly and can be present in the life balance dimension. They also recognize that physical wellness is critical, as is reflected in much of the literature on personal self-care. Dorociak et al. point out the importance of proactive, ongoing self-care as opposed to retroactive behaviors to counteract stress. In addition, while the PSCS was created for use with psychologists, the developers' goal is to develop a measure for other helping fields.

SELF-CARE AND TRANSFORMATIVE LEARNING

Fundamentally, as an educator, I believe that knowledge is socially constructed. This means I learn from each of my students and their view of the world, and what we are learning impacts how I interpret my understanding at every moment in the classroom. At the end of each class, I like to remind my students that we may be different than we were before this class because of the work we did together. As my students and I have the opportunities to encounter that which is both known and unknown to us, we are given a chance to alter our understanding of it. This learning never occurs in a vacuum. Students have the opportunity to interact with written knowledge in textbooks, journals, and manuals. They also engage in conversations about this knowledge with professors, peers, supervisors, personal support systems, clients, and patients. These encounters hold the potential for a transformation that is not always obvious. Baumgartner (2012) writes about this slow, incremental process as transformative learning when students are able to critically self-reflect on their underlying assumptions about what it means to engage in the therapeutic relationship with clients.

Mezirow (1978), who first theorized transformative learning, discussed the concept of learning and meaning as transformative when one realizes past assumptions are no longer accurate in describing lived experiences. For those experiencing burnout, STS, or vicarious trauma, purpose, efficacy, and competencies can diminish and are often replaced with self-doubt, apathy, and depression-like symptoms. Thus, the perspective of being able to facilitate healing in others has been skewed to reflect a cynical outlook, not only in the work counselors and therapists do, but also on their *ability* to do that work. Coming back from this negative cognitive and emotional space can be difficult, and, ideally, self-care habits are formed early in professional careers to help combat the likelihood of impairment. However, for those who had little exposure to the idea of self-care, or had exposure but were not aware of the connection these actions can have in preventing or lessening STS, it is important to consider what can be done. Helping professionals have an opportunity to become more resilient in their awareness of the need to devote time and energy to caring for themselves, just as they do for clients.

RECONCEPTUALIZING SELF-CARE

The need for proactive self-care that is not simply reactive is imperative for professional counselors to remain healthy and effective (Sommer, 2008). When thinking about modalities to best facilitate this care, it is critical to realize the importance of a transformative practice. By this, I mean a reflective practice that becomes habitual for the individual, not just something done once in response to a particularly stressful situation. When individuals continue to be curious about what, how, and why they react to stressors as they do, there is always the potential for lifelong change. Practitioners should work to find those strategies that best fit their personhood. This chapter focuses on techniques that become more habitual and ritualistic and can lead to lifestyle changes to affect who we are as people and as providers of care. Even positive change can be hard or initially awkward, according to the transtheoretical model of Prochaska and Velicer (1997). Their work describes a process that includes pre-contemplation, contemplation, determination, action, relapse, and finally, maintenance of new behaviors.

In a recent class, I asked my mental health counseling students to identify forms of self-care specifically for counselors. They started with things like "be sure to take a lunch break," "pause between clients," and "have snacks during the day." While these are helpful and focus on basic human needs (Maslow, 1943), much more is needed to bring about changes in self-care. I asked them to consider what has helped or could help them increase resilience. The students quickly moved to second-order habit changes such as "seek lots of supervision," "see your own counselor," "honor professional boundaries," and "understand professional ethics." Throughout the semester, students were faced with challenges in their field placements. We discussed these as a class, focusing on what they did and could have done to help avoid STS. Peers provided powerful suggestions that students had not considered before which led to a much broader understanding of self-care options. It was clear they had absorbed the conversations we had about work-life balance and career sustaining self-care that goes beyond a reactive response to STS and burnout.

Supervision

Most professional counseling and therapy programs work to provide a fair amount of supervision and mentorship for students. However, when counselors move into a professional role, these opportunities for supervision wain, specifically for those who have been in the field for many years and are themselves considered mentors and supervisors of others. The need for lifelong supervision is essential to remain resilient and continue to learn and grow as a competent mental health professional (Sommer, 2008). Effective supervisors often become mentors and trusted peers who help counselors conceptualize how they are experiencing reactions to clients in a more effective way. While these interactions may seem insignificant at the time, they lead to a change in the counselor's understanding of both client and self. Mentors and supervisors are the ones most likely to challenge the professionals' underlying assumptions, prompting the reflective processes that may ultimately lead to transformative learning. According to Andersen and Dybbroe (2017), social workers who seek out mentorship find it helpful in facilitating introspection. Supervision, specifically for novice counselors, brings about important, new awareness in what can be a daunting profession (Bernard & Goodyear, 2014).

Several scholars ascribe to participation in trauma-sensitive supervision for preventative self-care (Etherington, 2000; Pearlman & Saakvitne, 1995; Sommer, 2008). Any counselor who has experience with supervisors realizes that the quality of the supervision can vary. Having a supervisor who helps the counselor to be proactive in awareness of STS and vicarious trauma is important. Suggestions for counselors include seeking a supervisor who has a strong theoretical grounding in trauma therapy with attention to both the unconscious and conscious elements of treatment (Pearlman & Saakvitne, 1995). Etherington (2000) reiterated the importance for supervisors to be alert to changes in supervisees' behaviors and reactions to clients, as well as to pay attention to symptoms of burnout, withdrawal from supervision or clients, or the intrusion of client issues in the student counselor's nonwork life. A strong supervisory relationship is one in which the counselor is willing to have conversations with the supervisor about the effect that clients have on the counselor. Supervision needs to be collaborative, creative, and constructive to be effective as a lifelong tool to help prevent burnout and STS for professional counselors and others in the mental health field.

Peer Support Groups

This category of self-care within supervision is often overlooked; however, it is generally common to have a sense of camaraderie with peers that might not exist with supervisors. The literature supports peer groups as an effective way for counselors and therapists to support each other by fostering open communication (Beel, Chilokoa, & Ladak, 2017). Belonging to a community of practice (CoP) that includes thoughtful peer supervision encourages those in the mental health care field to explore areas of compassion within their work and also helps to discourage STS and vicarious trauma. Peers provide a sense of familiarity and comfort, with less pressure related to assessment and evaluation. Peer supervision is also usually free, or much less expensive than dyadic or group supervision with a designated facilitator. In creating effective peer supervision, it is helpful to have individuals with various skill levels among group members.

Overall, productive peer supervision consists of a mixture of sharing experiences, gaining new knowledge, and discussing the integration of knowledge to experience. According to Yalom (2002), "What is essential is that the group offer a safe, trusting arena for sharing of the stresses of personal and professional life" (p. 254). Peer group members need to remember the ethical requirements of client confidentiality. If the supervision occurs within a defined workspace, there may be releases that allow for conversations about clients. However, focusing on counselor reactions rather than those of the clients can increase the likelihood of having a transformative experience. Questions such as, "What came up for you as you were working with that client who was abused?" and "Why is that significant for you?" focus on the counselor's actions and thoughts. According to master psychology clinicians Norcross and Guy (2007):

> Our leaderless group of psychologists provides a format where each of us can express feelings and deal with life and work without trying to solve any specific problem or task, and without competing. It provides a point of balance for much of the rest of my life. We've been meeting for 90 minutes a week for several years. We deal with all kinds of stuff from the world of practice as well as personal things. (p. 76)

Supervision, whether it is with a superior at work, a paid supervisor, or a peer group, provides an opportunity for counselors to connect with those within the field, explore their own perceptions of events, and revise the meaning they have made of their experiences.

Continuing Education

Continuing education (CE) is required for all licensed counselors and therapists, as it is for most other professionals in health care and helping roles. While the exact requirements vary based on state and specialty, there are opportunities to choose CE that provides instruction in self-care. Counseling professionals can seek out opportunities that are likely to provide challenge to current belief systems, as well as support for trying out unfamiliar approaches. The key is, whenever possible, a counselor can purposefully choose CE that will lead to alternative perspectives and an expanded sense of self and what is possible in counseling.

Mindful Awareness and Meditation

Mindful awareness, or mindfulness, has been described as "knowledge and awareness of one's experience in the present moment" (Richards, Campenni, & Muse-Burk, 2010, p. 251). While there are various forms of meditation, all involve the goal of being more mindful. With recent research in neuroscience, it has become clear that mindful practices may be transformative at various mental and physical levels (Tang, Holzel, & Posner, 2015). Taylor (2008) wrote about holistic approaches to transformative learning that emphasize the importance of relationships, including imaginative relationships that include meditation. Mindfulness enables a person to focus attention on the present moment in a purposeful and non-judgmental manner (Kabat-Zinn, 1990). When one has cultivated this skill, it becomes easier to make a conscious choice about where we focus our attention moment to moment. Mezirow (1991) described transformative learning as changing one's frame of reference to be "more inclusive, differentiating, permeable, critically reflective, and integrative of experience" (p. 163). Ideally, with practice, mindful awareness leads to increased awareness and permits openness of thoughts, emotions, and reactions to stress and stressful situations, thus allowing us to be curious about these reactions as opposed to embodying them (Brown & Ryan, 2003; Kabat-Zinn, 1990).

Much like understanding or deconstructing other difficult concepts, mindfulness can initially be challenging to master as practitioners attempt to alter an ingrained emotional reaction. Reactivity is a schema that most know too well. With time and patience, mindful awareness can be an excellent resource for self-care as it allows us to examine our personal reactions, but not attach or respond to them as unhelpful triggers. Research across helping professions emphasizes mindfulness as a helpful tool (Sazima, 2016;

Schussler, Jennings, Sharp, & Frank, 2016). Through mindful practices, individuals have the opportunity to sit with their thoughts and observe the reactions, sensations, and environmental influences taking place while also taking away some of their emotional power by not being reactive to them. At the heart of mindfulness is the essence of self-care. It is the ability to reflect on a situation and withhold judgment of self and others. Mindfulness involves a multidimensional process to reorient the mind, body, and spirit to slow down, metaphorically jumping either "off of" or "out of" unhealthy cycles of repetitive thoughts or actions. Once the skills have been learned and regularly practiced, mindful awareness can be employed at any time.

Somatic awareness is a form of mindfulness that focuses on consciousness of one's body and what it tells us. Syndromes such as burnout can lower bodily defenses and immune system responses among those affected (Mommersteeg, Heijnen, Kavelaars, & van Doornen, 2006). Taylor's (2008) discussion of a more inclusive, holistic perspective of transformative learning recognizes that at times there are other ways of knowing such as somatic awareness and intuition. Somatic symptoms provide information that other, traditional means of self-perception do not. Practicing mindful awareness, specifically listening to what one's body communicates, can be helpful in recognizing or preventing stress. Siegel (2010) describes the brain's ability to rewrite important ways of knowing based on ideas of mindfulness. If counselors and therapists can learn to utilize mindful awareness as a lifelong tool within personal and professional situations, the opportunities for growth are tremendous.

Wellness as Self-Care

Counselors, like many others in the health care and helping professions, are not always good at taking care of themselves or "practicing what they preach." In 1998, Whitmer, Sweeney, and Myers created *The Wheel of Wellness* to provide a visual model of their research based on the components identified as comprising wellness. Later, Myers and Sweeney (2004) created the Wellness Evaluation of Lifestyle (WEL) scale, revising and renaming the model as *The Indivisible Self: An Evidence-Based Model of Wellness.* Both models were based on Alfred Adler's (1927) concepts of individual psychology that explored the whole self and one's purpose within life. In their research, Myers and Sweeney identified five second-order factors and one unidimensional, higher-order factor which they called "wellness." The five second-order factors were identified through factor analysis as comprising various parts of the self that contributed to wellness: essential self, creative self, coping self, social self, and physical self.

The essential self was found to consist of four components: spirituality, self-care, gender identity, and cultural identity. The five components of thinking, emotions, control, positive humor, and work addressed the creative self, while the coping self was composed of realistic beliefs, stress management, self-worth, and leisure. The social self included friendship and love. The final component, the physical self, was discovered to be no less important than the other factors and included exercise and nutrition. Myers and Sweeney (2004) also identified contextual variables within their model since the self is both influenced by and has an influence on the surrounding world. Drawing upon the work of Bronfenbrenner (1999) and his ecological model, Myers and Sweeney adopted four contextual elements from his work into their model of wellness: local, institutional, global, and chronometrical. The chronometric dimension recognizes that people change over time, an important quality supportive of the wellness that can be achieved through self-care.

The importance of exploring a model of wellness relates to being purposeful about personal attention. For counselors and therapists to care for themselves optimally, they must be willing to focus on themselves as care providers. This shift in focus, specifically for those who work with clients in high trauma situations, can be difficult. Myers and Sweeney's (2004) model provides a conceptual framework for counselors to examine all aspects of wellness and to explore their own wellness traits through the WEL scale.

Intrapersonal Work as Self-Care

Within the central tenets of transformative learning, deep personal work includes critical self-reflection and self-awareness of the assumptions that individuals use to guide their actions (Mezirow, 1991, 2012). According to Mezirow, transformative learning can lead to growth of the person as one becomes more open, more discriminating, and more integrative in making sense of experience in the world. While this process can occur through specific, dramatic, and intense episodes that Mezirow called "disorienting dilemmas," it can also occur gradually, through a long-term process of gradual changes in the meaning that a person makes of his or her experience.

As a counselor educator, I believe that self-awareness, intrapersonal work, and deep reflection form the cornerstone for personal and system transformation. Self-awareness allows for deep introspection, provides the opportunity for second order change, and can result in the transformation of a system of thinking, not just a single behavior. The nature of this change makes it more difficult to go back to the way things were prior to a revision in one's perspective or worldview. Resources that discuss the importance of intrapersonal self-care do not always point out the transformative potential for this type of work. While I attempt to create this type of brave, transformative learning space in every class, I particularly intend this awareness for those with a clinical or cultural counseling focus, where students are challenged more directly and often to look at intrapersonal meaning making.

Due to the solitary elements involved in intrapersonal learning, the traditional understanding of transformative learning, while still valid, deserves exploration. A psychodevelopmental view of transformative learning reflects a "continuous, incremental, and progressive growth" (Taylor, 2008, p. 7) over time. When also considering the neurobiological perspective that the structure of the brain changes during the learning process (Siegel, 2010), the likelihood for transformative learning occurring in an intrapersonal way becomes clear. Taylor (2008) discussed a psychoanalytic view of transformative learning as "a process of individuation, a lifelong journey of coming to understand oneself through reflecting on the psychic structures that make up an individual's identity" (p. 7). Young and Cashwell (2018) discuss the importance of mental health professionals seeking their own personal care. One study found that 84% of psychologists sought counseling or psychotherapy (Pope & Tabachnick, 1994). Interestingly, only 13% of those individuals had been required to participate in counseling within their academic training experience.

As counselors, we recognize that our profession can be similar to a one-sided friendship; clients receive the benefits of having someone to listen to them. That does not mean the practitioner does not learn, grow, and evolve with each therapeutic relationship. As counselors, therapists, and social workers, we need to allow ourselves to be cared for in this same way by seeking out our own counseling. When counselors participate in the therapeutic process as the client, the relationship does not need to be reciprocal. Being in a therapeutic relationship in which one is the client provides an opportunity to work on meaning making, optimize the potential for transformative learning, and foster resilience (Sommers-Flanagan & Sommers-Flanagan, 2018).

Self-Talk

The negative messages or faulty logic that one engages in internally are often much worse than what one would say to another person. Within professional counseling, gaining awareness and insight into this phenomenon is called *cognitive restructuring*. Learning to recognize when this is happening through self-monitoring is the first step to greater self-awareness. A simple change in the internal message can make a big difference in the ownership a person takes for things outside of his or her control. Research within the field of cognitive behavioral theory (CBT) shows the longitudinal difference in mental health when one alters negative self-talk to become more positive self-talk through cognitive restructuring. Changing a thought from the negative, such as "I am bad," to a more positively reframed expression, "that was not a good decision, but I usually make better ones," can alter the subsequent behavioral and emotional responses based merely on a shift in thought or perspective (Sommers-Flanagan & Sommers-Flanagan, 2018).

Expressive and Creative Arts

The field of expressive and creative arts provides an opportunity for students to transform in their understanding of themselves through classes that engage the more creative, right side of one's brain. These include use of modalities such as journal writing, storytelling, creation of sounds, and experiences in bodily movement. By putting pen (e.g., ink, crayons, or paint) to paper (e.g., fabric, wood, tile, and more), learners can suspend cognition to interact with aspects of the self that are less frequently engaged in an academic environment. For those who tend to be analytical, this is a particularly powerful and transformative form of self-care and self-expression. Ganim and Fox (1999) have suggested that to go deeper into our feelings, to get to the heart and soul of self-understanding, we need to use a different language that by its nature is not analytical or judgmental but reveals our feelings, rather than interprets them. They refer to this language as the body-mind's inner imagery (p. 10). As with most activities that involve tapping into parts of our body, mind, and spirit with which we may be less familiar, a level of trust is needed, and often a guide to help one get started. Dirkx (2006) wrote about the importance of "inviting the whole person...as an affective, intuitive, thinking, physical, spiritual self" when experiencing transformative learning (p. 46).

Meeting Body Needs

Within Dorociak et al.'s (2017) PSCS domains of life balance and daily balance, the authors did not find that physical activity prompts related to bodily needs were salient enough to warrant a separate domain. However, they did believe that various bodily needs related to professional self-care reside within these domains. A healthy lifestyle is important, but Norcross and Guy (2007) point out that helpers often neglect bio-behavioral basics such as adequate diet, sleep, rest, exercise, and human contact.

There are numerous resources that highlight different ways to take care of the body. One can do simple things such as eat healthy food, get appropriate amounts of sleep, go for walks during work breaks, drink plenty of water, and limit one's exposure to traumatic images outside of work. In addition, if a person has a family history of addiction and access to various medications within the workplace, that individual needs to be cognizant of the potential signs for burnout that might lead the person to self-medicate. Taking care of one's body also helps to create and sustain resilience, since a healthy body helps to ward off illness.

Religion and Spirituality

Research supports the connection between religion, spirituality, and meaning making (Diener, Tay, & Myers, 2011; Steger & Frazier, 2005; Wong, 1998). For many, spirituality and religion are essential factors in wellness and self-care; they allow individuals to believe in something greater than themselves. However, research shows when significant traumatic events occur, such as a serious diagnosis, a person's perception of the world can shift (Jim, Richardson, Golden-Kreutz, & Andersen, 2006; Park, 2010). In inimical times, meaning making can become difficult (Park, 2010) and reliance on religion or a spiritual direction can waver. For those who are struggling with compassion fatigue from experiencing a client's trauma, a person may experience a loss of control that can easily lead to a lack of meaning. In the face of such powerlessness, spirituality can provide a resource for stability when other options are not available (Park, Edmondson, & Hale-Smith, 2013). Counselors, therapists, and their clients who are facing traumatic or difficult situations can seek solace by relying on spiritual and religious beliefs and practices. Having an understanding that something is beyond oneself, whatever that may be, can be transformative (Batson, Schoenrade, & Ventis, 1993). It symbolizes the antithesis of loneliness if one is able to tap into a broader sense of meaning or belonging in the world. When faced with burnout symptoms that result in physical and mental health issues, such as exhaustion, depersonalization, depression, or anxiety, the concept of a higher power or omnipotent Other can bring comfort.

Relational Work as Self-Care

Ample research exists to support that the quality of the relationship between helping professionals and their clients has a positive impact on the perception of service (Trueland, 2009). Within the PSCS (Dorociak et al., 2017), the dimension of professional support was found to be one of five used to assess professional self-care. Participating in healthy relationships has been found to lead to more congruent, engaged professionals and provide benefits for their personal lives (Schwartzhoffer, 2010). Supportive relationships can also help professional helpers ward off the influences of burnout and compassion fatigue by having others who can both understand and provide alternatives to a skewed perspective. In addition, when one examines findings on compassion fatigue, there is research to show that relationships with others alleviate stress symptoms (Dorociak et al., 2017; Norcross & Guy, 2007; Schwartzhoffer, 2010).

In my work as a professional counselor, I often saw adolescents who were survivors of childhood sexual abuse that occurred months or years ago. One of the primary things we talked about was recognizing who was to blame for the abuse. In the beginning of our professional relationship, none of my clients placed blame solely on the perpetrator. More than one survivor put 90% of the responsibility on themselves. On a regular basis, I heard comments such as: "I should have said no"; "I should have known"; "Maybe he didn't mean it"; and "I ruined his life." All of these were statements made by incest survivors. Statistically, 30% of perpetrators are family members, and 90% are individuals known to the family (Finkelhor, 2012; Whealin, 2007). By the time we ended our counseling relationship, most of these clients had gained a new perspective, not only on the nature of their abuse and who was responsible for it, but also of themselves. When they had family support in addressing the past abuse, this growth often happened much more quickly.

One suggestion made within the literature to help counselors and therapists deal with vicarious trauma is to ask family and friends to have frank and honest conversations with them about how they are perceived, particularly with respect to what the counselor brings home from work (Norcross & Guy, 2007). This honesty can lead to meaningful conversations about how much of what occurs at work creates stress that requires support from others at home. It can also provide a trusted mirror into something we may not see in ourselves and enable us to become mindful of our personal situation. Much like the deep work that can occur in personal counseling and supervision, inquiring with a friend or family about the influences we have on others can be critical to self-awareness.

CONCLUSION

As a professor and former professional mental health counselor, when I think of transformation, I visualize the slow, sometimes painful process that often comes through counseling to realize a transformed perspective. Working with a client each week, and seeing that individual come to personal awareness around an issue that has caused great pain can be an honor. At times, I am the only one who is lucky enough to see the resilience that takes hold to give new or revised meaning to the experience. I see a version of this in the classroom, too. I have students write letters to their future selves at the beginning of their clinical work. They are fearful, anxious, and often full of self-doubt. A year later, as they prepare to graduate, they open these letters and discuss the transformation in their perspectives. There are different reactions to this experience: some laugh, some cry, and some simply smile. They are still nervous about their transition into the field of counseling practice, but they now have tools, experience, and greater awareness that come from using many of the self-care suggestions above. Often, they do not see these changes while they are occurring.

This growth can be found within the psychodevelopmental view of transformative learning that Taylor (2008) describes. Personal growth and awareness can arise unexpectedly for some; for others, it is much more intentionally achieved through deliberate and consistent efforts by working toward change over time. A reactive response to the stressors and trauma of the work environment often creates an uphill battle for those in the helping professions, including counselors and therapists. With resultant feelings of exhaustion, depersonalization, depression, or anxiety, professional helpers can experience lowered self-efficacy, detachment, depletion of emotional reserves, or cynicism towards those they seek to help. This is not only risky for our own well-being, but also for our clients who have put their lives in our care. It is time we do a better job of living our values, hopes, and dreams for our clients through our own lives by recognizing that self-care can no longer be seen as a luxury.

REFERENCES

Adler, A. (1927). *Understanding human nature.* Garden City, NY: Garden City.

American Counseling Association. (ACA). (2014). *Code of ethics.* Alexandria, VA: Author. Retrieved from https://www.counseling.org/resources/aca-code-of-ethics.pdf

American Psychological Association. (2010). *Ethical principles of psychologists and code of conduct.* Washington, DC: Author. Retrieved from http://www.apa.org/ethics/code/

Andersen, L. L., & Dybbroe, B. (2017). Introspection as intra-professionalism in social and health care. *Journal of Social Work Practices, 31*(1), 21–35. https://doi.org/10.1080/02650533.2016.1142952

Baird, S., & Jenkins, S. R. (2003). Vicarious traumatization, secondary traumatic stress, and burnout in sexual assault and domestic violence agency staff. *Violence and Victims, 18*(1), 71–86. https://doi.org/10.1891/vivi.2003.18.1.71

Barnett, J. E., Baker, E. K., Elman, N. S., & Schoener, G. R. (2007). In pursuit of wellness: The self-care imperative. *Professional Psychology: Research and Practice, 38*(6), 603–612. https://doi.org/10.1037/0735-7028.38.6.603

Batson, C. D., Schoenrade, P., & Ventis, W. L. (1993). *Religion and the individual: A social-psychological perspective.* New York, NY: Oxford University Press.

Baumgartner, L. M. (2012). Mezirow's theory of transformative learning from 1975 to present. In E. W. Taylor & P. Cranton (Eds.), *The handbook of transformative learning: Theory, research, and practice* (pp. 99–115). San Francisco, CA: Jossey-Bass.

Beel, C., Chilokoa, M., & Ladak, S. (2017). Critical reflection on peer supervision underpinning inter-agency work: EPs working experientially with a youth offending services. *Educational and Child Psychology, 34*(3), 109–118.

Bernard, J. M., & Goodyear, R. K. (2014). *Fundamentals of clinical supervision* (5th ed.). Boston, MA: Allyn & Bacon.

Bronfenbrenner, U. (1999). Environments in developmental perspective: Theoretical and operational models. In S. L. Friedman & T. D. Wachs (Eds.), *Measuring environment across the lifespan: Emerging methods and concepts* (pp. 3–28). Washington, DC: American Psychological Association.

Brown, K. W., & Ryan, R. M. (2003). The benefits of being present: Mindfulness and its role in psychological well-being. *Journal of Personality and Social Psychology, 84*(4), 822–848.

Christopher, J. C., Christopher, S. E., Dunnagan, T., & Schure, M. (2006). Teaching self-care through mindfulness practices: The application of yoga, meditation, and qigong to counselor training. *Journal of Humanistic Psychology, 46*(4), 494–509.

Coetzee, S. K., & Klopper, H. C. (2010). Compassion fatigue within nursing practice: A concept analysis. *Nursing and Health Sciences, 12*(2), 235–243. https://doi.org/10.1111/j.1442-2018.2010.00526.x

Crowe, C. (2015). Burnout and self-care considerations for oncology professionals. *Journal of Pain Management, 8*(3), 191–195.

Diener, E., Tay, L., & Myers, D. G. (2011). The religion paradox: If religion makes people happy, why are so many dropping out? *Journal of Personality and Social Psychology, 101*(6), 1278–1290. https://doi.org/10.1037/a0024402

Dirkx, J. M. (2006). Authenticity and imagination. *New Directions for Adult and Continuing Education,* Fall(111), 27–39. https://doi.org/10.1002/ace.225

Dorociak, K. E., Rupert, P. A., Bryant, R. B., & Zahniser, E. (2017). Development of the professional self-care scale. *Journal of Counseling Psychology, 64*(3), 325–334. https://doi.org/10.1037/cou0000206

Etherington, K. (2000). Supervising counsellors who work with survivors of childhood sexual abuse. *Counselling Psychology Quarterly, 13*(4), 377–389.

Figley, C. R. (1995). *Compassion fatigue: Coping with secondary traumatic stress disorder in those who treat the traumatized.* New York, NY: Routledge.

Finkelhor, D. (2012). *Characteristics of crimes against juveniles.* Durham, NH: Crimes Against Children Research Center. Retrieved from http://www.d2l.org/wp-content/uploads/2017/01/all_statistics_20150619.pdf

Ganim, B., & Fox, S. (1999). *Visual journaling: Going deeper than words.* Wheaton, IL: Quest Books.

Gündüz, B. (2012). Self-efficacy and burnout in professional school counselors. *Educational Sciences: Theory & Practice, 12*(3), 1761–1767.

Hodgkinson, P., & Shepherd, M. (1994). The impact of disaster support work. *Journal of Traumatic Stress Studies, 7*(4), 587–600.

Ivicic, R., & Motta, R. (2017). Variables associated with secondary trauma among mental health professionals. *Traumatology, 23*(2), 196–204. http://dx.doi.org/10.1037/trm0000065

Jenkins, S. R., & Baird, S. (2002). Secondary traumatic stress and vicarious trauma: A validation study. *Journal of Traumatic Stress, 15*(5), 423–433.

Jim, H. S., Richardson, S. A., Golden-Kreutz, D. M., & Andersen, B. L. (2006). Strategies used in coping with a cancer diagnosis predict meaning in life for survivors. *Health Psychology, 25*(6), 753–761. https://doi.org/10.1037/0278-6133.25.6.753

Joinson, C. (1992). Coping with compassion fatigue. *Nursing, 22*(4), 118–120.

Kabat-Zinn, J. (1990). *Full catastrophe living: Using the wisdom of your body and mind to face stress, pain, and illness.* New York, NY: Dell.

Killian, K. D. (2008). Helping till it hurts? A multimethod study of compassion fatigue, burnout, and self-care in clinicians working with trauma survivors. *Traumatology, 14*(2), 32–44. https://doi.org/10.1177/1534765608319083

Lyndall, S., & Bicknell, J. (2001). Trauma and the therapist: The experience of therapists working with the perpetrators of sexual abuse. *Australasian Journal of Disaster and Trauma Studies, 5,* 543–551.

Maslach, C., Jackson, S. E., & Leiter, M. P. (1996). *Maslach burnout inventory* (3rd ed.). Palo Alto, CA: Consulting Psychologists Press.

Maslach, C., Schaufeli, W. B., & Leiter, M. P. (2001). Job burnout. *Annual Review of Psychology, 52,* 397–422.

Maslow, A. H. (1943). A theory of human motivation. *Psychological Review, 50*(4), 370–394.

Mayorga, M. G., Devries, S. R., & Wardle, E. A. (2015). The practice of self-care among counseling students. *Journal of Educational Psychology, 8*(3), 21–28.

McCann, L., & Pearlman, L. (1990). Vicarious traumatization: A framework for understanding the psychological effects of working with victims. *Journal of Traumatic Stress Studies, 3*(1), 131–149.

Mezirow, J. (1978). Perspective transformation. *Adult Education, 28*(2), 100–110. http://dx.doi.org/10.1177/074171367802800202

Mezirow, J. (1991). *Transformative dimensions of adult learning.* San Francisco, CA: Jossey-Bass.

Mezirow, J. (2012). Learning to think like an adult: Core concepts of transformation theory. In E. W. Taylor, P. Cranton, & Associates (Eds.), *The handbook of transformative learning: Theory, research, and practice* (pp. 73–95). San Francisco, CA: Jossey-Bass.

Mommersteeg, P. M. C., Heijnen C. J., Kavellars, A., & van Doornen, L. J. P. (2006). Immune and endocrine function in burnout syndrome. *Psychosomatic Medicine, 68*(6), 879–886.

Myers, J. E., & Sweeney, T. J. (2004). The indivisible self: An evidence-based model of wellness. *Journal of Individual Psychology, 60*(3), 234–245.

National Association of Social Workers. (2008). *Code of ethics.* Retrieved from http://www.socialworkers.org/pubs/Code/

Newell, J. M., & Nelson-Gardell, D. (2014). A competency-based approach to teaching professional self-care: An ethical consideration for social work educators. *Journal of Social Work Education, 50*(3), 427–439. Retrieved from https://eric.ed.gov/?id=EJ1033201

Norcross, J. C., & Guy, J. D. (2007). *Leaving it at the office: A guide to psychotherapist self-care.* New York, NY: Guilford Press.

Park, C. L. (2010). Making sense of the meaning literature: An integrative review of meaning making and its effects on adjustment to stressful life events. *Psychological Bulletin, 136*(2), 257–301. http://dx.doi.org/10.1037/a0018301

Park, C. L., Edmondson, D., & Hale-Smith, A. (2013). Why religion? Meaning as motivation. In K. I. Pargament (Ed.), *APA handbook of psychology, religion, and spirituality* (Vol. 1; pp. 157–171). Washington, DC: American Psychological Association.

Pearlman, L., & Saakvitne, K. (1995). *Trauma and the therapist.* New York, NY: W. W. Norton.

Pope, K. S., & Tabachnick, B. G. (1994). Therapists as patients: A national survey of psychologists' experiences, problems, and beliefs. *Professional Psychology: Research and Practice, 25*(3), 247–258.

Prochaska, J. O., & Velicer, W. F. (1997). The transtheoretical model of health behavior change. *American Journal of Health Promotion, 12*(1), 38–48.

Richards, K. C., Campenni, C. E., & Muse-Burke, J. L. (2010). Self-care and well-being in mental health professionals: The mediating effect of self-awareness and mindfulness. *Journal of Mental Health, 32*(3), 247–264.

Saakvitne, K. W., & Pearlman, L. A. (1996). *Transforming the pain: A workbook on vicarious traumatization for helping professionals who work with traumatized clients.* New York, NY: W. W. Norton.

Salyers, M. P., Fukui, S., Rollins, A. L., Firmin, R., Gearhart, T., Noll, J. P., . . . Davis, C. J. (2014). Burnout and self-reported quality of care in community mental health. *Administration and Policy in Mental Health and Mental Health Services Research, 42*(1), 61–69.

Sazima, G. (2016). Incorporating meditation training into an outpatient psychiatry practice. *Psychiatric Times, 33*(3), 1–5.

Schauben, L. J., & Frazier, P. A. (1995). Vicarious trauma: The effect on female counselors of working with sexual violence survivors. *Psychology of Women Quarterly, 19*(1), 49–64.

Schussler, D. L., Jennings, P. A., Sharp, J. E., & Frank, J. L. (2016). Improving teacher awareness and well-being through CARE: A qualitative analysis of the underlying mechanisms. *Mindfulness, 7*(1), 130–142. Retrieved from http://dx.doi.org/10.1007/s12671-015-0422-7

Schwartzhoffer, R. V. (2010). *Psychology of burnout: Predictors and coping mechanisms.* New York, NY: Nova Science.

Sheehy Carmel, M. J., & Friedlander, M. L. (2009). The relation of secondary traumatization to therapists' perceptions of the working alliance with clients who commit sexual abuse. *Journal of Counseling Psychology, 56*(3), 461–467. https://doi.org/10.1037/a0015422

Siegel, D. (2010). *Mindsight: The new science of personal transformation.* New York, NY: Bantam Books.

Sommer, C. A. (2008). Vicarious traumatization, trauma-sensitive supervision, and counselor preparation. *Counselor Education and Supervision, 48*(1), 61–71. https://doi.org/10.1002/j.1556-6978.2008.tb00062.x

Sommer, C., & Cox, J. (2005). Elements of supervision in sexual violence counselors' narratives: A qualitative analysis. *Counselor Education and Supervision, 45*(2), 119–134.

Sommer, C., & Cox, J. (2006). Sexual violence counselors' reflections on supervision: Using stories to mitigate vicarious traumatization. *Journal of Poetry Therapy, 19*(1), 3–16.

Sommers-Flanagan, J., & Sommers-Flanagan, R. (2018). *Counseling and psychotherapy theories in context and practice: Skills, strategies, and techniques* (3rd ed.). Hoboken, NJ: Wiley.

Steger, M. F., & Frazier, P. (2005). Meaning in life: One link in the chain from religiousness to well-being. *Journal of Counseling Psychology, 52*(4), 574–582.

Tang, Y., Holzel, B., & Posner, M. (2015). The neuroscience of meditation. *Nature Reviews Neuroscience, 16*(4), 213–225. https://doi.org/10.1038/nrn3916

Taylor, E. W. (2008, September). Transformative learning theory. *New Directions for Adult and Continuing Education, 2008*(119), 5–15. https://doi.org/10.1002/ace.301

Trueland, J. (2009). Compassion through human connection. *Nursing Standards, 23*(48), 19–21.

Wee, D., & Myers, D. (2002). Stress response of mental health workers following disaster: The Oklahoma City bombing. In C. R. Figley (Ed.), *Treating compassion fatigue* (pp. 57–83). New York, NY: Brunner-Routledge.

Whealin, J. (2007). *Darkness to light: Child sexual abuse statistics.* National Center for Post Traumatic Stress Disorder, U.S. Department of Veterans Affairs. Retrieved from http://www.d2l.org/wp-content/uploads/2017/01/all_statistics_20150619.pdf

Whitmer, J. M., Sweeney, T. J., & Myers, J. E. (1998). *The wheel of wellness.* Greensboro, NC: Author.

Wise, E. H., Hersh, M. A., & Gibson, C. M. (2012). Ethics, self-care and well-being for psychologists: Re-envisioning the stress-distress continuum. *Professional Psychology: Research and Practice, 43*(5), 487–494. https://doi.org/10.1037/a0029446

Wong, P. T. P. (1998). Implicit theories of meaningful life and the development of the personal meaning profile. In P. T. P. Wong & P. S. Fry (Eds.), *The human quest for meaning: A handbook of psychological research and clinical applications* (pp. 111–140). Mahwah, NJ: Routledge.

World Health Organization. (2009, January). Self-care in the context of primary healthcare. In *Report of the Regional Consultation* (pp. 1–72). Bangkok, Thailand. Retrieved from http://apps.searo.who.int/PDS_DOCS/B4301.pdf

Yalom, I. D. (2002). *The gift of therapy: An open letter to new therapists and their patients.* New York, NY: HarperCollins.

Young, J. S., & Cashwell, C. S. (2017). *Clinical mental health counseling: Elements of effective practice.* Thousand Oaks, CA: SAGE.

CHAPTER 16

INFORMAL LEARNING IN A COMMUNITY-BASED HEALTH EDUCATION PROGRAM

The Transformative Experience of One Interprofessional Team

Maureen Coady
Saint Francis Xavier University

ABSTRACT

While nonformal education (e.g., workshops, certificates) and learning are a central focus of the professional development literature, informal and transformative learning have received less practical or theoretical consideration. The aim of this study was to surface informal learning, and its effects, as a team of health providers navigated interprofessional learning in a community-based cardiac rehabilitation/education program. The study reveals that informal learning and critical reflection helped the participants to adjust and to make meaning of a complex competency in a new and unfamiliar setting.

Transformative Learning in Healthcare and Helping Professions Education, pages 323–343
Copyright © 2019 by Information Age Publishing
323

> The learning journey involved not only new learning and unlearning, but also synergistic moments when individual transformation contributed to collective knowing and group transformation.

A major assumption associated with professional practice is that professionals continue to learn following their preservice education programs. Indeed, as individuals participate in professional practice, they acquire knowledge, gain skills, and increase occupational sensibilities across their professional careers through practical experiences and informal learning, as well as formal study (Coady, 2015, 2016; Daley & Cervero, 2016). Despite a growing emphasis on expert knowledge and formalized continuing professional education (CPE), there is a significant and growing body of research emphasizing that most professional learning occurs outside of planned programming, in practice experience (Billett, 2009; Boud & Hagar, 2012; Crowley, 2014; Daley & Cervero, 2016; Eraut, 2004, 2007; Kinsella & Pitman, 2012; Knox, 2016; Reich, Rooney, & Boud, 2014; Wilson & Cervero, 2014). Through informal learning, professionals acquire and sustain new knowledge and understanding that informs their practice.

In this circumstance, professional development is realized through interaction in the professional's own social network and communities (Cross & Parker, 2004; deLaat & Schreurs, 2013; Fenwick & Nerland, 2014; Servage, 2008). More recent scholarship extends this thinking, highlighting that the learning involved is situated and influenced by the sociocultural context of work (Daley & Cervero, 2016) and the professionals' identity—the values, experience, and understandings they bring to practice (Dirkx, 2008; Dirkx, Gilley, & Mayunich-Gilley, 2004). Reflective practice is closely related to this idea of learning from experience, providing a sophisticated process of integrating personal and professional knowledge with the demands of the situation as part of an intelligent and creative approach to practice (Bolton, 2014; Kinsella & Pitman, 2012; Thompson & Pascal, 2012).

The professional development literature does acknowledge the value of informal learning, highlighting how tacit knowledge and growing wisdom complement standard CPE offerings. Beyond this, however, the professional development literature largely ignores this dimension (deLaat & Schreurs, 2013; Eraut, 2004; Nisbet, Lincoln, & Dunn, 2013). Reich et al. (2014) assert the dominance of codified, propositional knowledge makes it more difficult for the more complex and informal aspects of learning in practice to be realized. Others, including Cross and Parker (2004) and Eraut (2004, 2007), claim that it is the spontaneous and largely invisible nature of informal learning that enables it to be so taken for granted and not recognized as learning, while deLaat and Schreurs (2013) point out the challenges in mapping and analyzing informal learning. The effect is that informal learning remains invisible and *what* is learned through and in practice—the kinds of knowledge, skills, and dispositions developed through informal learning in practice—is much less understood than *how* it is learned (Boud & Hagar, 2012; Coady, 2016; Milligan, Littlejohn, & Margaryan, 2014; Reich et al., 2014).

Transformative learning is similarly overlooked in the professional development and workplace learning literature (Choy, 2009; Jones & Charteris, 2017; Webster-Wright, 2009, 2010). In professional learning contexts, transformative learning involves individuals and groups transforming and constructing professional identities and socially meaningful knowledge and skills (Cranton & King, 2003; Crowley, 2014). This kind of learning demands critical reflection that potentially leads to more creative and innovative ways of being (as in communities of practice) that address troubling workplace challenges and practices (Jones & Charteris, 2017; Servage, 2008; Watkins, Marsick, & Faller, 2012). Despite this potential, little is known about this dynamic process of collective group learning and change in practice, or about how it is best facilitated (Cranton, 2006; de Groot, Endedijk, Jaarsma, Simons, & van Beukelen, 2014; Jones & Charteris, 2017; Shapiro, Wasserman, & Gallegos, 2012). In fact, a recent critical review of transformative learning literature reveals that most of the research on transformative learning continues to focus on individual learning, rather than on team or group learning (Taylor & Snyder, 2012). Even less is known about the interconnectedness of individual and group transformation; for example, whether individual transformation within a group or organization can contribute to overall group learning that is transformative (de Groot et al., 2015; Jones & Charteris, 2017).

These circumstances provide a strong rationale for making informal learning and transformative learning in professional practice and workplaces more visible. In surfacing informal learning as a way of meaning-making in everyday practice, the opportunity exists for a deeper and more unified understanding of how informal learning can work together with nonformal and formal education to support the development of professional knowledge, skills, dispositions, and, potentially, transformative learning (Colley, Hodgkinson, & Malcolm, 2003).

This chapter will provide an example of informal learning within one interprofessional team that resulted in enhanced knowledge and skills among healthcare professionals in service to the community, with implications for transformative learning at the group level.

THE HEALTH AND INTERPROFESSIONAL
LEARNING CONTEXT

Learning to work in new ways and new environments is always challenging and unpredictable and involves significant learning and change (Davies, 2000). Increasingly, health professionals are being encouraged to work in interprofessional collaborative teams to ensure that people have access to holistic and comprehensive care. Doing so involves integrating the clinical knowledge and experience of all team members and balancing an emphasis on clinical expertise with a focus on enabling people as competent managers of their health and health problems (Curran, 2010). Recognized barriers to interprofessional learning include the biomedical values and hierarchical and discipline-specific training of health professionals that have not oriented them to these interactive and participatory concepts and ideals (Chatalasingh & Reeves, 2014; Daley & Cervero, 2016; Hill, 2016). Learning to become a collaborative practitioner, therefore, is a complex and longer-term process, often involving a transformation of professional identity in order that the larger cognitive and value maps can be built for teamwork and collaboration (Freeth, Hammick, Reeves, Koppel, & Barr, 2005; Silver & Leslie, 2009).

The emphasis on health professionals' learning to work collaboratively extends beyond clinical practice to community settings in which interprofessional teams educate people about their health in order to reduce chronic disease. In this environment, these health professionals are challenged to work beyond their established and individualized clinical boundaries (Daley, 2006; McNair, Brown, Stone, & Sims, 2001) and within a social, rather than medical, model of health that acknowledges health as influenced by community and populations determinants (Wilkinson & Marmot, 2003). In this context, practicing professionals with little training or a history of working in collaborative teams, or with groups in community settings, are likely to feel challenged (Lewy, 2010; McNair et al., 2001). While their role often includes education, health professionals often lack sufficient knowledge about adult learning and appropriate curriculum design (Bryan, Kreuter, & Brownson, 2009; Hill, 2011, 2016; Stuttaford & Coe, 2007). In a community-based context, therefore, they must think more broadly than individual health, and they must learn not only about collaboration, but also about program planning and design and adult learning processes appropriate to diverse groups and community-based settings.

STUDY BACKGROUND AND METHODS

The Community Cardiovascular Hearts in Motion (CCHIM) is a cardiac health education and rehabilitation program operating in a single health district in Nova Scotia, Canada since 2008. The program is made available to referred cardiac patients having experienced, or at high risk of experiencing, a cardiac event. It is a group program that is community-based and available 2 full days a week for 12 weeks. Staff employ a motivational interviewing (MI) approach—a person-centered counseling style for addressing the common problem of patient ambivalence about change. Motivational interviewing pays attention to readiness for change and is designed to strengthen an individual's motivation by exploring reasons for change within an atmosphere of acceptance and compassion (Rollnick, Miller, & Butler, 2008). Motivational interviewing is appropriate in a social model of health because it attends to both individual and social determinants of health.

Between 2008 and 2014, when this research was undertaken, the CCHIM program had been offered in 12 rural communities in the district using an MI approach (Coady, 2013). Within these years, 150 participants from the district participated in the program. The interprofessional team who facilitated the program was comprised of a nurse, a dietician, a physiotherapist who worked full time in the program, and a part-time health motivator. A single case study methodology was appropriate because it focused not only on the learning of the health professionals, but also on context-specific factors and situations (Merriam & Tisdell, 2016). Data were collected in a single month and involved a single focus group with three participants followed by two individual interviews. A cardiac nurse practitioner provided oversight to the program and was also interviewed for this research to provide relevant background and institutional insights. The research was approved by the district health ethics board and the university where the researcher was employed.

TEAM LEARNING

Informal learning is learning that occurs as a result of individuals making sense of the experiences they encounter in their daily lives. This learning can be achieved through self-directed or incidental learning and can result from socialization (Livingstone, 2005). In this study, the "daily lives" of the healthcare team was their experience delivering the CCHIM program. The learning of interest was that which was realized from delivering the CCHIM program using an MI strategy over 6 years. Team members received some early training in MI, but no formal training in interprofessional collaboration. They were asked to focus on learning from and *in* practice (i.e., the CCHIM experience) and to consider any changes in overall outlook or practice, individually or collectively, that may have resulted from that experience.

A thematic analysis (Merriam & Tisdell, 2016) of group and individual interviews revealed professional learning in four key areas: collaboration and teamwork, adult learning and curriculum design, cultural competency (i.e., working with diverse populations), and reflective practice. Below, I explore the individual and team learning associated with these themes. The voices of team members (using pseudonyms) are brought into focus in order to bring their ideas to life. Discussion of transformative learning—learning that transforms one's worldview (Mezirow, 2009)—is interwoven into this discussion of informal learning.

Learning Collaboration

All the members of the CCHIM facilitation team were experienced clinicians with a work history primarily in acute care settings. They were knowledgeable in individualized clinical teaching but had limited experience facilitating group programs in community settings. Most of the team members had volunteered for this assignment and linked their motivation with professional values and interests, ranging from wanting to be part of a more comprehensive and holistic approach to care to wanting to shift their focus in practice from illness care to health promotion and wellness in community settings. For example, Susan, a dietician, linked her motivation with her professional values and beliefs:

> I see health as having many dimensions, but I work in the nutrition side of things, which is just one aspect related to heart disease, and so I was attracted to the idea of working as a collaborator in a more integrated approach. I thought we could have more of an impact if we addressed all aspects of a person's response to a heart condition, and to be able to see the results of that kind of an approach first-hand. I thought that would be very rewarding, and it has been.

As a rule, an adult's readiness to learn is closely related to the developmental tasks of his or her social role (Merriam, Caffarella, & Baumgartner, 2007). In theory, therefore, a high degree of perceived readiness to work in a collaborative team should mitigate some of the recognized barriers to interprofessional learning (Curran, 2010; Davies, 2000). Yet, when reflecting back on their experiences, team members described their early understanding and enthusiasm for teamwork as naive. In practice, while feeling ready for this change, they recalled hidden and sometimes open value conflicts associated with who would lead and how power and decision-making were to be shared. Mary, a physiotherapist, describes her initial unease when these unexpected power dynamics challenged her professional identity.

> We are all taught to lead, and our training teaches us to value our own clinical expertise most, so we had conflicts in the beginning. Over time in practice, however, I learned that my professional expertise was only one part of the

overall picture. So, there was this sense of losing power initially, and then acceptance, and learning to value other people's clinical expertise, and in some cases letting others lead. Patsy [nurse], for example, was the only one who had worked in cardiac care, so by times it was important for her to lead. Other times it was me who needed to lead . . . it depended on what or who we were dealing with.

This confirms the view offered by Wenger-Trayner, Fenton-O'Creevy, Hutchinson, Kubiak, and Wenger-Trayner (2015) that without a shared history, the boundaries of professional practice are places of potential misunderstanding and confusion arising from different "'regimes of competency,' commitments, values, repertoires and perspectives" (p. 17). Interprofessional learning is challenging because it involves professionals working across their traditional boundaries and structures, frames of thought, and habits (Gilbert, 2005).

For Mary, the physiotherapist, this meeting of perspectives was also a moment of unexpected transformative learning. The early conflicts seem to have triggered her to critically reflect, and to realize that such boundary encounters were an inevitable part of learning how to work interprofessionally. She had reached what Berger (2004) described as her "growing edge"—that liminal space where individuals come to terms with the limitations of their knowing, and which provides an impetus to stretch their thinking. Mary's comments suggest that in critically examining her assumptions, she was able to reframe her thinking and to value other professional perspectives in their shared practice. In transformative learning terms, she had "experienced a deep structural shift in her basic premise of thought, feelings and actions" (O'Sullivan, Morrell, & O'Connor, 2002, p. xvii).

Mary's comment that "it depends on what or who we were dealing with" signifies a patient-centered approach, which is an integral goal of social models of health and interprofessional care. Care that is truly interprofessional and patient-centered considers patients' cultural traditions, their personal preferences and values, their family situations, and their lifestyles (Zeighan & Ton, 2011). Patients and their loved ones are an integral part of the care team who collaborate with healthcare professionals in making clinical decisions (Epstein & Street, 2011).

Despite these initial power struggles, however, Bill, the team health motivator, emphasized that over time, and with positive results in their programming, a shared commitment to making the program work and a greater openness and willingness to work in new ways became evident.

We wanted to move people along the sickness spectrum towards wellness. Our goal was to support them [patients] in reaching their goals, which was a different starting point for most of us . . . so the challenge was trying to figure out where we positioned ourselves, what working together looked like, and in each different circumstance, to find our individual place... it was a disorienting experience and a big learning curve, but eventually there was a strong collective will that developed to talk about and to solve problems together... it just takes will if people decide they want to work together.

Bill is highlighting how time and the shared experience of working together contributed to a readiness for new learning. Recent studies suggest that prior experience of working together in the workplace contributes significantly to improved professional identities and attitudes towards teamwork (Maharajan et al., 2017).

Like Bill, Patsy, the team nurse, described how the experience of finding their way together helped her and others to critically reflect on and reconstruct their previous meaning perspectives and to stretch themselves to reenvision their practice:

> You don't think of it when you are working in a hospital with others, where everything is based on power and protocol. Working as a team outside of that environment the rules weren't so clear. In time, we realized that we had a lot more freedom and could be creative and imaginative; there was this synergy working with others where we could experiment with our own ideas. We learned to think more creatively and expansively, and I think we have all realized the limitations of our earlier clinical boxes.

Clearly, these processes of coming to understand collaboration and MI through interaction in practice involved learning to release power, which helped team members to more fully realize the benefits and efficiencies of teamwork and patient-centered care (McNair et al., 2001). Patsy, the team nurse, described how this progressive learning unfolded, and the transformative impact in outlook she experienced:

> Early on I struggled to know my place and what to do and when. But, we were together every day trying to figure things out about a client or community. Over time our way of working became rather intuitive... we learned that collaboration meant our scope of practice should overlap and so if I noticed someone should follow up with Susan, I would, say, catch her by the end of the day, and if someone else needs a medication adjustment they could see me, and so over time we learned that collaboration was about trust and respect, good communication, and just trying to do the best together for the people. My entire outlook shifted with that understanding of how to work, and I can now see how much more we can accomplish when we work together as a team.

These highlights reveal the CCHIM team as a "community of knowers" who made meaning from their experiences and constructed new knowledge through interactions in practice. As their accounts reveal, an emergent mutual interest in achieving good patient outcomes led them to overcome recognized barriers to communication and to value respectful dialogue. Much of the literature on interprofessional learning suggests that clear communication, trust, and respect for each other's perspective are central to developing collaborative team relationships (Nancarrow et al., 2013). A trusting environment for learning and promoting autonomy and collaboration are ideal conditions for fostering transformative learning (Taylor, 2009).

Learning Group Facilitation and Program Planning and Design

According to Hill (2011), curriculum that is based on the needs of adult learners can be more effective in conveying much needed information and helping adults see the necessity of behavioral and lifestyle changes. The CCHIM program provided participants with access to educational information related to heart health, nutrition, physical activity, and access to exercise programs and pharmacotherapy when needed. Yet, while the team members brought this health knowledge and some experience in one-to-one clinical teaching, they had no training in adult education learning theory and facilitation methods and had limited or no experience with curriculum design. As such, aspects of team teaching and curriculum design were new and of concern to them.

The initial training and some early mentoring in MI did help the team to orient their group teaching and facilitation style. MI is a patient centered, self-management approach based on a philosophy that individuals living with a chronic disease have the knowledge, skills, judgment, and ability to be experts in the management of their own health and wellness (Edwards, Jumper-Thurman, Plested, Oetting, & Swanson, 2000). As an empowerment approach, the role of the health professional in MI is to help people understand their lifestyle problems and to increase their readiness to make positive change in their everyday lives (Brobeck, Bergh, Odencrants, & Hildingh, 2011).

Initially, CCHIM team members felt very positive about MI. It provided a clear structure for dialogue with program participants that they were interested to test out. Yet, just as was their experience with collaborative concepts, some members felt challenged to embrace MI's spirit fully because it required a commitment to a certain degree of clinical detachment from outcomes (Rollnick et al., 2008). For some, recognizing and honoring the client's autonomy and right to make choices that may not result in the desired health improvements was challenging to accept. It was at odds with their preexisting perceptions of their roles as repositories of knowledge and skill, responsible for providing helpful advice to be acted upon by clients. Learning to share power and decision-making with clients, it seems, was equally as challenging as learning to share power with the team.

Susan, the team dietician, described how in using the MI approach, she gradually came to understand the limitations of her previous "power-over" and behaviorist orientation in practice. "Power-over describes social relationships in which one party is made to do what another party wishes them to, despite their resistance, and even if it may not be in their best interests" (Laverack, 2009, p. 12). In realizing the potentially silencing effect of her previous thinking, Susan was opening herself up to a new way of thinking and working. Here, she described progressive insights that enabled her to embrace MI, and the transformative impact of this shift:

> The whole readiness thing was a big shift for me, liberating but difficult for me and probably for most of us in our practice habits. You are usually the person who has what they need, and so sensitively telling them what they need to know or do . . . so it felt like you had no control when you couldn't do that. But, gradually I realized people need time to be ready to change and I can't control that, so now I position myself differently and work first with those who are ready and try to provide encouragement to the others until they are ready.

Having shifted her thinking, Susan was able to change her expectations of participants and to adopt a more learner-centered approach, which shifts the focus of instruction from the teacher to the learner (Weimer, 2013). In the context of healthcare, this is a major shift in thinking that is recognized to be difficult for providers to manage (Castro, Van Regenmortel, Vanhaecht, Sermeus, & Van Hecke, 2016). However, where it occurs, such a shift in perspective can enable health professionals to think differently about their relationship and role with patients. It enables them to adopt a more patient-centered approach and strategies that help patients to "shed their passive role and play an active part in the decision-making process about their health and quality of life" (Castro et al., p. 1923). Patient empowerment is consistent with a population and social model of health which attempts to increase the autonomy, power, and influence of oppressed groups such as the poor, working class residents, women, and ethnic minorities.

Repeated implementations of the program provided many opportunities for ongoing reflection and dialogue leading to insights about adult and group learning, which Susan and others tested out. For example, in observing and reflecting on different learning styles, Mary described how the team progressively adapted the curriculum and instructional strategies, with positive results:

> I saw that some people wanted lots of information; for others, less was bet-
> ter... some didn't want things written down but preferred the verbal instruc-
> tion or visual aids. I could even see a difference in their learning when I
> would stop using a power point screen to just an informal circle and discuss-
> ing with them with a flip chart... I think we have moved; 80% of our stuff now
> is around a circle. You had to get a sense of what worked and what didn't with
> them, and that was always different... different from one person to another,
> and one group and community to another. If I looked at the materials I used
> now versus back then, they are completely different. I think they are better
> and the participants make them better.

Like Susan, Mary's insights suggest a significant shift in her thinking towards creating a learner-centered curriculum, where the aim is developing the learner's autonomy and independence by putting responsibility for
the learning path in their hands (Weimer, 2013).

Bill, the health motivator, reinforced that a variety of learning strategies and formats became appropriate. He described his learning of how
small group formats fostered deeper understanding and learning in the
program. He also highlighted that group work provided participants with
important social support, which helped them learn:

> You see them learning from each other, the dialogue, the interactions that
> go back and forth between them, and you realize that is where change in
> knowledge and attitudes occurs.... You can see how they can make sense of
> something together, while supporting one another, and this adds value to our
> teaching... so over time we tried to orchestrate different kinds of interactive
> activities that they could learn from and also have some fun with. I realized
> there was much more to teaching than the content we were delivering.

Patients with chronic conditions often have to adjust their aspirations,
lifestyle, and employment, and many grieve about their predicament before adjusting to it; social support can play a key role in a decision to change
health-related behaviors (Baumgartner, 2011). Baumgartner describes how
group and experiential learning activities help learners feel safe, relaxed,
and willing to take risks, especially for those who may have had negative
experiences in traditional classroom environments. Bill's comment suggests that in group activities participants were able to express themselves
and build deeper relationships with their peers and teachers. Emotion is
therefore integral to living with a chronic disease, and clinicians can play
an important part by providing outlets and opportunities for expression of
emotions (Turner & Kelly, 2000). Patsy, the team nurse, acknowledged the
emotional and spiritual dimensions of living with a chronic condition and
how the team learned to consider and respond to these dimensions in their
program facilitation:

We saw repeatedly that change was very threatening and that people have strong emotional responses to the need for change—shame, anger, fear, and defensiveness—particularly in the early stages of the program. So, we needed to be accepting of that, and we created spaces where that could be acknowledged and supported and we hoped that would lead to a readiness to change. For all of us it was a lesson on how complex reaching a point of readiness for change can be.

It is likely that Mary's learning circles and Bob's use of group work provided emotionally safe spaces where program participants were able to enhance their self-esteem and self-efficacy (Bandura, 1997). In these safe spaces, they were able to express their thoughts and ideas and share their feelings and apprehensions, and in doing so, to believe they could take control of and manage their health choices. English and Tisdell (2010) have found that it is in these emotional and spiritual dimensions of learning that adults can learn alternate and varied ways of being, and acquire new insights about themselves. In these emotionally safe learning environments, individuals are able to express emotions with security and confidence to try something new (Merriam et al., 2007).

Learning Cultural Competency

In the context of healthcare, cultural competency involves providers and organizations effectively delivering healthcare services that meet the social, cultural, and linguistic needs of patients and their loved ones. Culturally competent healthcare systems contribute to a higher quality of care and improved health outcomes and to minimizing health disparities (Zieghan & Ton, 2011). In the CCHIM, the team learned to be more culturally sensitive as they moved from one community to another with the CCHIM program. Over time they realized the extent to which individuals and communities often have distinctively different health beliefs and values around illness. As health educators they realized they needed to use multiple methods to provide health education that was culturally relevant and helpful in supporting participants in managing chronic disease (Hill, 2011, 2016). As Bill, the health motivator, suggested, over repeated implementations of the program, the team learned that familiarity with the local context and culture enhanced learning of the participants in the CCHIM program:

We learned that one size doesn't fit all. You get more of a sense of this outside the facilities. The heritage here is predominantly Acadian, Scottish, and Irish, and the demographics are very different from one community to another. . . . We learned we needed to bring context into the discussion, so people can think about health in relation to that reality, and their social circumstances. We were either quite familiar with the community or made a point to know more before we went in, and it seemed that participants appreciated and responded well when we started to talk about that.

With this knowledge, the team found that demonstrating a respect for the history and culture of communities was important in fostering participant learning in the program. As Mary, the physiotherapist remembers, people appreciated spaces where they had the opportunity to talk about health in the context of their collective culture and history. As she highlights, when this occurred, participants in the CCHIM program were able to make connections with their health, thereby increasing their health literacy:

> People in this region have a strong sense of their history and heritage and their beliefs are rooted in it [history]. Providing spaces where they could talk about this sometimes led to new insights. For example, translating hardship related to economic times in the region into an understanding of their resilience and coping skills helped people to understand the wider and historical influences on their health, and their capacity to act to improve individual and community health.

In these situations, the team was increasing their cultural knowledge and realizing that culturally responsive teaching involves including the patients' experience, worldview, and cultural references in all aspects of learning (Gay, 2010).

Learning Reflective Practices

A reflective capacity is regarded as an essential characteristic for maintaining professional competency across a lifetime of practice (Kinsella & Pitman, 2012). It is the ability to reflect on our actions so as to engage in a process of continuous learning in and from practice—what Schön (1983) referred to as "a dialogue of thinking and doing through which I become more skillful" (p. 31). Taken literally, according to Schön (1987), reflective practice refers to the process of thinking about the work we undertake and reflecting on our actions either at the time (reflection-*in*-action) or at some point after an action (reflection-*on*-action). This reflection can involve intentional, self-directed and unanticipated incidental learning. Within this reflective cycle, according to Argyris & Schön (1978), practitioners may become aware of and act on discrepancies between their beliefs (i.e., their espoused theories) and what they do (i.e., theories in action). It is a cyclical and ongoing process of knowledge construction that can be undertaken individually or in groups, and which can generate new learning in and from practice.

Yet, despite this potential, and while reflective practice is recognized as a process for continuous professional learning in and from practice experience, it is not widely practiced in the health professions (Mann, Gordon, & MacLeod, 2009). According to Boud (2010), health professionals do not engage in reflective practices for a number of reasons, including a lack of awareness and experience; they may not know how to engage in reflective practice and may not see its value within their busy practice environments. Moreover, Boud contends that reflection on tacit knowledge can be perceived by practitioners as challenging the status quo, the professional knowledge base of experienced and expert professionals. In an environment where instrumental practice knowledge is highly valued, this can create a fear of change.

Clearly, however, the CCHIM team recognized that a reflective capacity would support their ongoing learning in and from practice. Repeated implementations of the program provided an opportunity to reflect and to continually refine and adapt their approaches to foster individual and group learning successes. Susan, the dietician, described the emergence and value of these reflective dialogues, and the corresponding shift in her identity as part of a collaborative team:

> Like the participants, we learned to stretch ourselves because there was so much new learning and we knew pretty quickly that we needed to work together. So, it was about having a conversation with someone about why something didn't work, and how we might change our approaches, and then we could test something new out with the next group, and it became [a] more formalized cycle of talking and reflecting on our experience, and this enabled us to collectively solve almost any problem we came across. I feel inspired because I have a sense of my own contribution to these processes of change. Like with our groups, cooperation and trust built up in the team over time.

Her comments suggest that the team realized parallels between their own readiness for learning and change and that of their participants, from whom they were learning a great deal about teaching. Successive iterations of the program also provided continued opportunities for deeper critical reflection that enabled team members to transform long-held beliefs and values. As their accounts suggest, despite the emotional challenges and discomfort involved with change, critically reflective dialogues—both individual and collective—helped them locate the ongoing motivation required to navigate the significant shifts in identity from autonomous to interdependent professional (Billett & Somerville, 2004; Boud, 2010).

This inclination towards reflective and critically reflective practices for the purpose of sharing knowledge and creating meaning highlights the creation of a learning community within the CCHIM team. Using the definition of Wenger-Trayner et al. (2015), the CCHIM team can be seen as a community of practice (CoP); a group of professionals engaged in collective learning. Although not always formalized, the team used reflective practices to improve their work and engaged in critically reflective dialogues to develop shared norms and values and to assume and act from their collective knowledge base and sense of shared responsibility. Such critically reflective dialogues, according to Servage (2008), function to examine practice "with others as trusted members of a community, and always against the standards of excellence defined by a shared vision" (p. 65). Servage found that critically reflective dialogues, to the extent that they engage professionals in deep learning of this nature, offer significant potential as sites for transformative learning.

SIGNIFICANCE AND IMPLICATIONS

This case study reinforces scholarly thinking that experiences we have in work-based practice settings are resources for genuine learning, learning which lives on and has implications for future practice experiences (Kinsella & Pitman, 2012). The CCHIM experience highlights that informal learning can support the development of adaptive capacities as professionals navigate transitions in response to new practice demands. With limited formal or nonformal training in MI and group process or adult learning methods, the CCHIM team navigated informal learning (i.e., incidental, self-directed, and reflective learning) that helped them to adapt to a new setting to progressively build on their relationships and develop new knowledge and skills. In a cyclical process of ongoing reflective and constructivist learning and dialogue, the team members were able to make meaning of their experience and construct new knowledge to improve their practice as they learned what worked and did not work related to interprofessional care, MI, and aspects of teaching and curriculum planning.

The CCHIM experience also highlights significant professional learning that was transformative. Through their interactions in day-to-day practice and critically reflective dialogue, team members developed strong and supportive interprofessional relationships. Dialogue, according to Shapiro et al. (2012), is the essential medium "for critical reflection to be put into action, where experience is reflected on, assumptions and beliefs are questioned, and habits of mind are ultimately transformed" (p. 355). Trust in these relationships contributed to the CCHIM team's ability to progressively overcome uncertainty and complexity, as well as to value conflicts and to transform their professional identities from autonomous to interdependent professionals. According to Taylor (2007), developing a sense of trust in the process of transformative learning allows individuals to navigate discomfort while on the edge of knowing, in the process of gaining new insights and understandings (p. 187). Over the course of their time and by reflecting on their work together, team members such as Susan (dietician) gradually became aware of the limitations of their previous frames of references and habits of mind, and they were able to let go of long-held professional values and assumptions assimilated through socialization into their individual professions. These new insights and shifts in identity included progressively understanding the nature of shared decision-making, and what it means to give up professional power as the provider in order to enable patients to assume more responsibility for their own well-being. The strong and supportive interprofessional relationships that developed among team members also contributed to the team's ability to be creative and to innovate. As the chapter reveals, ongoing dialogue and reflective capacity enabled progressive new insights and action related to interprofessionality, MI, and culturally responsive teaching, including strategies to enhance health literacy.

This study provides insights on how informal learning occurs in unstructured situations in professional practice and through reflection and collegial team dialogue. As the CCHIM experience reveals, progressive informal learning can provide a significant and powerful opportunity for enhancing learning related to professional identity formation, competency development, and, potentially, transformative learning. However, barriers to informal learning and reflection in this context also bear investigation, given that informal learning is clearly linked to transformation and professional development. For example, in the CCHIM experience, time and shared experiences were contributing factors to reflective capacity and transformative learning. The opportunity for a dedicated interprofessional team to work through repeated iterations of the same program over 6 years afforded much time for reflection, dialogue, collective knowing, and transformative learning to occur. In other health settings, a rushed environment and the heavy demands of clinical work might be impediments to dialogue, critical reflection and transformative learning. Healthcare agencies and districts might well put resources into strengthening the opportunity for such learning through providing time for group discussion and exchange and CPE related to reflective learning. Although this study did not explore the possibilities for rewarding this type of learning in the workplace, it might be worth examining in the future.

REFERENCES

Argyris, C., & Schön, D. (1978). *Organizational learning: A theory of action perspective.* Reading, MA: Addison Wesley.

Bandura, A. (1997). Self-efficacy and health behaviour. In A. Baum, S. Newman, J. Wienman, R. West, & C. McManus (Eds.), *Cambridge handbook of psychology, health and medicine* (pp. 160–162). Cambridge, England: Cambridge University Press.

Baumgartner, L. (2011). The role of adult learning in coping with chronic illness. *New Directions for Adult and Continuing Education, 2011*(130), 1–17. https://doi.org/10.1002/ace.297

Berger, J. G. (2004). Dancing on the threshold of meaning: Recognizing and understanding the growing edge. *Journal of Transformative Education, 2*(4), 336–351. https://doi.org/10.1177/1541344604267697

Billett, S. (2009). Personal epistemologies, work and learning. *Educational Research Review, 4*(3), 210–219.

Billett, S., & Somerville, M. (2004). Transformations at work: Identity and learning. *Studies in Continuing Education, 26*(2), 309–326.

Bolton, G. (2014). *Reflective practice: Writing and professional development* (4th ed.). London, England: SAGE.

Boud, D. (2010). Relocating reflection in the context of practice. In H. Bradbury, N. Frost, & M. Zukas (Eds.), *Beyond reflective practice: New approaches to professional lifelong learning* (pp. 25–37). New York, NY: Routledge.

Boud, D., & Hagar, P. (2012). Rethinking continuing professional development through changing metaphors and location in professional practices. *Studies in Continuing Education, 34*(1), 17–30. https://doi.org/10.1080/0158037X.2011.608656

Brobeck, E., Bergh, H., Odencrants, S., & Hildingh, C. (2011). Primary healthcare nurses' experiences with motivational interviewing in health promotion practice. *Journal of Clinical Nursing, 20*(23–24), 3322–3330. https://doi.org/10.1111/j.1365-2702.2011.03874

Bryan, R., Kreuter, M., & Brownson, R. (2009). Integrating adult learning principles into training for public health practice. *Health Promotion Practice, 10*(4), 557–563.

Castro, E. M., Van Regenmortel, T., Vanhaecht, K., Sermeus, W., & Van Hecke, A. (2016). Patient empowerment, patient participation and patient-centeredness in hospital care: A concept analysis based on a literature review. *Patient Education and Counseling, 99*(12), 1923–1939. https://doi.org/10.1016/j.pec.2016.07.026

Chatalasingh, C., & Reeves, S. (2014). Leading team learning: What makes interprofessional teams learn to work well together. *Journal of Interprofessional Care, 28*(6), 513–518. https://doi.org/10.3109/13561820.2014.900001

Choy, S. (2009). Transformative learning in the workplace. *Journal of Transformative Education, 7*(1), 65–84. https://doi.org/10.1177/1541344609334720

Coady, M. (2013). Adult health learning and transformation: A case study of a Canadian community-based health education program. *Adult Education Quarterly, 63*(4), 321–337. https://doi.org/10.1177/0741713612471419

Coady, M. (2015). From Houle to Dirkx: Continuing professional education (CPE). A critical "state of the field" review. *Canadian Journal for Studies in Adult Education, 27*(3), 27–40.

Coady, M. (Ed.). (2016). Contexts, practices, and challenges: Critical insights from continuing professional education (CPE). *New Directions for Adult and Continuing Education, 2016*(151). San Francisco, CA: Jossey-Bass.

Colley, H., Hodkinson, P., & Malcolm, J. (2003). *Informality and formality in learning: A report for the Learning and Skills Research Centre.* London, England: Learning and Skills Research Centre. Retrieved from https://core.ac.uk/download/pdf/91282.pdf

Cranton, P. (2006). *Understanding and promoting transformative learning: A guide for educators of adults* (2nd ed.). San Francisco, CA: Jossey-Bass.

Cranton, P., & King, K. P. (2003). Transformative learning as a professional development goal. *New Directions for Adult and Continuing Education, 2003*(98), 31–38. https://doi.org/10.1002/ace.97

Cross, R., & Parker, A. (2004). *The hidden power of social networks: Understanding how work really gets done in organizations.* Boston, MA: Harvard University Press.

Crowley, S. (Ed.). (2014). *Challenging professional learning.* London, England: Routledge.

Curran, V. (2010). *Interprofessional education for collaborative patient-centred practice: Research synthesis paper.* Ottawa, Canada: Health Canada. Retrieved from https://pdfs.semanticscholar.org/3fb5/206cc62ef10868a1fdca047420b1220 66bc3.pdf

Daley, B. (2006). Aligning health promotion and adult education for healthier communities. In S. Merriam, B. Courtenay, & R. Cervero (Eds.), *Global issues and adult education: Perspectives from Latin America, Southern Africa, and the United States* (pp. 231–242). San Francisco, CA: Jossey-Bass.

Daley, B. J., & Cervero, R. M. (2016). Learning as the basis for continuing professional education. *New Directions for Adult and Continuing Education,* Fall(151), 19–29. https://doi.org/10.1002/ace.20192

Davies, C. (2000). Getting health professionals to work together. *British Medical Journal, 320*(7241), 1021–1022.

de Groot, E., Endedijk, M., Jaarsma, D. C., Simons, P. R., & van Beukelen, P. (2014). Critically reflective dialogues in learning communities of professionals. *Studies in Continuing Education, 36*(1), 15–37. https://doi.org/10.1080/015803 7X.2013.779240

deLaat, M., & Schreurs, B. (2013). Visual informal professional development networks: Building a case for learning analytics in the workplace. *American Behavioral Scientist, 57*(10), 1421–1438.

Dirkx, J. (2008). Care of the self: Mythopoetic dimensions of professional preparation and development. In T. Leonard & P. Willis (Eds.), *Pedagogies of the imagination: Mythopoetic curriculum in educational practice* (pp. 65–83). New York, NY: Springer.

Dirkx, J., Gilley, J. W., & Maycunich-Gilley, A. (2004). Change theory in CPE and HRD: Toward a holistic view of learning and change in work. *Advances in Developing Human Resources, 6*(1), 35–51. https://doi.org/10.1177/1523422303260825

Edwards, R., Jumper-Thurman, P., Plested, B., Oetting, E., & Swanson, L. (2000). Community readiness for change. *Journal of Community Psychology, 28*(3), 291–307.

English, L. M., & Tisdell, E. J. (2010). Spirituality and adult education. In C. Kasworm, A. Rose, & J. Ross-Gordon (Eds.), *Handbook of adult and continuing education* (pp. 285–293). Thousand Oaks, CA: SAGE

Epstein, R. M., & Street, R. L. (2011). The values and value of patient-centered care. *Annals of Family Medicine, 9*(2), 100–103. https://doi.org/10.1370/afm.1239

Eraut, M. (2004). Informal learning in the workplace. *Studies in Continuing Education, 26*(2), 247–273. https://doi.org/10.1080/158037042000225245

Eraut, M. (2007). Learning from others in the workplace. *Oxford Review of Education, 33*(4), 403–422.

Fenwick, T., & Nerland, M. (Eds.). (2014). *Reconceptualising professional learning: Sociomaterial knowledge, practices and responsibilities.* New York, NY: Routledge.

Freeth, D., Hammick, M., Reeves, S., Koppel, I., & Barr, H. (2005). *Effective interprofessional education: Development, delivery and evaluation.* Oxford, England: Blackwell.

Gay, G. (2010). *Culturally responsive teaching: Theory, research and practice* (2nd ed.). New York, NY: Teachers College Press.

Gilbert, J. (2005). Interprofessional education for collaborative, patient-centred practice. *Nursing Leadership, 18*(2), 32–38.

Hill, L. (Ed.). (2011). Adult education for health and wellness. *New Directions for Adult & Continuing Education, 2011*(130). https://doi.org/10.1002/ace.297

Hill, L. (2016). Interactive influences on health and adult education. *New Directions for Adult & Continuing Education, 2016*(149), 41–51. https://doi.org/10.1002/ace.20175

Jones, M., & Charteris, J. (2017). Transformative professional learning: An ecological approach to agency through critical reflection. *Reflective Practice, 18*(4), 496–513. https://doi.org/10.1080/14623943.2017.1307729

Kinsella, E., & Pitman, A. (Eds.). (2012). *Phronesis as professional knowledge: Practice wisdom in the professions.* Rotterdam, Netherlands: Sense.

Knox, A. (2016). *Improving professional learning: Twelve strategies to enhance performance.* Sterling, VA: Stylus.

Laverack, G. (2009). *Public health: Power, empowerment and professional practice.* New York, NY: Palgrave.

Lewy, L. (2010). The complexities of interprofessional learning/working: Has the agenda lost its way? *Health Education Journal, 69*(1), 4–12.

Livingstone, D. W. (2005). Expanding conceptions of work and learning: Research and policy implications. In K. Leithwood, D. W. Livingstone, A. Cumming, N. Bascia, & A. Datnow (Eds.), *International handbook of educational policy* (pp. 977–996). New York, NY: Kluwer.

Mann, K., Gordon, J., & MacLeod, A. (2009). Reflection and reflective practice in health professions education: A systematic review. *Advances in Health Science Education, 14*(4), 595–621. https://doi.org/10.1007/s10459-007-9090-2

Maharajan, M. K., Rajiah, K., Khoo, S. P., Chellappan, D. K., De Alwis, R., & Chui, H. C., . . . Lau, S. Y. (2017). Attitudes and readiness of students of healthcare professions towards interprofessional learning. *PLoS ONE, 12*(1), e0168863. https://doi.org/10.1371/journal.pone.0168863

McNair, R., Brown, R., Stone, N., & Sims, J. (2001). Rural interprofessional education: Promoting teamwork in primary health care education and practice. *Australian Journal of Rural Health, 9*(suppl 1), S19–S26.

Merriam, S. B., & Tisdell, E. J. (2016). *Qualitative research: A guide to design and implementation* (4th ed.). San Francisco, CA: Jossey-Bass.

Merriam, S., Caffarella, R., & Baumgartner, L. (2007). *Learning in adulthood: A comprehensive guide* (3rd ed.). San Francisco, CA: Jossey-Bass.

Mezirow, J. (2009). Transformative learning theory. In J. Mezirow & E. Taylor (Eds.), *Transformative learning in practice: Insights from community, workplace, and higher education* (pp. 18–33). San Francisco, CA: Jossey-Bass.

Milligan, C., Littlejohn, A., & Margaryan, A. (2014). Workplace learning in informal networks. *Journal of Interactive Media in Education, 2014*(1), p. Art.6. https://doi.org/10.5334/2014-06

Nancarrow, S., Booth, A., Aris, S., Smith, T., Enderby, P., & Roots, A. (2013). Ten principles of good interdisciplinary teamwork. *Human Resources for Health, 11*(19). Retrieved from https://human-resources-health.biomedcentral.com/track/pdf/10.1186/1478-4491-11-19

Nisbet, G., Lincoln, M., & Dunn, S. (2013). Informal professional learning: An untapped opportunity for learning and change within the workplace. *Journal of Interprofessional Care, 27*(6), 469–475.

O'Sullivan, E., Morrell, A., & O'Connor, M. (2002). *Expanding the boundaries of transformative learning: Essays on theory and praxis.* New York, NY: Palgrave.

Reich, A., Rooney, D., & Boud, D. (2014). Dilemmas in continuing professional learning: Learning inscribed in frameworks or elicited from practice. *Studies in Continuing Education, 37*(2), 131–141. https://doi.org/10.1080/0158037X.2015.1022717

Rollnick, S., Miller, W. R., & Butler, C. (2008). *Motivational interviewing in health care: Helping patients change behaviour.* New York, NY: Guilford Press.

Servage, L. (2008). Critical and transformative practices in professional learning. *Teacher Education Quarterly, 35*(1), 63–77.

Schön, D. A. (1983). *The reflective practitioner: How professionals think in action.* New York, NY: Routledge.

Schön, D. A. (1987). *Educating the reflective practitioner: Toward a new design for teaching and learning in the professions.* San Francisco, CA: Jossey-Bass.

Shapiro, S. A., Wasserman, I. L., & Gallegos, V. G. (2012). Group work and dialogue: Spaces and processes for transformative learning in relationships. In E. W. Taylor & P. Cranton (Eds.), *The handbook of transformative learning* (pp. 355–373). San Francisco, CA: Jossey-Bass.

Silver, I. L., & Leslie, K. (2009). Faculty development for continuing interprofessional education and collaborative practice. *Journal of Continuing Education in the Health Professions, 29*(3), 172–177.

Stuttaford, M., & Coe, C. (2007). The "learning" component of participatory learning and action in health research: Reflections from a local sure start evaluation. *Qualitative Health Research, 17*(10), 1351–1360. https://doi.org/10.1177/1049732307306965

Taylor, E. (2007). An update of transformative learning theory: A critical review of the empirical research (1999–2005). *International Journal of Lifelong Education, 26*(2), 173–191.

Taylor, E. (2009). Fostering transformative learning. In J. Mezirow & E. Taylor (Eds.), *Transformative learning in practice: Insights from community, workplace, and higher education* (pp. 3–18). San Francisco, CA: Jossey-Bass.

Taylor, E. W., & Snyder, M. J. (2012). A critical review of research on transformative learning theory, 2006–2010. In E. W. Taylor & P. Cranton (Eds.), *The handbook of transformative learning* (pp. 37–56). San Francisco, CA: Jossey-Bass.

Thompson, N., & Pascal, J. (2012). Developing critically reflective practice. *Reflective Practice, 13*(2), 311–325. https://doi.org/10.1080/14623943.2012.657795

Turner, J., & Kelly, B. (2000). Emotional dimensions of chronic disease. *Western Journal of Medicine, 17*(2), 124–138.

Watkins, K. E., Marsick, V. J., & Faller, P. G. (2012). Transformative learning in the workplace: Leading learning for self and organizational change. In E. W. Taylor & P. Cranton (Eds.), *The handbook of transformative learning* (pp. 373–388). San Francisco, CA: Jossey-Bass.

Webster-Wright, A. (2009). Reframing professional development through understanding authentic professional learning. *Review of Educational Research, 79*(2), 702–739. https://doi.org/10.3102/0034654308330970

Webster-Wright, A. (2010). *Authentic professional learning: Making a difference through learning at work.* London, England: Springer.

Weimer, M. (2013). *Learner-centered teaching: Five key changes to practice* (2nd ed.). San Francisco, CA: Jossey-Bass.

Wenger-Trayner, E., Fenton-O'Creevy, M., Hutchinson, S., Kubiak, C., & Wenger-Trayner, B. (Eds.). (2015). *Learning in landscapes of practice: Boundaries, identity and knowledgeability in practice-based learning.* New York, NY: Routledge.

Wilkinson, R., & Marmot, M. (2003). *Social determinants of health: The solid facts.* Geneva, Switzerland: World Health Organization. Retrieved from http://www.euro.who.int/__data/assets/pdf_file/0005/98438/e81384.pdf

Wilson, A., & Cervero, R. (2014). Continuing professional education in the United States: A strategic analysis of current and future directions. In B. Kapplinger & S. Robak (Eds.), *Changing configurations of adult education in transitional times: International perspectives in different countries* (pp. 211–222). New York, NY: Peter Lang.

Zeighan, L., & Ton, H. (2011). Adult educators and cultural competence within health care systems: Change at the individual and structural levels. *New Directions for Adult & Continuing Education, 2011*(130), 55–64. https://doi.org/10.1002/ace.410

ABOUT THE EDITORS

Teresa (Terry) J. Carter, MA, EdD, is professor emerita of Virginia Commonwealth University (VCU) in Richmond, Virginia. Dr. Carter spent 6 years as associate dean of Professional Instruction and Faculty Development in the School of Medicine at VCU prior to her retirement in 2018, and served as director of TiME (Teaching in Medical Education), a graduate certificate program for VCU physicians and faculty in the Health Sciences. From 2005 until 2012, she directed the MEd in adult learning program and mentored PhD students studying adult learning in the School of Education. Dr. Carter holds a master's degree in education and human development and a doctorate in human and organizational learning, both from The George Washington University. Her scholarly publications and presentations have emphasized transformative learning among professionals in the workplace, reflective practice, mentoring, and the scholarship of teaching and learning. She has professional experience in whole system interventions, organization development practice, and large and small group teaching methods. In 2009, she received the student-nominated Charles P. Ruch Award for Excellence in Teaching.

Carrie J. Boden, PhD, is professor of Occupational, Workforce, and Leadership Studies at Texas State University. Her research is primarily focused in the areas of teaching and learning strategies, mentoring, and transformative learning. She is the founding editor of the Adult Higher Education Alliance book series and has presented papers in over 30 states and foreign countries and recently published articles in journals such as *International Journal of Adult Vocational Education and Technology*, *Journal of Nutrition Education and*

Transformative Learning in Healthcare and Helping Professions Education, pages 345–346
Copyright © 2019 by Information Age Publishing
All rights of reproduction in any form reserved.

Behavior, and *The Reference Librarian.* Her awards include Alpha Chi Favorite Professor, Texas State University Award for Excellence in Online Teaching, and Distinguished Teaching Fellowship from the Academy of Teaching and Learning Excellence. Dr. Boden serves as a director on the board for the Adult Higher Education Alliance and series editor for Adult Learning in Professional, Organizational, and Community Settings.

Kathy Peno, PhD, is professor of adult education at the University of Rhode Island. She prepares professional adult educators who teach in adult literacy, the military, higher education, corporations, and the healthcare fields. Her scholarship focuses on professional learning and skill development from novice to expert, with a focus on mentoring, in particular. She has written, consulted and presented extensively on workforce development, professional development and mentoring as a vehicle for continuous performance improvement in organizations. A former treasurer and board member of AAACE, she now serves as president of the Adult Higher Education Alliance (AHEA) and is treasurer/executive committee member of the coalition of lifelong learning organizations (COLLO). She holds a master's and PhD in adult learning and human resource development from the University of Connecticut.

ABOUT THE CONTRIBUTORS

Bryan Adkins, MBM, EdD, is the CEO of Denison Consulting, a global research, diagnostic, and organizational development firm known for linking organizational culture and leadership practices to business performance. In addition to providing leadership to the firm, he provides consulting support to leaders and organizations from across the globe. His professional background includes leadership positions within the manufacturing, professional, and not-for-profit sectors. Dr. Adkins holds a master's degree in business management from Penn State University and received his doctorate in human and organizational learning from The George Washington University. He presents to a variety of organizations including The British Academy of Management, The Academy of Management, and Society for Industrial & Organizational Psychologists (SIOP). His work has been published in journals and books including *The Journal of Organizational Behavior, Advances in Global Leadership*, and *Corporate Learning: Proven and Practical Guidelines for Building a Sustainable Learning Strategy* (Wiley, 2005).

Scott T. Armistead, MD, Diploma of International Medicine and Public Health (DIMPH), is an assistant professor of Family Medicine and Population Health at Virginia Commonwealth University (VCU). He also serves as the Richmond area director for the Christian Medical and Dental Association (CMDA). Prior to working at VCU, Dr. Armistead served with his family at Bach Christian Hospital in northern Pakistan from 1999–2015. He enjoys mentoring students at VCU interested in careers in underserved populations and international mission, and started VCU's International Medical Mission Elective in 2017. Dr. Armistead has been a speaker for The Insti-

Transformative Learning in Healthcare and Helping Professions Education, pages 347–357
Copyright © 2019 by Information Age Publishing

tute for International Medicine, and was honored with INMED's Comninellis Award for Compassionate Medical Care. He has recently published a book review on a new biography of Dr. Albert Schweitzer. Dr. Armistead is a 2018 graduate of the VCU Teaching in Medical Education Faculty Fellows program. He received VCU's Practice of Clinical Medicine Course Best Teacher Award for 2017–2018.

Amy D. Benton, PhD, LCSW, is an associate professor of social work at Texas State University. She received a PhD in social welfare from University of California, Berkeley, and a Master of Science in social work from the University of Texas at Austin. Prior to earning her doctorate, Dr. Benton worked for 10 years in the nonprofit sector. Her primary areas of interest are management and administration of child welfare and human service agencies, worker support, development, and retention, and policy. Dr. Benton is currently principal investigator of the Behavioral Health Workforce Education & Training project in the School of Social Work at Texas State, providing training and support to advanced MSW students in order to increase the number of social workers prepared to provide trauma-informed, culturally sensitive, evidence-based behavioral health prevention and intervention practices in integrated care settings.

Ellen L. Brock, MD, MPH, Professor emeritus in the Department of Obstetrics and Gynecology at Virginia Commonwealth University, was appointed as the first medical director for the VCU Center for Human Simulation and Patient Safety in 2008. Dr. Brock received the MD degree from the Medical University of South Carolina and completed residency training in obstetrics and gynecology at Virginia Commonwealth University. She received the MPH degree with a special interest in international health from VCU, and has worked internationally in healthcare delivery and education. From 1987 until 2016, Dr. Brock served with distinction as faculty in the Department of Obstetrics and Gynecology, where she established a record of excellence in patient care, teaching, and service.

Christopher K. Brown Jr., MS, is a current medical student at the Virginia Commonwealth University (VCU) School of Medicine in Richmond, Virginia. Prior to attending medical school in 2016, Mr. Brown studied integrated science and technology, concentrating in environmental management at James Madison University. He worked as a teaching fellow at a Pre-K–12 grade school in Richmond, Virginia, and completed a Master of Science degree in biomedical sciences at Eastern Virginia Medical School. His volunteer efforts prior to and during medical school have focused on medically underserved communities, in particular, the homeless population. He was selected for the International, Inner City, Rural Preceptorship, a longitudinal program for medical students at VCU who hold a commitment to working with underserved communities. His research regarding attitudinal barriers to health insurance enrollment among vulnerable populations was presented at the first annual VCU Medical Education Symposium in 2017, for which he received the Best Trainee Presentation award. He continues to work towards a career that addresses health disparities faced by vulnerable populations.

Ashley Castleberry, PharmD, MEd, is an associate professor at the University of Texas at Austin College of Pharmacy in Austin, Texas. Prior to this appointment in 2018, Dr. Castleberry spent 6 years as an assistant professor and director of assessment at the University of Arkansas for Medical Science (UAMS) College of Pharmacy in Little Rock, Arkansas. After completing her Doctor of Pharmacy degree from UAMS, she obtained a master's in higher education for health professions teaching and learning from the University of Arkansas at Little Rock. Her scholarly publications and presentations focus on metacognition, student success, interprofessional education, assessment, and objective structured clinical examinations. She has extensive training and experience in large and small group facilitation and is the recipient of several awards for teaching excellence.

Maureen Coady, MAdEd, PhD, is an associate professor and chair of the Department of Adult Education at Saint Francis Xavier University (StFX) in Antigonish, Nova Scotia, Canada. Dr. Coady's research and scholarship focuses on the links between health and learning, and the role adult education and community development can play in enabling improved individual and community health. Her more recent work focuses on continuing professional education and learning (CPE). She is particularly interested in how health professionals can work in more empowering ways with people. She has been published in *Adult Education Quarterly* and *Canadian Journal for the Study of Adult Education* and various texts that focus on health education and learning in the professions. Most recently, in 2016, she edited a special edition of *New Directions for Adult and Continuing Education* in which she focused on continuing professional education, not only for health professionals, but for all those engaged in professional occupations.

Deborah J. DeWaay, MD, FACP, is associate dean of Undergraduate Medical Education and associate professor of internal medicine at the University of South Florida Morsani College of Medicine. She completed her undergraduate degree from Grinnell College in 1998, and her MD from the University of Iowa. She completed a residency and chief year in internal medicine at the Medical University of South Carolina (MUSC). Her specialty is general internal medicine with a focus in hospital medicine. She has served as the associate vice-chair of education for the Department of Medicine at MUSC. Dr. DeWaay has won numerous teaching awards, including the MUSC Department of Medicine Excellence in Teaching Award and the Leonard Tow Humanism in Medicine Award. She is a member of the Gold Humanism in Medicine and Alpha Omega Alpha Honor Medical Societies. Since 2016, she has served as the associate dean for undergraduate medical education at USF. In this role, Dr. DeWaay has been focusing on streamlining the assessment and evaluation system and creating a state of the art curriculum map.

Mary L. Falk, MSN, RN, CCRN, is a clinical instructor at Virginia Commonwealth University (VCU) School of Nursing and a Clinician III Registered Nurse at VCU Health System in Richmond, Virginia. Her background in nursing includes extensive clinical experience with the cardiothoracic and vascular surgery patient populations in both the progressive and critical care environments, and she has recently engaged in clinical practice as an in-patient palliative care nurse. As a nurse educator, she works with undergraduate baccalaureate nursing students across the spectrum of the curriculum from the fundamentals level to the critical care level, with a heavy focus in the clinical environment of these courses. Her scholarly presentations and publications focus on teaching and learning, particularly emphasizing the importance of developing empathy in nursing students. Ms. Falk holds a master's degree in nursing from the University of Virginia. She has been recognized as the recipient of multiple awards for excellence in teaching and clinical practice.

Doug Franzen, MD, MEd, is an assistant professor at the University of Washington in Seattle, Washington. Dr. Franzen has been the associate residency director for the Emergency Medicine residency program at the University of Washington since 2013. Prior to that, he served as the emergency medicine clerkship director and as an assistant dean at Virginia Commonwealth University School of Medicine in Richmond, Virginia. He practices clinical emergency medicine and is actively involved in teaching and advising medical students and residents. He holds a master's degree in education from the Virginia Commonwealth University School of Education. Dr. Franzen's scholarly work focuses on the assessment of medical students and residents. He has also contributed a range of educational materials including books, websites, and online videos on a wide variety of topics in Emergency Medicine.

Frank A. Fulco, MD, RPh, is a graduate of the West Virginia University Schools of Pharmacy and Medicine. Dr. Fulco trained in Virginia Commonwealth University's combined internal medicine and pediatrics residency program and served as chief medical resident in 2000–2001. He joined the faculty as an assistant professor in internal medicine within VCU's Department of Internal Medicine, and currently serves as an associate program director, site director, and academic hospitalist at the Hunter Holmes Mc-Guire Veterans' Affairs Medical Center in Richmond, VA. Dr. Fulco has received numerous awards for teaching excellence in the Department of Internal Medicine, including the prestigious Irby-James Award for Excellence in Clinical Teaching in 2011. He is also a recent graduate of the graduate certificate program in medical education from the School of Education at Virginia Commonwealth University.

Adam M. Garber, MD, is an assistant professor of internal medicine and academic hospitalist at Virginia Commonwealth University. He is the acting internship course director for fourth-year medical students across the School of Medicine and also within the Department of Internal Medicine at VCU. Dr. Garber received his undergraduate degree from the University of Virginia, graduated from the Virginia Commonwealth University School of Medicine in 2010, and completed his residency at Duke University Medical Center. Dr. Garber also teaches first and second year medical students in the Principles of Clinical Medicine course, serves as a medical student advisor, and is a resident mentor in the Hospitalist Medicine program at VCU.

Marsha R. Griffin, MD, FAAP, is professor of pediatrics and director of the Community for Children program at the University of Texas Rio Grande Valley School of Medicine on the Texas/Mexico border. In response to the extreme poverty and social injustices on the border, Dr. Griffin has spent the last 10 years preparing physicians-in-training to recognize and address social injustices. Within the context of fighting for others, she finds that young physicians are themselves transformed. In 2018, Dr. Griffin received the American Academy of Pediatrics' highest award, the Clifford G. Grulee Award, for her advocacy for *all* children and for her outstanding service to the American Academy of Pediatrics. Prior to her medical education at the University of Texas Health Science Center at San Antonio (UTHSCSA) and pediatric residency training at Baylor/Texas Children's Hospital and UTHSCSA, she produced documentary films for marginalized teens and developed housing services for street children, Somalian refugees, former addicts, alcoholics, and the homeless in Minnesota. She also studied social justice issues at United Theological Seminary in New Brighton, Minnesota.

Reena H. Hemrajani, MD, is an associate professor of medicine at Emory University in Atlanta, Georgia. She serves as an assistant division director for faculty development for the division of hospital medicine, and in this role, she coordinates and supports the formal mentorship program in the division. She also serves as an associate program director for Emory's internal medicine residency program. Prior to this, she was on faculty at Virginia Commonwealth University (VCU) from 2013 through 2017 as an associate program director overseeing core faculty in their development as educators and focusing on evaluation and assessment of resident performance. She has completed additional training through the Stanford Faculty Development Program in 2015 and obtained a graduate certificate in the Teaching in Medical Education program in 2017. Dr. Hemrajani has a passion for inpatient clinical medicine, graduate medical education, and faculty development.

Charity Johansson, PT, PhD, is a professor of physical therapy in the School of Health Sciences at Elon University in Elon, North Carolina. She earned her master's degree in physical therapy from Stanford University and her doctorate in adult and higher education from the University of North Carolina at Chapel Hill. Dr. Johansson has received multiple awards for her teaching and scholarship. A board-certified clinical specialist in geriatrics, she also maintains a small private clinical and coaching practice. In addition to her coauthored books, *Mobility in Context: Principles of Patient Care Skills* (F. A. Davis, 2012) and *Transforming Students: Fulfilling the Promise of Higher Education* (Johns Hopkins University Press, 2014), Dr. Johansson's scholarly work includes numerous national and international presentations, book chapters, and peer-reviewed articles on geriatrics, psychosocial aspects of healthcare, and education.

Cameron Kiosoglous, PhD, has coached on eleven U.S. rowing national teams and is a four-time U.S. Olympic coach at the 2004, 2008, 2012, and 2016 Olympic Games. Cam began his coaching in Canberra, Australia in 1991 and moved to the United States in 2000. He completed his PhD in adult education at Virginia Tech with a focus on sports coaching development in 2013. He has presented at a variety of national and international conferences and published in journals in the area of sports coaching development and performance improvement. He is currently an adjunct professor at Drexel University in the School of Education.

Bennett B. Lee, MD, MPH, is an associate professor in the Division of General Internal Medicine within the Department of Internal Medicine at Virginia Commonwealth University. Dr. Lee is a 1988 graduate of Williams College and a 1994 graduate of the School of Medicine at Virginia Commonwealth University. In 2000, he earned a master's degree in public health from Boston University, where he also completed fellowship training in general and preventive medicine in 2001. He served as an associate residency program director, and his research interests include medical education. Currently, Dr. Lee directs the third-year medical student clerkship in Ambulatory Care in the VCU School of Medicine.

Judith E. Livingston, PhD, MCHES, is assistant professor, Department of Pediatrics, Long School of Medicine, UT Health San Antonio (UTHSA). In 2017, she received her PhD in adult, professional, and community education from Texas State University to augment her knowledge and 35 years of experience in educational programming, grant-writing, and project management in academic medicine, public health, and nonprofit sectors. Dr. Livingston has a master's degree in health education and is a master certified health education specialist (MCHES). She has been a member of the UTHSA faculty since 2008. For the past decade, she has been integral to the work of Community for Children, a social justice education program on the Texas/Mexico border for physicians-in-training. Prior to coming to UTH-SA, she served as director, Texas Department of Health Newborn Screening Follow-up program; director, Science and Preventive Medicine Department/Texas Medical Association; director of education/Harris County Medical Society; and public health educator for the Harris County Health Department. The overarching theme of her career has been promoting the health of children, families, and communities through education.

Elaine M. Silva Mangiante, PhD, is an assistant professor of teacher education at Salve Regina University in Newport, RI. Dr. Silva Mangiante holds a doctorate degree in science education from the University of Rhode Island/Rhode Island College. Formerly, she served as a professional development specialist with The Education Alliance at Brown University for educational reform in high-poverty districts, as well as a science specialist and mathematics curriculum coordinator for a K–8 school where she mentored early career teachers. Currently, as a university teacher educator, Dr. Silva Mangiante's specific research interests include examining how teachers working in high-poverty school districts plan for reform-based science education and create a collaborative climate for elementary students' scientific discourse and engineering problem-solving. Her scholarly publications and presentations focus on effective teaching practices for science and engineering design education in urban schools, elementary science pedagogy for critical thinking, elementary students' negotiation of engineering design ideas, purposeful ongoing mentoring, and teacher development from novice to expert. Though her work, she has received several awards for both her teaching and research.

Scott C. Matherly, MD, is assistant professor of gastroenterology in the Department of Internal Medicine at Virginia Commonwealth University (VCU) where he teaches in the Gastroenterology and Metabolism course for second-year medical students. Dr. Matherly is a 2017 graduate of the teaching in medical education graduate certificate program for faculty in the School of Medicine at VCU. Since 2014, he has been the recipient of numerous teaching awards for his innovative work with students, including the development of process oriented guided inquiry learning (POGIL) modules and collaborative methods of team-based learning instruction. Dr. Matherly graduated from the University of South Carolina School of Medicine and completed his residency training at Johns Hopkins University in Baltimore, Maryland before fellowship training at VCU. His specialties include gastroenterology, hepatology, and nutrition, with clinical expertise in end-stage liver disease, cirrhosis, hepatocellular cancer, and liver transportation.

Kelly E. McCarthy, MBA, PhD is the assistant director of assessment at the University of South Florida Morsani College of Medicine in Tampa, Florida. Dr. McCarthy has spent the last decade of her career working in secondary and postsecondary education. In her current role, she works collaboratively with basic science and clinical faculty to develop valid and reliable multiple-choice examinations. She also serves as an adjunct professor for the University of South Florida College of Education. Dr. McCarthy's teaching contributions have been recognized both regionally and nationally; she was awarded Teacher of the Year in 2013 and was a Noyce Master Teacher Fellow nominee in 2014. Dr. McCarthy holds a master's degree in business administration and a doctorate degree in curriculum and instruction from the University of South Florida. Her research interests include professional development, mentoring, and learner autonomy.

Emily R. Miller, Doctor of Osteopathy (DO), is a clinical assistant professor of pediatrics in the Section of Pediatric Endocrinology and Diabetes at Michigan State University/Helen Devos Children's Hospital. Dr. Miller is a 2010 graduate of the Ohio University College of Osteopathic Medicine in Athens, Ohio. She completed her residency training in general pediatrics at the University of Tennessee in 2013 prior to completing her fellowship training in Pediatric Endocrinology and Diabetes at Virginia Commonwealth University in 2016. Dr. Miller has been board certified in Pediatrics since 2013 and Pediatric Endocrinology and Diabetes since 2017. In addition to managing pediatric patients with endocrine and metabolism disorders, she teaches medical students and residents in her specialty and serves as a resident mentor for the general pediatrics program.

Amanda J. Minor, PhD, is an assistant professor at Salve Regina University, in Newport, Rhode Island. Dr. Minor serves as a counselor educator and internship coordinator within the Holistic Clinical Mental Health Counseling program. She is passionate about training future counselors to be culturally competent, ethical, social change agents who help create a more just and harmonious world. She holds a master's degree in educational psychology, specializing in community counseling and couple and family counseling from Southern Illinois University and a doctorate in counselor education and counseling from Idaho State University. Her scholarly work is related to diversity and equity, creative pedagogy, best practices within counselor education, and civic engagement. She has worked as a licensed professional counselor with survivors of sexual abuse and their families. In addition to her role as a Counselor Educator, she currently works as a counselor with survivors of domestic violence and serves as a board member for Sankofa Community Connections.

Marion Nesbit, PhD, senior faculty at Lesley University in Cambridge, MA and consulting psychologist, earned her doctoral degree from The University of Texas at Austin in an APA model, clinical and organizational scholar-practitioner program. She completed additional studies in law. Dr. Nesbit's professional roles have included law-driven statewide education program development and professional training in Texas, 3 decades as core faculty and administrator in higher education, and consulting. She has taught interdisciplinary courses in psychology, human development, leadership and organizations, work–family relationships, and research. She has led faculty and institutional committees and initiatives involving budgeting, planning, personnel, organizational development, assessment, and evaluation. Dr. Nesbit's interdisciplinary research focus encompasses studies of leadership and collaboration, and she has presented nationally and internationally. She received several fellowships and served as visiting faculty at Harvard Medical School to conduct research involving program leadership and children's health. Dr. Nesbit has chaired 500+ interdisciplinary, creative-constructivist graduate students' thesis committees and chaired doctoral committees for professional trailblazers. An award recipient, Dr. Nesbit has dedicated service to education and health-related organizations.

Christine Lynn Norton, PhD, LCSW, is an associate professor of social work at Texas State University. She received a PhD in social work from Loyola University Chicago, a Master of Arts in social service administration from the University of Chicago, and a Master of Science in experiential education from Minnesota State University-Mankato. She is a licensed clinical social worker and a board approved supervisor in the State of Texas. She has over 20 years of experience working with youth and young adults in a variety of settings, including therapeutic wilderness programs, juvenile justice, schools, mentoring, and campus support programs. She is a research scientist with the Outdoor Behavioral Healthcare Center and she helped launch the Foster Care Adventure Therapy Network, an international group of programs and practitioners who utilize adventure therapy with current and former foster care youth and young adults. She was also a Fulbright Scholar in Taiwan.

Pamela O'Callaghan, PhD, is the director of the Academic Support Center at the University of South Florida Morsani College of Medicine in Tampa, Florida. Dr. O'Callaghan received her PhD from the University of Houston, Houston, Texas in educational psychology—individual differences in 2009. She joined the USF faculty in 2014 from the University of Texas Medical

Branch in Galveston, Texas where she served as director of academic support services and career counseling. Her career has been focused on providing academic advising, U.S. medical licensing examination preparation, and career counseling to medical students. Her research concentrates on teaching and learning in medicine, including support for struggling learners, as well as, the development of clinical reasoning and remediation curriculum. Dr. O'Callaghan began her teaching career in Kenya, West Africa as a U.S. Peace Corps volunteer.

John G. Pierce Jr., MD, is an associate professor and chairman of Women's Health and the Medical Specialties at Liberty University College of Osteopathic Medicine (LUCOM). Dr. Pierce earned his undergraduate and medical degrees from the University of Florida, completed his internal medicine residency at Carolinas Medical Center, and then finished his obstetrics and gynecology residency at the University of Florida Health Science Center, Jacksonville. Prior to his tenure at LUCOM, he was an associate professor at Virginia Commonwealth University (VCU) School of Medicine in the Departments of Obstetrics/Gynecology and Internal Medicine. During his 16 years at VCU, he was extensively involved in education, serving as the OB/GYN clerkship director for 9 years and OB/GYN residency program director for 3 years. He is passionate about teaching and clinical care, and has received multiple clinical and teaching awards. He is married to his wife, Nicole, and is dedicated to his four children.

Michael J. Schultz, EdD, is the director of Organizational Climate and Staff Support at the State of Connecticut's Department of Children and Families. Dr. Schultz is a licensed psychologist and family therapist with more than 30 years of professional experience in public and private settings as an administrator, clinician, researcher, supervisor, and university professor. Dr. Schultz holds a master's degree in counseling psychology from Lesley University in Cambridge, Massachusetts and a doctorate degree in counseling psychology and family systems medicine from the University of Massachusetts. His scholarly publications and presentations focus on family systems therapies, organizational psychology, trauma and secondary trauma, outdoor adventure-based group work, global stress and race relations. Dr. Schultz has extensive experience providing systemic assessments and interventions with a variety of professional groups such as schools, healthcare organizations, law enforcement agencies, mental health centers, and community programs experiencing crises and intensive interpersonal conflict.

Wendy L. Ward, PhD, ABPP, is a professor with tenure at the University of Arkansas for Medical Sciences College of Medicine. She is also an APA Fellow with over 25 years of professional experience. Dr. Ward serves in two institution-level positions (across five colleges and the Graduate School at

UAMS) as the director of Interprofessional Faculty Development and associate director of Professional Wellness with extensive experience in faculty affairs. Her career began in collaborative, team-based care initially with obese youth, leading to program development such that she now oversees faculty and fellows in 38 subspecialty clinics at Arkansas Children's Hospital. Her research interests are in the following areas: interprofessional education, faculty development, integrated behavioral health, faculty affairs, professional wellness, pediatric obesity, and sleep disorders.

Michael D. Webb, DDS, MEd, is the chair of Pediatric Dentistry and Orthodontics and Dentofacial Orthopedics at the East Carolina University School of Dental Medicine in Greenville, NC. Prior to being named chair, Dr. Webb was the founding program director for the Residency in Pediatric Dentistry at ECU. Dr. Webb received his Doctor of Dental Surgery degree from the Northwestern University Dental School. He then completed a residency in pediatric dentistry at The Children's Hospital of Pittsburgh and a residency in dental anesthesiology at the University of Pittsburgh School of Dental Medicine. Dr. Webb also holds a certificate in health care administration from St. Joseph's College and a master's in education from Virginia Commonwealth University with a concentration in adult learning. In addition to lecturing at the local, national, and international levels, Dr. Webb has practiced pediatric dentistry and dental anesthesiology in both academic and private practice settings.

Patrice B. Wunsch, DDS, MS, is a professor at Virginia Commonwealth University (VCU), School of Dentistry. Dr. Wunsch has spent the past 3 years mentoring pediatric dentistry residents and dental students. Prior to this, she was the program director for Advanced Education in Pediatric Dentistry since her arrival at VCU in 2011. From 2003 to 2011, Dr. Wunsch provided care for patients and mentored pediatric dentistry residents at a hospital-based dental clinic, part of the University of Maryland Medical System. In 2007, she was promoted to chief of dental services and was responsible for the clinical operations of the dental clinic and operating rooms. Dr. Wunsch earned her dental degree from Marquette University in 1986. She became a member of the armed services by serving as an army dental officer from 1986 to 1991. In 2002, she completed her training in pediatric dentistry and earned a Master of Science in oral biology. More recently, she has earned a graduate certificate in teaching in medical education at VCU School of Medicine. Dr. Wunsch has given numerous presentations locally and nationally. She has a number of publications with her primary focus on pulp therapy, early childhood caries, and dental anomalies.

66156293R00220

Made in the USA
Columbia, SC
16 July 2019